COLONOSCOPY

Edited by **Paul Miskovitz**

Colonoscopy
Edited by Paul Miskovitz

Published by InTech

Janeza Trdine 9, 51000 Rijeka, Croatia

Publishing Process Manager Igor Babic

Technical Editor Teodora Smiljanic

Cover Designer InTech Design Team

Additional hard copies can be obtained from orders@intechopen.com

Colonoscopy, Edited by Paul Miskovitz
p. cm.
ISBN 978-953-307-568-6

For EU product safety concerns:
IN TECH d.o.o., Prolaz Marije Krucifikse Kozulić 3, 51000 Rijeka, Croatia,
info@intechopen.com or visit our website at intechopen.com.

Meet the editor

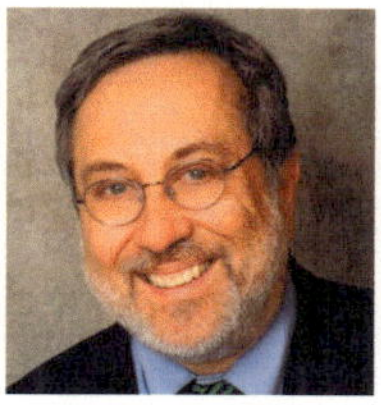

Dr. Paul Miskovitz is Clinical Professor of Medicine in the Division of Gastroenterology and Hepatology, Department of Medicine, Weill Cornell Medical College and Attending Physician at the New York—Presbyterian Hospital Weill/Cornell Campus in New York. The author of a variety of articles on gastroenterology, hepatology and internal medicine topics, co-developer of several medical computer software programs, the co-author of three books in the field of gastroenterology, Dr. Miskovitz currently maintains a clinical consultative practice for gastroenterology, hepatology, gastrointestinal endoscopy and gastrointestinal parasitology, and teaches at the Weill Cornell Medical College in New York City and Doha, Qatar. In the Fall of 2009 Dr. Miskovitz was the recipient of a CINE Golden Eagle Award in the Professional Advertising and Promotion Division, Public Service Announcements, for participation in the CBS Cares Colonoscopy Sweepstakes, a very successful PSA designed to increased public awareness nationwide with regard to colorectal cancer screening using colonoscopy.

Contents

Preface

To publish a book on colonoscopy suitable for an international medical audience, drawing upon the expertise and talents of many outstanding world-wide clinicians, is a daunting task. To edit such a book is a comparable challenge. The use of the Internet for both medical research and communication greatly helps with this international endeavor.

The field of colonoscopy within the larger realm of gastrointestinal endoscopy is, so to speak, a moving target. New developments in videocolonoscope instruments and ancillary equipment, infection risk and control, the use of patient antibiotic prophylaxis, the doctrine of informed consent, procedural technique, the need for terminal ileal intubation, documentation including the use of the electronic health record, patient selection for the procedure, patient preparation, and moderate sedation and monitoring are being made and reported daily in both the medical and the lay press. The rigors developed from the discipline of medical outcomes research are rapidly being applied to the field, hand in hand with questions about procedural reimbursement issues being raised by government and private insurers as well as by patients themselves. Just as over the last several decades colonoscopy has largely supplanted the use of barium enema x-ray study of the colon, new developments in gastrointestinal imaging such as computerized tomographic colonography (CT colonography, "virtual" colonoscopy) and video transmitted capsule study of the colonic lumen and new discoveries in cellular and molecular biology that may facilitate the early detection of colon cancer, colon polyps and other gastrointestinal pathology threaten to relegate the role of colonoscopy as a diagnostic screening technique to the side lines of medical practice.

The field has certainly come a long way since the winter of 1974 when as a fourth year medical student at Cornell University Medical College doing a gastroenterology elective rotation at the then New York Hospital in New York City I was given the opportunity (courtesy of my mentors) to look down the "teaching head" of the colonoscope and actually see pathology within the lumen of the large bowel of a patient I was following on the wards! I trust you will find the efforts of the talented and renowned physicians who have contributed to this endeavor to convey a sense of the history, the present state-of-the art and ongoing confronting issues, and the predicted future of this discipline both rewarding and worthy of your time and consideration.

July 2011

Paul Miskovitz MD, AGAF
Clinical Professor of Medicine
Division of Gastroenterology and Hepatology
Department of Medicine
Weill Cornell Medical College
New York, New York, U.S.A.
Faculty Lecturer in Gastroenterology and Hepatology
Weill Cornell Medical College-Qatar
Doha, Qatar
Faculty Lecturer in Gastroenterology and Hepatology
The American Austrian Foundation
Salzburg-Weill Cornell Seminars
Salzburg, Austria
Attending Physician
New York-Presbyterian Hospital
Weill Cornell Campus
New York, New York, U.S.A.
Consulting Gastroenterologist
Hospital for Special Surgery
New York, New York, U.S.A.

A Brief Overview of Selected Aspects of Colonoscopy: Past, Present and Future

Paul Miskovitz, MD, AGAF
Clinical Professor of Medicine
Division of Gastroenterology and Hepatology
Department of Medicine
Weill Cornell Medical College
New York, New York USA
Faculty Lecturer in Gastroenterology and Hepatology
Weill Cornell Medical College-Qatar
Doha, Qatar
Faculty Lecturer in Gastroenterology and Hepatology
The American Austrian Foundation
Salzburg-Weill Cornell Seminars
Salzburg, Austria
Attending Physician
New York-Presbyterian Hospital
Weill Cornell Campus
New York, New York, USA
Consulting Gastroenterologist
The Hospital for Special Surgery
New York, New York, USA

1. Introduction

All the organs of the body were having a meeting, trying to decide who should be the one in charge. "I should be in charge," said the brain, "Because I run all the body's systems, so without me nothing would happen." "I should be in charge," said the blood, "Because I circulate oxygen all over so without me you'd all waste away." "I should be in charge," said the stomach," Because I process food and give all of you energy." "We should be in charge," said the legs, "because we carry the body wherever it needs to go." "We should be in charge," said the eyes, "Because we allow the body to see where it goes." "We should be in charge," said the colon and rectum, "Because we're responsible for waste removal." All the other body parts laughed at the colon and rectum and insulted them, so in a huff, they shut down tight. Within a few days, the brain had a terrible headache, the stomach was bloated, the legs got wobbly, the eyes got watery, and the blood became toxic. They all decided that the colon and rectum should be the boss. The moral of the story? ***The importance of the colon and rectum to patient well-being has been affirmed and colonoscopy has come of age!***

As editor of this book it is my intent in this brief introductory book chapter to provide a sampling of some of the varied topics related to the discipline of colonoscopy. By whetting the reader's appetite for this subject one will better enjoy the many superb multi-authored chapters written with an international perspective that follow.

2. The historical development of colonoscopy

In the last half century the field of gastroenterology has recruited ever increasing numbers of well-motivated and capable physician trainees. During the period 1950–70, investigations of the colon were largely restricted to barium radiographic studies, stool examinations, and the performance of rigid sigmoidoscopy. [Old habits such as performing diagnostic contrast enema studies of the colon die hard, however (Matsukawa et al., 2007).] In contrast, the modern-day gastroenterologist undergoes advanced training in gastroenterology and hepatology, unlike his predecessors has a wide armamentarium of services to offer and medications to use in clinical care, and is expected to develop a high level of skill in performing endoscopic procedures including colonoscopy and interpreting diagnostic studies such as CT enterography, magnetic resonance cholangiopancreatography, and capsule endoscopy. Because of patient demand and the financial considerations inherent in maintaining a clinical practice, the average practicing gastroenterologist however, may find that he has his plate full of endoscopic procedures, particularly screening colonoscopy to the possible detriment of teaching, research and perhaps other aspects of clinical care (Ganz, 2004).

The development that irreversibly altered the field of gastroenterology forever, by allowing the widespread use of endoscopes to peer into gastrointestinal orifices (and later, body cavities), occurred in the 1950s and 1960s when Drs. Basil Hirschowitz. William Wolff, Hiromi Shinya, Bergein Overholt and others used the principles of fiberoptics to develop and apply to gastroenterology the 'fiberscope' (Modlin, 2000, Wolf, 1989). Fiberoptic colonoscopes arrived on the scene in the 1970's (Achord, 2005). At first, the procedure was thought to be technically difficult in a way similar to the simultaneously developed biliary and pancreatic procedure endoscopic retrograde cholangiopancreatography (ERCP). Due to a lack of complete understanding of the intraluminal colonic anatomy, early attempts at using colonoscopy often required the aid of fluoroscopy. Because of this, the widespread acceptance of colonoscopy as a diagnostic and later therapeutic procedure was delayed despite the introduction of colonoscopic polypectomy (Dr. Hiromi Shinya in New York City using a home-made wire threaded through a thin plastic catheter with an assistant hand-holding the connection between the active cord of an electrosurgical unit and a hemostat clamped on the wire after the polyp was ensnared) and the demonstration of superior diagnostic results for colonoscopy when compared to barium enema studies and rigid sigmoidoscopy (Wolff & Shinya, 1971). Developments in colonoscopy have continued at a rapid pace with one major one occurring in 1983 when Welch Allyn® Inc. inserted an image sensor or charge-coupled device into the distal tip of an endoscope (Sivak & Fleischer, 1984). Light was still transmitted down the endoscope through a fiberoptic bundle but the light falling on the charge-coupled device is converted into an array of electrical charges that are reconstructed on a video monitor. As electronic solid-state sensors had only previously been able to produce black and white images, modifications were required to reproduce the image in color. This was achieved by two techniques: either the rapid sequential use of the primary colors, red, green and blue, at the light source or by the use of color-chip imaging where the solid-state sensor has colored microfilters fixed to its surface. By the 1990's, videocolonoscopy, through developments at Olympus®, Pentax® and Fujinon®, had largely replaced fiberoptic colonoscopy with the video image projected onto monitors and thus facilitating teaching and allowing the findings to be shared "live" with endoscopy staff and other physicians. It was not long before the findings of the procedure were able to be "captured" by video recording devices and entered into the electronic health record. From an international perspective the development of gastrointestinal endoscopy over the last four decades in Malaysia has recently been chronicled (Goh, 2011).

As we will see, the future of (particularly therapeutic) colonoscopy seems assured, with new developments on the horizon.

3. Credentialing of colonoscopists

The provision of high-quality colonoscopy by well trained colonoscopists should be the goal of any institution whether it be an academic university medical center, hospital, ambulatory endoscopy center, physician's office, subspecialty society, government regulatory agency, or health insurance provider (ASGE, 1998, Parry & Williams, 1991, Marshall, 1995, Chak et al., 1996, ASGE, 1999, Wexner et al., 2001). Issues include uniformity of standards, training and determination of competence, the learning of new procedures, monitoring of colonoscopic performance and the need for continuing education (Cohen, 2011). This area has come under increased scrutiny in both training programs (Sedlack, 2010) and for application and re-application for hospital colonoscopy privileges (Wexner et al., 2002, Obstein et al., 2011). Polypectomy rate has been proposed as a useful quality measure with a high degree of correlation with the rate of detection of colorectal adenomas (Williams et al., 2011). Gastrointestinal procedure oriented meetings and sponsored courses (American Society of Gastrointestinal Endoscopy meeting held during the annual Digestive Disease Week and the annual course held in New York City sponsored by the New York Society for Gastrointestinal Endoscopy to name two of many available in the United States) are well attended and produce enduring materials that are circulated well beyond the population of the course attendees. Advanced DVD and Internet courses are becoming increasingly popular among those performing colonoscopies.

4. Indications for colonoscopy

Colonoscopy has made gains in popularity as a medical diagnostic procedure. It has been popularized by the publication of a patient-oriented paperback guide book,

Colonoscopy for Dummies, (Dobie & Burke, 2011) and in a television media public service announcement campaign to make people aware of the importance of screening for colorectal cancer in the United States, launched by the Columbia Broadcasting System's CBS Cares® Program (http://www.cbs.com/cbs cares/topics/?sec=colorectal cancer, http://www.cbs.com/cbs cares/video/?cid=822059380)). A colonoscopy has even become the prize of a popular sweepstakes (http://promotions.mardenkane.com /cbs/cbscares/rules.cfm). Nevertheless, it is prudent to keep in mind the proven utility of the procedure.

Colonoscopy is most useful in diagnosing and treating patients with neoplasms, strictures or colonic mucosal disease previously diagnosed on radiological imaging. Other uses include the evaluation of patients with gastrointestinal hemorrhage (hematochezia and occult bleeding) (Davila et al., 2005, Miskovitz & Steinberg, 1982, Miskovitz et al., 1987, Khalid et al., 2011, Kistler et al., 2011), unexplained iron deficiency anemia (Goddard et al., 2011), screening and surveillance for colonic neoplasms (Davila et al., 2006, Denberg et al., 2005, Wilschut et al., 2011, Lasser et al., 2011)), diagnosis and surveillance of inflammatory bowel disease (Leighton et al., 2006, Basseri et al., 2011), evaluation of chronic diarrhea (with or without stool microbiology sampling, intubation of the terminal ileum for Crohn's disease and multiple mucosal biopsies to diagnose microscopic colitis) (Eisen et al., 2001, Miskovitz & Rochwarger, 1993, Jaskiewicz et al., 2006, Misra et al., 2010), constipation (Qureshi et al., 2005), foreign body removal (Safioleas et al., 2009), decompression of megacolon and sigmoid volvulus (Eisen et al., 2002), and the treatment of anorectal disorders (Eisen et al., 2001). "Open access colonoscopy", a program designed to make colorectal cancer screening more convenient and available has been the subject of some debate (Rex, 2010-2011, Feld, 2010-2011). In this situation, patients without significant gastrointestinal symptoms have a screening colonoscopy without the inconvenience or cost of a preliminary office visit. Its purpose is to provide colonoscopy for screening purposes to a wider audience with less waiting time.

World-wide, colorectal cancer is the third most commonly diagnosed cancer in males and the second in females, with more than 1.2 million new cases and more than 600,000 deaths estimated to have occurred from colorectal cancer in 2008 (Jemal et al., 2011). Despite more than three decades of experience with using colonoscopy for colorectal cancer screening controversies about the procedure do exist (Smith, 2011a, Helwick, 2011a, Helwick, 2011b, Smith, 2011b). The field of colorectal cancer screening and prevention in women has recently been reviewed (Krishnan & Wolf, 2011) as has the overuse of screening colonoscopy in the Medicare (federal government subsidized health insurance for older people) population in the United States (Goodwin et al., 2011). The upper age limit for colorectal cancer screening by colonoscopy has recently drawn attention (Habbema et al., 2011, Naravadi et al., 2011). Recently proposed cascade colorectal screening guidelines from the World Gastroenterology Organization (Winawer et al., 2011) advocate that each country, region or healthcare setting needs to determine whether colorectal cancer screening is a legitimate consideration based upon other healthcare priorities. This group endorses enhanced colorectal screening worldwide, especially in developing countries where the colorectal cancer incidence and mortality is rising.

As chapters in this book will illustrate, the indications for colonoscopy are expanding with advancements in technology.

5. Contraindications to and risks of colonoscopy

Contraindications to performing colonoscopy must take into account that this procedure represents a somewhat stressful physiological experience for the patient. Hypotension, cardiac dysrhythmias (including bradyarrhythmias from increased vagal stimulation), abdominal distention with compromise of diaphragmatic function, and oxygen desaturation, are a few among the many complications that may occur during the procedure. For this reason, patient selection for the procedure should take into account any bleeding diathesis the patient may have, the cardiovascular (recent myocardial infarction or recent evaluation of the patient's cardiac status) and pulmonary status of the patient along with concomitant conditions such as infection (contraindicated in acute diverticulitis), severe ulcerative, ischemic, infective or Crohn's colitis (contraindicated). It has become customary to use the American Society of Anesthesiologists 1963 derived and subsequently amended preoperative physical status classification system (ASA I→ASA VI) (American Society of Anesthesiologists http://www.asahq.org/clinical/physicalstatus.htm) in classifying patients undergoing the procedure. The clinician must also exercise judgment in deciding to convert a planned colonoscopy into a flexible fiberoptic sigmoidoscopy if findings in the rectosigmoid suggest that the planned procedure be terminated.

Colonoscopy is not without its risks (Miskovitz & Gibofsky, 1995). Perforation is perhaps the most dreaded, occurring more frequently in therapeutic colonoscopy than in diagnostic colonoscopy. Statistics from the last two decades of the last century reveal a perforation rate of approximately 1 in 2,500 procedures (Sieg et al., 2001) and a mortality rate of 1 in 15,000 procedures (Waye et al., 1996), deaths often being related to the management of perforations. Immediate laparoscopic surgery is the best treatment although there may be a role for conservative therapy with surgical observation, intravenous fluids and the use of antibiotics in select cases (Kavin et al., 1992). Hemorrhage, related to biopsy, polypectomy or balloon dilatation is another risk of the procedure occurring on up to 1.5% of cases (often with a delay up to four weeks). The risk of hemorrhage can be lessened by the sole use of coagulation current (as opposed to "cutting" current), slow transection of the polyp stalk, the submucosal injection of saline and or epinephrine at the polyp site, the use of endoscopically placed clips and loops, and the treatment of bleeding sites with biopolar electrocautery. A recent outpatient colonoscopy study proposes that the use of a 14-day time period for reporting would capture all perforations and the majority (96%) of post-procedure hemorrhages that required hospital admission (Rabeneck et al., 2011).

As with many decisions in clinical medicine, the decision to perform colonoscopy on a patient is a balance between the risks and benefits of the procedure, made easier by a careful medical history, physical examination and a review of available laboratory data. These same factors are utilized in obtaining informed consent for the procedure from the patient and/or the patient's family.

6. Informed consent for colonoscopy

The concept of informed consent (and its corollary, informed refusal) for colonoscopy involves an assessment of the competence of the patient, disclosure of, in an understandable way, the information necessary to allow the patient to make an informed decision regarding the role of colonoscopy in his care, and the documentation of these proceedings in the medical record (Stunkel et al., 2010). It is an intrinsic part of the doctor-patient relationship and an ethical obligation on the part of the physician in the practice of medicine. In the United States, the doctrine of medical informed consent is often traced to a 1914 New York court decision centered about the observation that since most surgical operations involve some use of force, there must be consent. Because the nature of surgery is outside the experience of most patients, the consent must be granted only after the patient is properly informed. The most famous description of informed consent is a quote from Justice Benjamin Cardozo who, in 1914, stated that: "*Every human being of adult years and sound mind has a right to determine what shall be done with his own body; and a surgeon who performs an operation without his patient's consent commits an assault for which he is liable in damages*" (*Schloendorff v Society of New York Hospital*, 1914).

Without going into detail regarding the subsequent legal history of the development of the doctrine of informed consent and its applications, nor the legal consequences of not obtaining proper informed consent for colonoscopy, recent international reviews have concluded there is room for improvement in this area (Banic et al., 2008, Bai et al., 2007). Novel approaches to facilitating the obtaining of informed consent have even included the use of video presentations (Agre, 1994) and more recently by referring patients to peer-reviewed Internet educational websites for information about colonoscopy, preparation and procedure-associated risk prior to the patient's arrival in the unit. As colonoscopy is often performed under intravenous ("conscious") sedation, the issue of withdrawal of informed consent by a patient experiencing pain has recently drawn attention (Ward et al., 1999). Of interest is that patient recall post-procedure of having given informed consent for colonoscopy appears to be similar whether the consent is obtained immediately or several days before the procedure. (Elfant et al., 1995).

7. Bowel preparation for colonoscopy

Proper and safe patient bowel preparation for colonoscopy is essential (Beck, 2010). It is generally accepted that inadequate bowel preparation for colonoscopy can result in missed lesions, cancelled procedures, increased procedural time, and a potential increase in complication rates. Bowel preparation itself may also be associated with complications (Korkis et al., 1992). An evidence based medicine summary of bowel preparations for colonoscopy has recently been published by the United States Department of Health and Human Services, Agency for Healthcare and Quality, National Guideline Clearinghouse and is accessible through the Internet (Wexner et al., 2006, http://asge.org/ PublicationsProductsIndex.aspx?id=352). Consideration is given to the elderly, those with documented or suspected underlying inflammatory bowel disease, those with diabetes mellitus, the pediatric population and the admittedly rare pregnant patient who requires colonoscopy. A new trend is to look at the timing of the bowel preparation with regard to its efficacy (Gurudu et al., 2010, Eun et al., 2011). Others have recommended a split-dose bowel preparation as effective and better accepted by patients in terms of tolerance (Huffman et al., 2010). Suffice to say that "one size does not fit all" in this matter.

8. Antibiotic prophylaxis for selected patients undergoing colonoscopy

The value of antibiotic prophylaxis for patients undergoing colonoscopy has been the subject of much debate. In the past, the rationale for antibiotic prophylaxis was to prevent patients with high-risk cardiac conditions from developing infective endocarditis and from those with prosthetic devices in place (vascular grafts, ventriculo-peritoneal shunts, prosthetic joints, etc.) from developing infected hardware. Recently, the practice of antibiotic prophylaxis for colonoscopy has substantially changed due in part to the low incidence of infective endocarditis following this procedure and the lack of evidence based medicine data supporting the benefit of antibiotic prophylaxis. It is also recognized that the widespread use of antibiotics can be associated with the development of resistant organisms, *Clostridium difficile* colitis, added expense, and the risk of drug toxicity. Recent guidelines for the use of antibiotic

Heart Association and the American Society for Gastrointestinal Endoscopy, respectively (Wilson et al., 2007, ASGE Standards of Practice Committee, 2008). Although the recommendation in these published guidelines are largely consistent with one another, they substantially differ from prior guidelines, the largest change being that both sets of guidelines no longer consider and gastrointestinal procedure high risk for bacterial endocarditis, thus lifting the recommended routine use of antibiotics for bacterial endocarditis including for those patients with high risk cardiac conditions such as prosthetic heart values and prior history of bacterial endocarditis). Although antibiotics are not recommended for patients receiving peritoneal dialysis who are undergoing colonoscopy with or without polypectomy, it may be reasonable to drain the peritoneum before performing the colonoscopy to minimize the risk of developing bacterial peritonitis.

9. Antithrombotic agents in patients undergoing colonoscopy

P4atients requiring colonoscopy with or without biopsy and/or polypectomy are often taking antithrombotic agents including anticoagulants such as warfarin, heparin, and low molecular weight heparin, and antiplatelet agents such as aspirin, non-steroidal anti-inflammatory drugs, thienopyridines such as clopidrogel and ticlopidine, and glycoprotein IIb/IIIa receptor inhibitors. Indications for the use of these medications include atrial fibrillation, acute coronary syndrome, deep venous thrombosis hypercoagulable states and endoprotheses such as coronary artery stents. When bleeding does occur in patients taking these agents it is most commonly from the gastrointestinal tract (Choudari et al., 1994). Risk stratification for these patients can be relegated to two categories. Low risk procedures include diagnostic colonoscopy including mucosal biopsy (Sieg et al., 2001, Parra-Blanco et al., 2000)) and high-risk procedures include colonoscopy with polypectomy and the dilatation of colonic benign or malignant strictures (guidelines extrapolated in part from experience reported in the upper gastrointestinal endoscopy literature) (Singh et al., 2005, Solt et al., 2003, DiSario et al., 1994). A comprehensive review of the types of antithrombotic therapies, their implications for patients undergoing colonoscopy, and recommendations and a management algorithm for such patients using these agents has recently been published (ASGE Standards of Practice Committee, 2009). Newer anticoagulants, for which current guidelines regarding their being held for endoscopic procedures are lacking, are reaching the market at an increasing rate. These include danaparoid, a low molecular weight heparinoid consisting of a mixture of heparan sulfate, dermatan sulfate, and chondroitin sulfate (Danhof et al., 1992, Nurmohamed, et al., 1991) which was recently removed from the US market due to shortages; the direct thrombin inhibitors recombinant hirudin (lepirudin), argatroban, desirudin and bivalirudin (Greinacher & Warkentin, 2008, Clarke, et al., 1991, Warkentin, et al., 2008); the recently available orally active direct thrombin inhibitor dabigatran etexlate (Schulman, et al., 2009); and the factor XA inhibitors idraparinux, rivaroxaban, and apixaban (Turpie, 2008).

10. Sedation for colonoscopy

The use of sedation for colonoscopy is undergoing changes both in the United States and worldwide (Heuss et al., 2005, Aisenberg et al., 2005, Aisenberg & Cohen, 2006, Cohen et al., 2006). Driven in part by insurance reimbursement, the desire to improve efficiency in the procedure facility, the availability of anesthesiologists to sedate and properly monitor patients for endoscopic procedures and the development of new, short acting anesthetics, the days of either unsedated colonoscopy and/or endoscopist administered benzodiazepine and opioid cocktail may well be numbered (Luginbühl et al., 2009). This topic has been nicely reviewed in a recent Internet-based international study of endoscopic sedation practices (Benson et al., 2008). The authors conclude that although benzodiazepine with an opioid is used 56% of the time for colonoscopy sedation by the 84 endoscopists from 46 countries who participated in the study, propofol was use 18% of the time (as opposed to an unsedated colonoscopy rate of 10%). A comparison of sedation practices worldwide showed that sedation is used for most colonoscopies and sedation practices did not differ significantly between developing and developed countries. Computer-assisted personalized sedation holds the promise of delivering safe and effective minimal to moderate propofol sedation to ASA class I and II patients undergoing colonoscopy with the medication provided by health care professionals who are not anesthesiologists (ASGE Technology Committee, 2011, Pambianco, et al., 2011). The effect that the untimely death of superstar Michael Jackson due to an off-label use of propofol by a non-anesthesiologist has had and will continue to have on the acceptance of the use of propofol outside of the operating room (and by those other than credentialed anesthesiologists) by insurance companies and regulatory agencies has been recently addressed (http://blogs.wsj.com/health/2009/08/06/ the-other-propofol-issue-when-insurance-should-pay-for-it/, http://thehappyhospitalist.blogspot.com/2009_08_01_archive.html, Coté, 2011)). As a counterpoint, the need for conscious sedation in routine adult cases has recently been challenged (Khalid et al., 2011).

The means for sedation of pediatric patients undergoing colonoscopy has also received attention (Fredette & Lightdale, 2008). Two general types of sedation are available for children undergoing colonoscopy: general anesthesia which entails increased costs and the need for hospital resources and intravenous sedation runs the risk of agitation (Thakkar et al., 2007). Increasingly, propofol, which can be given alone or in combination with other sedatives, administered by a dedicated anesthesiologist, is being used (Elisur et al., 2000). Wider concerns exist about the long-term effects of the use of anesthetics in infants and children (Rappaport et al., 2011, Blum, 2011))

11. Patient monitoring during colonoscopy

It is difficult to talk about sedation for colonoscopy without considering issues regarding patient monitoring during colonoscopy. Since the first colonoscopies were performed in the hospital setting, it has long been recognized that patients ("consciously") sedated for colonoscopy required proper peri-procedure monitoring (Bell et al., 1991). The availability of resuscitation equipment, airway suctioning equipment, EKG cardiac monitoring, and parenterally administered medications (including sedative reversal agents) in the procedure and recovery areas, having staff who were properly credentialed in state-of-the-art resuscitation methods, the presence of a qualified registered nurse to monitor the patient during the procedure, the obtaining and documenting of a preoperative history and performance and documenting of a preoperative physical examination, adequately maintained intravenous access, the use of oxygen enriched air by nasal cannula or face mask monitored by pulse oximetry, and more recently capnography monitoring of respiratory depression (Cacho et al., 2010), and the recording of vital signs from the procedure and in the recovery room became commonplace and the norm. As colonoscopy moved to the outpatient setting including ambulatory endoscopy facilities and doctors' offices, and the duration of the procedure lengthened due to therapeutic maneuvers, these standards became more formalized, often involving input from the anesthesiology community (particularly in situations where moderate or deep sedation were employed) with debate and at times even controversy as to the best method of sedation patients (from minimal sedation or anxiolysis through general anesthesia). Much of the impetus for this came from the simultaneously evolving practice of using anesthesiology services outside of the operating room such as in the emergency department, the intensive care unit, the bronchoscopy suite, doctors' and dentists' offices and the radiology suite.

Today, many feel that propofol is the agent of choice for sedation for colonoscopy (Luginbühl et al., 2009). The increasing demand for sedating and properly monitoring patients may not be met by anesthesiology departments because of staffing reductions, reimbursement issues which drive up health care costs, and challenges by health insurance companies (Aisenberg & Cohen, 2006). Currently, the use of propofol in this setting by non-anesthesiologists (gastroenterologist-directed propofol use) is controversial (Faigel et al., 2002), monitoring-intensive because of the level of sedation, and may violate the package insert for the use this drug in some locales. The answer to this dilemma in the future may be computer-assisted sedation systems that are currently under development and investigation (Hickle, 2001, Pambianco, 2008, Caruso et al., 2009, ASGE Technology Committee, 2011).

12. The electronic endoscopic record and colonoscopy

Electronic endoscopic medical record systems with report generating capabilities and patient flow management modules are increasingly becoming an integral part of the daily operation of many office, hospital and ambulatory endoscopy center endoscopy units (Savides et al., 2004, Petersen, 2006). Using pull-down template menus designed for standardization, data retrieval, and coding for billing purposes, rather than "old-fashioned" free-text entry, the costs for such programs vary significantly between vendors and may range between $5,000 and $45,000 (US) per room for software implementation with an additional requirement for an annual maintenance contract and telephone support. Besides providing a standardized procedure report these systems provide for ease of information retrieval particularly when generating endoscopy unit statistics and maintaining research-related databases (Groenen et al., 2006, Faigel et al., 2006). They are also of value in providing a means for patient recall to improve adherence to follow up recommendations after colonoscopic examinations (Leffler et al., 2011). Issues confronting the colonoscopist contemplating the implementation of such systems include the multitude of competing systems available to choose from (some of which are Internet based and others of which require a Virtual Private Network to access) and the necessity to integrate these systems with pre-existing electronic health records already in place in doctors' offices and hospitals. Although features of these systems may improve patient care and enhance endoscopy unit efficiency and productivity, further studies to document this are necessary (ASGE Technology Committee, 2008).

13. The future of colonoscopy

"Perhaps the best thing about the future is that it comes one day at a time"-U.S. Secretary of State Dean Acheson (1893-971)

"Prediction is extremely difficult, especially about the future"—Danish physicist Niels Bohr (1885-1962)

"640 K should be enough for anybody"-CEO of Microsoft® Corporation Bill Gates, 1981

The future of colonoscopy has been the subject of much speculation (Sawhney, 2011, Marshall, 2011). Before reviewing the future of colonoscopy it would be prudent to review where we are today. Currently, colonoscopy is useful for diagnosis, polypectomy and biopsy, hemostasis, endoscopic mucosa resection, endoscopic submucosal dissection, decompression of the colon, treatment of radiation proctitis, stenting for malignancy, stenting for benign strictures, the occasional treatment of hemorrhoids and rarely cecostomy placement. Sometimes advances in colonoscopy technique are subtle in nature such as the increasingly accepted use of carbon dioxide over air for colonic insufflation (Church & Delaney, 2002, Uraoka et al., 2009, Yamano et al., 2010). Other advances are more profound. Future developments in colonoscopy will likely center about five areas: new methods of imaging, new colonoscopes, new colonoscopy assisting devices, new therapeutic tools, and new territories to explore.

New imaging techniques to enhance our vision are already upon us and undergoing refinement. Chromoscopy providing morphological enhancement (Brown & Baraza, 2010, Kahi et al., 2010, Pohl et al., 2011), magnifying endoscopy (Filip et al., 2011), high definition endoscopy (Singh et al., 2010, Buchner et al., 2010), confocal laser endomicroscopy (Gheona et al., 2011), endocytoscopy (Singh et al., 2010), narrow band imaging with enhancement of mucosal fine structure and vasculature (Cash, 2010, Van den Broek et al., 2011, Chiu et al., 2011, Oka et al., 2011, Wada et al., 2011), multiband imaging (Fedeli et al., 2011), computed virtual chromoendoscopy (Chung et al., 2010), optical coherence tomography (Roy et al., 2009, Adler et al., 2009, Consolo et al., 2008), spectroscopy and fluorescence (Ortner et al., 2010), autofluorescence imaging (ASGE Technology Committee, 2011a) and molecular endoscopy (Buchner et al., 2010) are but some of the new imaging techniques being unfurled. Using these techniques the colonoscopist is deepening the depths of colonic mucosal interrogation to the level of the submucosa with image resolution approaching that of conventional pathology in essence becoming an *in vivo* pathologist! This is not unlike our current use of visualization over histology for diagnosing duodenal ulceration, gastrointestinal stromal neoplasms, lipomas and pancreatic rests.

New colonoscopes are under development (Rösch et al., 2007) including the Aer-O-Scope™ which is a pneumatic, skill-independent, self-propelling, self-navigating colonoscope providing an omni-directional view through a conic lens and mirror system (Pfeffer et al., 2006). The Third Eye® Retroscope® (Waye, 2010, Rex, 2009, Leufkens et al., 2010) provides a continuous retrograde (backward) view side-by-side with the usual forward view of the colonoscope. This is particularly useful in locating polyps hidden behind folds. A novel computer-assisted colonoscope (NeoGuide Endoscopy System) (Eickhoff et al., 2007) delivers a real-time, three-dimensional map of the tip position and insertion tube shape in addition to the video image of the colon lumen. Three-dimensional map images generated by the NeoGuide endoscopy system provide accurate information regarding tip position, insertion tube position, and colonic looping. The Invendoscope™ SC20 (http://www.invendo-medical.com/index eng.html, Rösch et al., 2008) has several features that are new to the field of colonoscopy. It is a single-use colonoscope with a working channel that is not pushed or pulled, but driven in and out of the colon. All endoscopic functions are performed using a handheld device and most importantly, it reduces potential forces on the colon wall to enable a gentle colonoscopy lessening the need for patient sedation. A recent study reports that for patients with a previously incomplete conventional optical colonoscopy, balloon colonoscopy performed by using the single-balloon enteroscope with an overtube was superior to a repeat attempt with a standard colonoscope in completing the examination (Keswani, 2011).

It is likely that current videocolonoscopes with only minor modifications will be widely used for the next 5-10 years with the ideal colonoscope of the future being a multi-modal instrument capable of switching from white light colonoscopy to magnification colonoscopy, multiband imaging and even endoscopic ultrasound. It is also quite likely that patient preference for capsule colonoscopy over conventional colonoscopy will drive the development of this modality (Sacher-Huvelin et al., 2010, Kuramoto et al., 2011).

One of the therapeutic tools that will undergo increased availability and usage in the future is stenting. This area, shared by both colonoscopists and interventional radiologists (Katsanos et al., 2010, Bonin & Baron, 2010), uses a minimally invasive procedure for palliation of inoperable malignant disease and for temporary bowel decompression, often as a bridge to surgery. Recent technological advances have been supported by an increasing number of publications detailing clinical experience with these devices (Farrell, 2007, Farrell & Sack, 2008).

Another therapeutic tool that will undergo refinements and increased availability is endoscopic mucosal resection, the technique of injecting fluid (saline or hydroxypropylmethylcellulose [HPMC]) into the submucosal space to create a submucosal cushion followed by resection of the lesion (De Melo et al., 2011, Moss et al., 2011). Wider acceptance of this technique will parallel outcomes research data and complications rates. Colonoscopic closure of colonic perforation with band ligation after enoclip failure (not for the faint at heart) has recently been reported (Han et al, 2011)!

Despite the lack of Medicare (government subsidized insurance for the elderly in the United States) coverage for the procedure and questions about its sensitivity and specificity, the use of CT colonography for colorectal cancer screening in United States hospitals appears to be on the rise, particularly in medical facilities that do not offer optical colonoscopy and may not be prepared to provide adequate follow up for patients with failed CT colonography (McHugh et al., 2011). This trend, if sustained, will undoubtedly impact upon the future of conventional colonoscopy.

The use dogs for colorectal cancer screening not withstanding (Sonoda et al., 2011), along with avoiding performing the procedure late in the day (Lee et al., 2011), although others would argue that time-dependent factors such as colonoscopist fatigue and decreased colon cleanliness can be addressed (Freedman et al., 2011), the future of colonoscopy seems secure and bright.

14. References

Achord, J.L. (2005) The history of gastrointestinal endoscopy, In: *Clinical Gastrointestinal Endoscopy*, Ginsberg, G.G., Kochman, M.L., Norton, I., Gostout, C.J., (Eds.), pp. 3-12, Elsevier Inc. ISBN 10: 0-7216-0282-7, London

Adler, D.C., Zhou, C., Tsai, T.H. Schmitt, J., Huang, Q., Mahimo, H., Fujimoto, J.G. (2009) Three-dimensional endomicroscopy of the human colon using optical coherence tomography. *Opt Express.* Vol.17, No.2, (January 2009) pp. 784-96. ISSN 1094-4087

Agre, P., Kurtz, R.C., Krauss, B.J., (1994) A randomized trial using videotape to present consent information for colonoscopy. *Gastrointest Endosc.* Vol.40, No.3, (May-June 1994) pp. 271-6. ISSN 0016-5107

Aisenberg, J., Brill, J.V., Ladabaum, U., Cohen, L.B. (2005) Sedation for gastrointestinal endoscopy: new practices, new economics. *Am J Gastroenterol.* Vol.100, No.5, (May 2005) pp. 996-1000. ISSN 0002-9270

Aisenberg, J., Cohen, L.B. (2006) Sedation in endoscopic practice. *Gastrointest Endosc Clin N Am.* Vol.16, No.4, (October 2006) pp. 695-708. ISSN 1052-5157

American Society of Anesthesiologists. "ASA Physical Status Classification System," Accessed 1/5/2011. Available from: http://www.asahq.org/clinical/physicalstatus.htm.

ASGE [No authors listed]. (1998) Guidelines for credentialing and granting privileges for gastrointestinal endoscopy. American Society for Gastrointestinal Endoscopy. *Gastrointest Endosc.* Vol.48, No.6, (December 1998) pp. 679-82. ISSN 0016-5107

ASGE [No authors listed]. (1999) Principles of training in gastrointestinal endoscopy. From the ASGE. American Society for Gastrointestinal Endoscopy. *Gastrointest Endosc.* Vol.49, No.6. (June 1999) pp. 845-53. ISSN 0016-5107

ASGE Standards of Practice Committee, Anderson, M.A., Ben-Menachem, T., Gan, S.I., Appalaneni, V., Banerjee, S., Cash, B.D., Fisher, L., Harrison, M.E., Fanelli, R.D., Fukami, N., Ikenberry, S.O., Jain, R., Khan, K., Krinsky, M.L., Lichtenstein, D.R., Maple, J.T., Shen, B., Strohmeyer, L., Baron, T., Dominitz, J.A. (2009) Management of antithrombotic agents for endoscopoic procedures. *Gastrointest Endosc.* Vol.70, No.6, (December 2009) pp. 1060-70. ISSN 0016-5107

ASGE Standards of Practice Committee, Banerjee, S., Shen, B., Baron, T.H., Nelson, D.B., Anderson, M.A., Cash, B.D., Dominitz, J.A., Gan, S.I., Harrison, M.E., Ikenberry, S.O., Jagannath, S.B., Lichtenstein, D., Fanelli, R.D., Lee, K., van Guilder, T., Stewart, L.E. (2008) Antibiotic prophylaxis for GI endoscopy. *Gastrointest Endosc.* Vol.67, No.6, (May 2008) pp. 701-8. ISSN 0016-5107

ASGE Technology Committee, Banerjee, S., Desilets, D., Diehl, D.L., Farraye, F.A., Kaul, V., Kethu, S.R., Kwon, R.S., Mamula, P., Pedrosa, M.C., Rodriguez, S.A., Wong Kee Song, L.M., Tierney, W.M. (2011) Computer-assisted personalized sedation. *Gastrointest Endosc.* Vol.73, No.3, (March 2011) pp. 423-427. ISSN 0016-5107

ASGE Technology Committee, Wong Kee Song, L.M., Banerjee, S., Desilets, D., Diehl, D.L., Farraye, F.A., Kaul, V., Kethu, S.R., Kwon, R.S., Mamula, P., Pedrosa, M.C., Rodriguez, S.A., Tierney, W.M. (2011a) Autofluorescence imaging. *Gastrointest Endosc.* Vol.73, No.4, (April 2011) pp. 647-50. ISSN 0016-5107

ASGE Technology Committee, Conway, J.D., Adler, D.G., Diehl, D.L., Farraye, F.A., Kantsevoy, S.V., Kwon, R., Mamula, P., Rodriguez, B. Shah, R.J. Song, L.M., Tierney, W.M. (2008) Endoscopic electronic medical records systems. *Gastrointest Endosc.* Vol.67, No.4, (April 2008) pp. 590-4. ISSN 0016-5107

Bai, Y., Gao, j., Yang, Y., Long, F., Jin, H., Li, C., Zou, D.W., Li, Z.S. (2007) A multicenter prospective survey on informed consent for gastrointestinal endoscopy in China. *Digestion.* Vol.76, No.3-4, (December 2007) pp. 203-6. ISSN 0012-2823

Banic, M., Kardum, D., Plesko, S., Petrovecki, M., Urek, M., Babic, Z., Kujundzic, M., Rotkvic, I. (2008) Informed consent for gastrointestinal endoscopy: a view of endoscopists in Croatia. *Dig Dis.* Vol.26, No.1, (February 2008) pp. 66-70. ISSN 0257-2753

Basseri, R.J., Basseri, B., Papadakis, K.A. (2011) Dysplasia and cancer in inflammatory bowel disease. *Expert Rev Gastroenterol Hepatol.* Vol.5, No.1, (February 2011) pp. 59-66. ISSN 1747-4124

Beck, D.E. (2010) Bowel preparation for colonoscopy. *Clin Colon Rectal Surg.* Vol.23, Vol.1, (February 2010) pp. 10-3. ISSN 1531-0043

Bell, G.D., McCloy, R.F., Charlton, J.E., Campbell, D., Dent, N.A., Gear, M.W., Logan, R.F., Swan, C.H. (1991) Recommendations for standards of sedation and patient monitoring during gastrointestinal endoscopy. *Gut.* Vol.32, No.7, (July 1991) pp. 823-7. ISSN 0017-5749

Benson, A.A., Cohen, L.B., Waye, J.D., Akhavan, A., Aisenberg, J. (2008) Endoscopic sedation in developing and developed countries. *Gut Liver.* Vol.2, No.2, (September 2008) pp. 105-12. ISSN 1976-2283

Blum, K. (2011) More data, but few answers for anesthesia safety in peds. *Anesthesiol News.* Vol.37, No.4, (April 2011) pp. 1, 26-8. ISSN 0747-4679

Bonin, E.A., Baron, T.H. (2010) Update on the indications and use of colonic stents. *Curr Gastroenterol Rep.* Vol.12, No.5, (October 2010) pp. 374-82. ISSN 1522-8037

Brown, S.R., Baraza, W. (2010) Chromoscopy versus conventional endoscopy for the detection of polyps in the colon and rectum. *Cochrane Database of Systematic Reviews*. Vol.6, No.10, (October 2010) pp. 1-30. ISSN 1469-493X

Buchner, A.M., Shahid, M.W, Heckman, M.G. Krishna, M., Ghabril, M., Hasan, M., Crook, J.E., Gomez, V., Raimondo, M., Woodward, T., Wolfsen, H.C., Wallace, M.B. (2010) Comparison of probe-based confocal laser endomicroscopy with virtual chromoendoscopy for classification of colon polyps. *Gastroenterology*. Vol.138, No.3, (March 2010) pp. 834-42. ISSN 0016-5085

Buchner, A.M., Shahid, M.W., Heckman, M.G., McNeil, R.B., Cleveland, P., Gill, K.R., Schore, A., Ghabril, M., Raimondo, M., Gross, S.A., Wallace, M.B. (2010) High-definition colonoscopy detects colorectal polyps at a higher rate than standard white-light colonoscopy. *Clin Gastroenterol Hepatol*. Vol.8, No.4, (April 2010) pp. 364-70. ISSN 1542-3565

Cacho, G., Pérez-Calle, J.L., Barbado, A., Lledó, J.L., Ojea, R. Fernández-Rodríguez, C.M. (2010) Capnography is superior to pulse oximetry for the detection of respiratory depression during colonoscopy. *Rev Esp Enferm Dig*. Vol.102, No.2, (February 2010) pp. 86-9. ISSN 1130-0108

Caruso, A., Bouillon, T.W., Schumacher, P.M., Zanderigo, E., Morari, M. (2009) Control of drug administration during monitored anesthesia care. *IEEE Tran Automation Sci Eng*. Vol.6, No.2, (April 2009) pp. 256-64. ISSN 1545-5955

Cash, B.D. (2010) Narrow-band imaging for colorectal polyps: it can be taught but will it be used? *Gastrointest Endosc*. Vol.72, No.3, (September 2010) pp. 577-9. ISSN 0016-5107

Chak, A.M., Cooper, G.S., Blades, E.W., Canto, M., Sivak, M.V. Jr. (1996) Prospective assessment of colonoscopic intubation skills in trainees. *Gastrointest Endosc*. Vol.44, No.1, (July 1996) pp. 54-7. ISSN 0016-5107

Chiu, H-M., Wang, H-P., Wu M-S., Lin, J-T. (2011) The clinical efficacy and future perspective of narrow band imaging for the diagnosis of colorectal neoplasm. *Dig Endosc*. Vol.23, Suppl.1, (May 2011) pp. 116-9. ISSN 1443-1661

Choudari, C.P., Rajgopal, C., Palmer, K.R. (1994) Acute gastrointestinal haemorrhage in anticoagulated patients: diagnoses and response to endoscopic treatment. *Gut*. Vol.35, No.4, (April 1994) pp. 464-6. ISSN 0017-5749

Chung, S.J., Kim, D., Song, J.H., Park, M.J., Kim, Y.S., Jung, H.C., Song, I.S. (2010) Efficacy of computed virtual chromoendoscopy on colorectal cancer screening: a prospective, randomized, back-to-back trial of Fuji Intelligent Color Enhancement versus conventional colonoscopy to compare adenoma miss rates. *Gastrointest Endosc*. Vol.72, No.1, (July 2010) pp. 136-42. ISSN 0016-5107

Church, J., Delaney, C. (2002) Randomized, controlled trial of carbon dioxide insufflation during colonoscopy. (2002) *Dis Colon Rectum*. Vo.46, No.3, (March 2003) pp. 322-6. ISSN 0012-3706

Clarke, R.J., Mayo, G., FitzGerald, G.A., Fitzgerald, D.J. (1991) Combined administration of aspirin and a specific thrombin inhibitor in man. *Circulation.* Vol.83, No.5. (May 1991) pp. 1510-8. ISSN 0009-7322

Cohen, J. (Editor) (2011) *Successful Training in Gastrointestinal Endoscopy.* pp. 1-416. Wiley-Blackwell, ISBN-10 978-1405196635, Hoboken, New Jersey

Cohen, L.B., Wecsler, J.S., Gaetano, J.N., Benson, A.A., Miller, K.M., Durkalski, V., Aisenberg, J. (2006) Endoscopic sedation in the United States: results from a nationwide survey. *Am J. Gastroenterol.* Vol.101, No.5, (May 2006) pp. 967-74. ISSN 0002-9270

Consolo, P., Strangio, G., Luigiano, C., Giacobbe, G., Pallio, S., Familiari, L. (2008) Optical coherence tomography in inflammatory bowel disease: prospective evaluation of 35 patients. *Dis Colon Rectum.* Vol.51, No.9, (September 2008) pp. 1374-80. ISSN 0012-3706

Coté, G.A. (2011) The debate for nonanesthesiologist-administered propofol sedation in endoscopy rages on: who will be the "King of Prop?" *Gastrointest Endosc.* Vol.73, No.4, (April 2011) pp. 773-6. ISSN 0016-5107

Danhof, M., de Boer, A., Magnani, H.N., Stiekema, J.C. (1992) Pharmacokinetic considerations on Orgaran (Org 10172) therapy. *Haemostasis* Vol.22, No.2, (February 1992) pp. 73-84. ISSN 0340-5338

Davila, R.E., Rajan, E., Adler, D.G., Egan, J., Hirota, W.K., Leighton, J.A., Qureshi, W., Zuckerman, M.J., Fanelli, R., Wheeler-Harbaugh, J., Baron, T.H., Faigel, D.O., Standards of Practice Committee. (2005) ASGE Guideline: the role of endoscopy in the patient with lower-GI bleeding. *Gastrointest Endosc.* Vol.62, No.5, (November 2005) pp. 656-60. ISSN 0016-5107

Davila, R.E., Rajan, E., Baron, T.H., Adler, D.G., Egan, J.V., Faigel, D.O., Gan, S.I., Hirota, W.K., Leighton, J.A., Lichtenstein, D., Qureshi, W.A., Shen, B., Zuckerman, M.J., VanGuilder, T., Fanelli, R.D.; Standards of Practice Committee, American Society of Gastrointestinal Endoscopy. (2006) ASGE guideline: colorectal cancer screening and surveillance. *Gastrointest Endosc.* Vol.63, No.4, (April 2006) pp. 546-57. ISSN 0016-5107

De Melo, S.W., Cleveland, P., Raimondo, M., Wallace, M.B., Woodward, T. (2011) Endoscopic mucosal resection with the grasp-and-snare technique through a double-channel endoscope in humans. *Gastrointest Endosc.* Vol.73, No.2, (February 2011) pp. 349-52. ISSN 0016-5107

Denberg, T.D., Melhado, T.V., Coombes, J.M., Beaty, B.L., Berman, K., Byers, T.E., Marcus, A.C., Steiner, J.F., Ahnen, D.J. (2005) Predictors of nonadherence to screening colonoscopy. *J Gen Intern Med.* Vol.20, No.11, (November 2005) pp. 989-95. ISSN 0884-8734

DiSario, J.A., Fennerty, M.B., Tietze, C.C., Hutson, W.R., Burt, R.W. (1994) Endoscopic balloon dilation for ulcer-induced gastric outlet obstruction. *Am J Gastroenterol.* Vol.89, No.6, (June 1994) pp. 868-71. ISSN 0002-9270

Dobie, K.A., Burke, C. (2011) *Colonoscopy for Dummies.* pp. 1-64, Wiley Publishing Inc., ISBN 978-0-47061661-1, Hoboken, New Jersey

Eickhoff, A., van Dam, J., Jakobs, R., Kudis, V., Hartmann, D., Damian, U., Weickert, U., Schilling, D., Riemann, J.F. (2007) Computer-assisted colonoscopy (the NeoGuide Endoscopy System): results of the first human clinical trial ("PACE study"). *Am J Gastroenterol.* Vol.102, No.2, (February 2007) pp. 261-6. ISSN 0002-927

Eisen, G.M., Baron, T.H., Dominitz, J.A., Faigel, D.O., Goldstein, J.L., Johanson, J.F., Mallery, J.S., Raddawi, H.M., Vargo, J.J., Waring, J.P., Fanelli, R.D., Wheeler-Harbaugh, J. (2002) Acute colonic pseudo-obstruction. *Gastrointest Endosc.* Vol.56, No.6, (December 2002) pp. 789-92. ISSN 0016-5107

Eisen, G.M., Dominitz, J.A., Faigel, D.O., Goldstein, J.L., Kalloo, A.N., Petersen, J.L., Raddawi, H.M., Ryan, M.E., Vargo, J.J. 3rd, Young, H.S., Fanelli, R.D., Hyman, N.H., Wheeler-Harbaugh, J., American Society for Gastrointestinal Endoscopy Standards of Practice Committee. (2001) Endoscopic therapy of anorectal disorders. *Gastrointest Endosc.* Vol.53, No.7, (June 2001) pp. 867-70. ISSN 0016-5107

Eisen, G.M., Dominitz, J.A., Faigel, D.O., Goldstein, J.A., Kalloo, A.N., Petersen, B.T., Raddawi, H.M., Ryan, M.E., Vargo, J.J. 3rd, Young, H.S., Fanelli, R.D., Hyman, N.H., Wheeler-Harbaugh, J.; American Society for Gastrointestinal Endoscopy. (2001) Use of endoscopy in diarrheal illnesses. *Gastrointest Endosc.* Vol.54, No.6, (December 2001) pp. 821-3. ISSN 0016-5107

Elfant, A.B., Korn, C., Mendez, L., Pello, M.J., Peikin, S.R. (1995) Recall of informed consent after endoscopic procedures. *Dis Colon Rectum.* Vol.38, No.1. (January 1995) pp. 1-3. ISSN0012-3706

Elitsur, Y., Blankenship, P., Lawrence, Z. (2000) Propofol sedation for endoscopic procedures in children. *Endoscopy.* Vol.32, No.10. (October 2000) pp. 788-91. ISSN 0013-726X

Eun, C.S., Han, D.S., Hyun, Y.S., Bae, J.H., Park, H.S., Kim, T.Y., Jeon, Y.C., Sohn, J.H. (2011) The timing of bowel preparation is more important than the timing of colonoscopy in determining the quality of bowel cleansing. *Dig Dis Sci.* Vol.56, No.2, (February 2011) pp. 539-44. ISSN 0163-2116

Faigel, D.O., Baron, T.H., Goldstein, J.L., Hirota, W.K., Jacobson, B.C., Johanson, J.F., Leighton, J.A., Mallery, J.S., Peterson, K.A., Waring, J.P., Fanelli, R.D., Wheeler-Harbaugh, J; Standards Practice Committee, American Society for Gastrointestinal Endoscopy. (2002) Guidelines for the use of deep sedation and anesthesia for GI endoscopy. *Gastrointest Endosc.* Vol.56, No.5. (November 2002) pp. 613-7. ISSN 0016-5107

Faigel, D.O., Pike, I.M., Baron, T.H., Chak, A., Coen, J. Deal, S.E., Hoffman, B., Jacobson, B.C., Mergener, K., Petersen, B.T., Petrini, J.L., Rex, D.K., Safdi, M.A; ASGE/ACG Taskforce on Quality in Endoscopy. (2006) *Am J Gastroenterol.* Vol.101, No.4, (April 2006) pp. 866-72. ISSN 0002-9270

Farrell, J.J. (2007) Preoperative colonic stenting: how, when and why? *Curr Opin Gastreoenterol.* Vol.23, No.5, (September 2007) pp. 544-9. ISSN 0267-1379

Farrell, J.J., Sack, J. (2008) Removable colonic stenting: time to expand the indications? *Gastrointest Endosc.* Vol.68, No.4, (October 2008) pp. 721-3. ISSN 0016-5107

Fedeli, P., Gasbarrini, A., Cammarota, G. (2011) Spectral endoscopic imaging: the multiband system for enhancing the endoscopic surface visualization. *J Clin Gastroenterol.* Vol.45, No.1, (January 2011) pp. 6-15. ISSN 0192-0790

Feld, A.D. (12/2010-1/2011) Open access. Risky business. *AGA Perspectives.* Vol.6, No.6, (December 2010-January 2011) pp. 5,7. ISSN 1554-3366

Filip, M., Iordache, S., Săftoiu, A., Ciurea, T. (2011) Autofluorescence imaging and magnification endoscopy. *World J Gastroenterol.* Vol.17, No.1, (January 2011) pp. 9-14. ISSN 1007-9327

Fredette, M.E., Lightdale, J.R. (2008) Endoscopic sedation in pediatric practice. *Gastrointest Endosc Clin N Am.* Vol.18, No.4, (October 2008) pp. 739-51. ISSN 1052-5157

Freedman, J.S., Harari, D.Y., Bamji, N.D., Bodian, C.A., Kornacki, S., Cohen, L.B., Miller, K.M., Aisenberg, J. (2011) The detection of premalignant colon polyps during colonoscopy is stable throughout the workday. *Gastrointest Endosc.* Vol.73, No.6, (June 2011) pp.1197-206. ISSN 0016-5107

Ganz, R.A. (2004) The development and the implementation of new endoscopic technology: what are the challenges? *Gastrointest Endosc.* Vol.60, No.4, (October 2004) pp. 592-8, ISSN 0016-5107

Gheonea, D.I., Cârţână, T., Ciurea, T., Popescu, C., Bădărău, A., Săftoui, A. (2011) Confocal laser endomicroscopy and immunoendoscopy for real-time assessment of vascularization in gastrointestinal malignancies. *World J Gastroenterol.* Vol.17, No.1, (January 2011) pp. 21-7. ISSN1007-9327

Goddard, A.F., James, M.W., McIntyre, A.S., Scott, B.B., on behalf of the British Society of Gastroenterology. (2011) *Gut.* (May 2011) [Epub ahead of print] pp. 1-8. ISSN 1468-3288

Goh, K-L. (2011) Development of gastrointestinal endoscopy in Malaysia: A historical perspective with special reference to the experience at the University of Malaya Medical Centre. *Dig Endosc.* Vol.23, Suppl.1, (May 2011) pp. 150-3. ISSN 1443-1661

Goodwin, J.S., Singh, A., Reddy, N., Riall, T.S., Kuo, Y.F. (2011) Overuse of screening colonoscopy in the Medicare population. *Arch Intern Med.* (May 2011) [Epub ahead of print] pp. E1-9. ISSN 0003-9926

Greinacher, A., Warkentin, E. (2008) The direct thrombin inhibitor hirudin. *Thromb Haemost.* Vol.99, No.5, (May 2008) pp. 819-29. ISSN 0340-6245

Groenen, M.J., Kuipers, E.J., van Berge Henegouwen, G.P., Fockens, P., Ouwendijk, R.J. (2006) Computerisation of endoscopy reports using standard reports and text blocks. *Neth J Med.* Vol.64, No.3, (March 2006) pp. 78-83. ISSN 0300-2977

Gurudu, S.R., Ratuapli, S., Heigh, R., DiBaise, J., Leighton, J., Crowell, M. (2010) Quality of bowel cleansing for afternoon colonoscopy is influenced by time of administration. *Am J Gastroenterol.* Vol.105, No.11, (November 2010) pp. 2318-22. ISSN 0002-9270

Habbema, J., Moore, E.A., Zauber, A.G. (2011) Until what age is colonoscopy indicated in elderly people without prior screening (abstract)? *Gastroenterology.* Vol.140, No.5, Supplement 1, (May 2011) pp. S-16. ISSN 0016-5085

Han, J-H., Park, S., Youn, S. (2011) Endoscopic closure of colon perforation with band ligation; Salvage technique after endoclip failure. *Clin Gastroenterol Hepatol.* Vol.9, No.6, (June 2011) pp. e54-5. (Available online at www.cghjournal.org.) ISSN 1542-3565

Helwick, C. (2011a) "Clouds" still hover over colonoscopy. *Gastroenterol Endosc News.* Vol.62, No.3, (March 2011) pp. 6-7. ISSN 0162-6566

Helwick, C. (2011b) Colorectal cancer screening: United States vs. Europe. *Gastroenterol Endosc News.* Vol.62, No.3, (March 2011) pp. 9-10. ISSN 0162-6566

Heuss, L.T., Froehlich, F., Beglinger, C. (2005) Changing patterns of sedation and monitoring during endoscopy: results of a nationwide survey in Switzerland. *Endoscopy.* Vol.37, No.2, (February 2005) pp. 161-6. ISSN 013726X

Hickle RS. (2001) Apparatus and method for providing a conscious patient relief from pain and anxiety associated with medical or surgical procedures. US Patent Application 2001: 20020017296.

http://blogs.wsj.com/health/2009/08/06/the-other-propofol-issue-when-insurance-should-pay-for-it/ (The other propofol issue: when insurance should pay for it-Accessed 4/17/2011)

http://promotions.mardenkane.com/cbs/cbscares/rules.cfm (Accessed 1/10/2011)

http://thehappyhospitalist.blogspot.com/2009_08_01_archive.html (Propofol during colonoscopy anesthesia by gastroenterologists and general practitioners-Accessed 4/17/2011)

http://www.asge.org/PublicationsProductsIndex.aspx?id=352 (Accessed 1/11/2011

http://www.cbs.com/cbs cares/topics/?sec=colorectal cancer (Accessed 1/15/2011)

http://www.cbs.com/cbs cares/video/?cid=822059380 (Accessed 1/15/2011)

http://www.invendo-medical.com/index_eng.html (Accessed 1/17/2011)

Huffman, M., Unger, R.Z., Thatikonda, C., Amstutz, S., Rex, D.K. (2010) Split-dose bowel preparation for colonoscopy and residual gastric fluid volume: an observational study. *Gastrointest Endosc.* Vol.72, No.3, (September 2010) pp. 516-22. ISSN 0016-5107

Jaskiewicz, K., Rzepko, R., Adrych, K., Smoczynski, M. (2006) Microscopic colitis in routine colonoscopies. *Dig Dis Sci.* Vol.51, No.2, (February 2006) p. 241-4. ISSN 0163-2116

Jemal, A., Bray, F., Center, M.M., Ferlay, J., Ward, E., Forman, D. (2011) Global cancer statistics. *CA: Cancer J Clin.* Vol61, No.2, (March-April 2011) pp. 69-90. ISSN 0007-9235

Kahi, C.J., Anderson, J.C., Waxman, I., Kessler, W.R., Imperiale, T.F., Li, X., Rex, D.K. (2010) High-definition chromocolonoscopy vs. high-definition white light colonoscopy for average-risk colorectal cancer screening. *Am J Gastroenterol.* Vol.105, No.6, (June 2010) pp. 1301-7. ISSN 0002-9270

Katsanos, K., Sabharwal, T., Adam, A. (2010) Stenting of the lower gastrointestinal tract: current status. *Cardiovasc Intervent Radiol.* (December 2010) [Epub ahead of print] ISSN 0174-1551

Kavin, H., Sinicrope, F., Esker, A.H. (1992) Management of perforation of the colon at colonoscopy. *Am J Gastroenterol.* Vol.87, No.2, (February 1992) pp. 161-7. ISSN 0002-9270

Keswani, R.N. (2011) Single-balloon colonoscopy versus repeat standard colonoscopy for previous incomplete colonoscopy: a randomized, controlled trial. *Gastrointest Endosc.* Vol.73, No.3, (March 2011) pp. 507-12. ISSN 0016-5107

Khalid, A.B., Majid, S., Salih, M., Hashmat, F., Jafri, W. (2011) Is full colonoscopic examination necessary in young patients with fresh bleeding per rectum? *Endoscopy.* (March 2011) [Epub ahead of print] ISSN 0013-726X

Khalid, O., Srivastava, R., Mulhall, A., Paladugu, A., Dryden, G., Lippman, S. (2011) Conscious sedation: Is it always needed for endoscopy? *Practical Gastroenterol.* Vol.35, No.2, (February 2011) pp. 10-15. ISSN 0277-4208

Kistler, C.E., Kirby, K.A., Lee, D., Casadei, M.A., Walter, L.C. (2011) Long-term outcomes following positive fecal occult blood test results in older adults. *Arch Intern Med.* (May 2011) [Epub ahead of print] pp. E1-8. ISSN 1538-3679

Korkis, A.M., Miskovitz, P.F., Yurt, R.W., Klein, H. (1992) Rectal prolapse after oral cathartics. *J Clin Gastroenterol.* Vol.14, No.4. (June 1992) pp. 339-41. ISSN 0192-0790

Krishnan, S. Wolf, J.L. (2011) Colorectal cancer screening and prevention in women. *Women's Health.* Vol.7, No.2, (March 2011) pp. 213-26. ISSN 1541-0331

Kuramoto, T., Umegaki, E., Kinoshita, S., Kojima, Y., Shindo, Y., Nishihara, H., Murano, M., Ohtsuka, N., Higuchi, K. (2011) Retrograde colon capsule endoscopy from anus using a new self-propelling capsule; the first human trial (abstract). *Gastrointest Endosc.* Vol.73, No.4S, (April 2011) pp. AB67(Su1552). ISSN 0016-5107

Lasser, K.E., Murillo, J., Lisboa, S., Casimir, A.N., Valley-Shah, L., Emmons, K.M., Fletcher, R.H., Ayanian, J.Z. (2011) Colorectal cancer screening among ethnically diverse, low-income patients. *Arch Intern Med.* Vol.171, No.10, (May 2011) pp. 906-12. ISSN 0003-9926

Lee, A., Iskander, J.M., Gupta, N., Borg, B.B., Zuckerman, G., Banerjee, B., Gyawali, C.P. (2011) Queue position in the endoscopic schedule impacts effectiveness of colonoscopy. *Am J Gastroenterol.* (March 2011) [Epub ahead of print] pp. 1-9. EISSN 1572-0241

Leffler, D.A., Neeman, N., Rabb, J.M., Shin, J.Y., Landon, B.E., Pallav, K., Falchuk, Z.M., Aronson, M.D. (2011) An alerting system improves adherence to follow-up recommendations from colonoscopy examinations. *Gastroenterol.* Vol.140, No.4, (April 2011) pp. 1166-73. ISSN 0016-5085

Leighton J.A., Shen, B., Baron, T.H., Adler, D.G., Davila, R., Egan, J.V., Faigel, D.O., Gan, S.I., Hirota, W.K., Lichtenstein, D., Qureshi, W.A., Rajan, E., Zuckerman, M.J., VanGuilder, T., Fanelli, R.D.; Standards of Practice Committee, American Society of Gastrointestinal Endoscopy. (2006) ASGE guideline: endoscopy in the diagnosis and treatment of inflammatory bowel disease. *Gastrointest Endosc.* Vol.63, No.4, (April 2006) pp. 558-65. ISSN 0016-5107

Leufkens, A.M., Demarco, D.C., Rastogi, A., Akerman, P.A., Azzouzi, K., Rothstein, R.I., Vieggaar, F.P., Repici, A., Rando, G., Okolo, P.I., Dewit, O., Ignjatovic, A., Odstrcil, E., East, J., Deprez, P.H., Saunders, B.P., Kalloo, A.N., Creel, B., Singh, V., Lennon, A.M., Siersema, P.D; The Third Eye Retroscope Randomized Clinical Evaluation [TERRACE] Study Group. (2011) Effect of a retrograde-viewing device on adenoma detection rate during colonoscopy: the TERRACE study. *Gastrointest Endosc.* Vol.73, No.3, (March 2011) pp. 480-9. ISSN 0016-5107

Luginbühl, M., Vuilleumier, P., Schumacher, P., Stüber, F. (2009) Anesthesia or sedation or gastroenterologic endoscopies. *Curr Opin Anaesthesiol.* Vol.22, No.4, (August 2009) pp. 524-31. ISSN 0952-7907

Marshall, J.B. (1995) Technical proficiency of trainees performing colonoscopy: a learning curve. *Gastrointest Endosc* Vol.42, No.4, (October 1995) pp. 287-91. ISSN 0016-5107

Marshall, J.B. (2011) Post-colonoscopy era ahead? Not immediately. *AGA Perspectives.* Vol.6, No.2, (April-May 2011) pp. 5,7. ISSN 1554-3366

Matsukawa, H., Shiraga, N., Tsugu, T., Adachi, M., Miyazawa, M., Kashiwazaki, K., Hibi, T. (2007) The use of water-soluble contrast enema without pretreatment for the diagnosis of colon disease. *Nippon Shokakibyo Gakkai Zasshi.* Vol.104, No.9, (September 2007) pp. 1344-51. ISSN 0446-6586

McHugh, M., Osei-Anto, A., Klabunde, C.N., Galen, B.A. (2011) Adoption of CT colonography by US hospitals. *J Amer Coll Radiol.* Vol.8, No.3. (March 2011) pp. 169-74. ISSN 15461440

Miskovitz, P. Gibofsky, A. (1995) Risk management in endoscopic practice. *Gastrointest Endosc Clin North Am.* Vol.5, No.2, (April 1995) pp. 391-401. ISSN 1052-5157

Miskovitz, P., Gordon, B., Yurt, R., Herbstman, C. (1987) Gastrointestinal bleeding in the critically ill immunosuppressed patient. In: *The Critically Ill Immunosuppressed Patient: Diagnosis and Management,* Parrillo, J.D. & Mazur, H.; (Eds.). pp. 189-213, Aspen Publishers, Inc. ISBN 0-87189-636-2, Rockville, MD.

Miskovitz P., Margulis, S.J., (1990) Risikogruppen und ihre Überwachung In: *Das kolorektale Karazinom und seine Präkanzerosen. Grundlagen, Diagnostik, interdisziplinäre Therapie und Operationstechnik,* Izbicki J.R., Wilker D.K., Schweiberer L. (Eds), pp. 139-45, Walter de Gruyter, ISBN 3110115751, Berlin & New York.

Miskovitz, P.F., Rochwarger, A. (1993) *The Evaluation and Treatment of the Patient with Diarrhea.* pp. 1-179. Andover Medical Publisher, ISBN 1563720590, Boston, Massachusetts

Miskovitz, P.F., Steinberg, H. (1982) Diverticula of the gastrointestinal tract. *Dis Mon.* Vol.29, No.3, (December 1982) pp. 1-61. ISSN 1557-8194

Misra, V., Misra, S.P., Dwivedi, M., Singh, P.A., Agarwal, V. (2010) Microscopic colitis in patients presenting with chronic diarrhea. *Indian J Pathol Microbiol.* Vol.53, No.1, (January-March 2010) pp. 15-19. ISSN 0337-4929

Modlin, I.M. (2000) *A Brief History of Endoscopy*. pp. 1-144. Multimed ISBN None, Milano, Italy

Moss A., Bourke, M.J., Williams, S.J., Hourigan, L.F., Brown, G., Tam, W., Singh, R., Zanati, S., Chen, R.Y., Byth, K. (2011) Endoscopic mucosal resection outcomes and prediction of submucosal cancer from advanced colonic mucosal neoplasia. *Gastroenterology.* (March 2011) [Epub ahead of print] ISSN 0016-5085

Naravadi, V., Balasubramanian, G., Madireddy, S., Shenoy, S., Guthrie, W., Verma, A.K., Anand, K. (2011) Screening for colorectal cancer above 75 years--Is it necessary (abstract)? *Gastroenterology.* Vol.140, No.5, Supplement 1, (May 2011) pp. S-16-S-17. ISSN 0016-5085

Nurmohamed, M.T., Fareed, J., Hoppensteadt, D., Walenga, J.M., ten Cate, J.W. (1991) Pharmacological and clinical studies with Lomoparan, a low molecular weight glycosaminoglycan. *Semin Thromb Hemost.* Vol.17 Suppl.2, pp. 205-13. ISSN 0094-6176

Obstein, K.L., Patil, V.D., Jayender, J., Estépar, R.S., Spofford, I.S., Lengyel, B.I., Vosburgh, K.G., Thomson, C.C. (2011) Evaluation of colonoscopy technical skill levels by use of an objective kinematic-based system. *Gastrointest Endosc.* Vol.73, No.2, (February 2011) pp. 315-21. ISSN 0016-5107

Oka, S., Tanaka, S., Takata, S., Kanao, H., Chayama, K. (2011) Clinical usefulness of narrow band imaging magnifying classification for colorectal tumors based on both surface pattern and microvessel features. *Dig Endosc.* Vol.23, Suppl.1, May 1011) pp. 101-5. ISSN 1443-1661

Ortner, M.A., Fusco, V., Ebert, B., Sukowski, U., Weber-Eibel, J., Fleige, B., Stolte, M., Oberhuber, G., Rinneberg, H., Lochs, H. (2010) Time-gated fluorescence spectroscopy improves endoscopic detection of low-grade dysplasia in ulcerative colitis. *Gastrointest Endosc.* Vol.71, No.2, (February 2010) pp. 312-8. ISSN 0016-5107

Pambianco, D.J. (2008) Future directions in endoscopic sedation. *Gastrointest Endosc Clin N Am.* Vol.18, No.4, (October 2008) pp. 789-99. ISSN 1052-5157

Pambianco, D.J., Vargo, J.J., Pruitt, R.E., Hardi, R., Martin J.F. (2011) Computer-assisted personalized sedation for upper endoscopy and colonoscopy: a comparative multicenter randomized study. *Gastrointest Endosc.* Vol.73, No.4. (April 2011) pp. 765-72. ISSN 0016-5107

Parra-Blanco, A., Kaminaga, N., Kojima, T., Endo, Y., Uragami, N., Okawa, N., Hattori, T., Takahashi, H., Fujita, R. (2000) Hemoclipping for postpolypectomy and postbiopsy colonic bleeding. *Gastrointest Endosc.* Vol.51, No.1, (January 2000) pp. 37-41. ISSN 0016-5107

Parry, B.R., Williams, S.M. (1991) Competency and the colonoscopist: a learning curve. *Aust N Z J Surg.* Vol.61, No.6, (June 1991) pp. 419-22. ISSN 0004-8690

Petersen, B.T. (2006) Promoting efficiency in gastrointestinal endoscopy. *Gastrointest Endosc Clin N Am.* Vol.16, No.4, (October 2006) pp. 671-85. ISSN 1052-5157

Pfeffer, J., Grinshpon, R., Rex. D., Levin, B., Rösch, T., Arber, N., Halpern, Z. (2006) The Aer-O-Scope: proof of the concept of a pneumatic, skill-independent, self-propelling, self-navigating colonoscope in a pig model. *Endoscopy.* Vol.38, No.2, (February 2006) pp. 1444-8. ISSN 0013726

Pohl, J., Schneider, A., Vogell, H., Mayer, G., Kaiser, G., Ell, C. (2011) Pancolonic chromoendoscopy with indigo carmine versus standard colonoscopy for detection of neoplastic lesions: a randomized two-centre trial. *Gut.* Vol.60, No.4, (April 2011) pp. 485-490. ISSN 0017-5749

Qureshi, W., Adler D.G., Davila, R.E., Egan, J. Hirota, W.K., Jacobson, B.C., Leighton, J.A., Rajan, E., Zuckerman, M.J., Fanelli, R., Wheeler-Harbaugh, J., Baron, T.H., Faigel, D.O. (2005) ASGE guideline: guideline on the use of endoscopy in the management of constipation. *Gastrointest Endosc.* Vol.62, No.2, (August 2005) pp. 199-201. ISSN 0016-5107

Rabeneck, L., Saskin, R., Paszat, L.F. (2011) Onset and clinical course of bleeding and perforation after outpatient colonoscopy: a population-based study. *Gastrointest Endosc.* Vol.73, No.3 (March 2011) pp. 520-523. ISSN 0016-5107

Rappaport, B., Mellon, R.D., Simone, A., Woodcock, J. (2011) Defining safe use of anesthesia in children. N Engl J Med. Vol.364, No.10, (March 2011) pp. 1-3. ISSN 0028-4793

Rex, D.K. (2009) Third eye retroscope: rationale, efficacy, challenges. *Rev Gastroenterol Disord.* Vol.9, No.1, (Winter 2009) pp. 1-6. ISSN 1533-001X

Rex, D.K. (12/2010-1/2011) Open access endoscopy is indispensable. *AGA Perspectives.* Vol.6, No.6, (December 2010-January 2011) pp. 4,6. ISSN 1554-3366

Rösch. T., Adler, A., Pohl, H., Wettschureck, E., Koch, M., Wiedermann, B., Hoepffner, N. (2008) A motor-driven single-use colonoscope controlled with a hand-held device: a feasibility study in volunteers. *Gastrointest Endosc.* Vol.67, No.7, (June 2008) pp. 1129-46. ISSN 0016-5107

Rösch, T., Eickhoff, A., Fritscher-Ravens, A., Eliakim, R., Arber, N. (2007) The new scopes—broadening the colonoscopy marketplace. *Digestion.* Vol.76, No.1, (October 2007) pp. 42-50. ISSN 0012-2823

Roy, H.K., Turzhitsky, V., Kim, Y., Goldberg, M.J., Watson, P., Rogers, J.D., Gomes, A.J., Kromine, A., Brand, R.E., Jameel, M., Bogovejic, A., Pradhan, P., Backman, V. (2009) Association between rectal optical signatures and colonic neoplasia: potential applications for screening. *Cancer Res.* Vol.69, No.10. (May 2009) pp. 4476-83. ISSN 0008-5472

Sacher-Huvelin, S., Coron, E., Gaudric, M., Planche, L., Benamouzig, R., Maunoury, V., Filoche, B., Frédéric, M., Saurin, J.C., Subtil, C., Lecleir, S., Cellier, C., Coumaros, D., Heresbach, D., Galmiche, J.P. (2010) Colon capsule endoscopy vs. colonoscopy in patients at average or increased risk of colorectal cancer. *Aliment Pharmacol Ther.* Vol.32, No.9, (November 2010) pp. 1145-53. ISSSN 0269-2813

Safioleas, M., Stamatakos, M., Safioleas, C., Chatziconstantinou, C., Papachristodoulou, A. (2009) The management of patients with retained foreign bodies in the rectum: from surgeon with respect. *Acta Chir Belg.* Vol.109, No.3, (May-June 2009) pp. 352-5. ISSN 0001-5458

Savides, T.J., Chang, K., Cotton, P. (2004) Possible features of current electronic endoscopic information systems: what to look for. *Gastrointest Endosc Clin N Am.* Vol.14, No.4, (October 2004) pp. 735-43. ISSN 1052-5157

Sawhney, M.S. (2011) The future of endoscopy, post-colonoscopy. *AGA Perspectives.* Vol.7, No.2, (April-May 2011) pp. 4,6. ISSN 1554-3366

Schloendorff v Society of New York Hospital, 105 N.E. 92, N. Y., (1914)

Schulman, S., Kearon, C., Kakkar, A.K., Mismetti, P., Schellong, S., Eriksson, H., Baanstra, D., Schnee, J., Goldhaber, S.Z.; RE-COVER Study Group. (2009) Dabigatran versus warfarin in the treatment of acute venous thromboembolism. *N Engl J Med.* Vol.361, No.24, (December 2009) pp. 2342-52. ISSN 0028-4793

Sedlack, R.E. (2010) The Mayo Colonoscopy Skills Assessment Tool: validation of a unique instrument to assess colonoscopy skills in trainees. *Gastrointest Endosc.* Vol.72, No.6. (December 2010) pp. 1125-33. ISSN 0016- 5107

Sieg, A., Hachmoeller-Eisenbach, U., Eisenbach, T. (2001) Prospective evaluation of complications in outpatient GI endoscopy: a survey among German gastroenterologists. *Gastrointest Endosc.* Vol.53, No.6, (May 2001) pp. 620-7. ISSN 0016-5107

Singh, R., Chen Yi Mei, S.L., Tam, W., Raju, D., Ruszkiewicz, A. (2010) Real-time histology with the endocytoscope. *World J Gastroenterol.* Vol.16, No.40, (October 2010) pp. 5016-9. ISSN 1007-9327

Singh, V.V., Draganov, P., Valentine, J. (2005) Efficacy and safety of endoscopic balloon dilation of symptomatic upper and lower gastrointestinal Crohn's disease strictures. *J Clin Gastroenterol.* Vol.39, No.4, (April 2005) pp. 284-90. ISSN 0192-0790

Sivak, M.V. Jr., Fleischer, D.E. (1984) Colonoscopy with a VideoEndoscope: preliminary experience. *Gastrointest Endosc.* Vol.30, No.1, (February 1984) pp. 1-3. ISSN 0016-5107

Smith, M.J. (2011a) Is colonoscopy the optimal method for colorectal cancer screening? *Gastroenterol Endosc News.* Vol.62, No.3, (March 2011) pp. 1,5,7. ISSN 0162-6566

Smith, M.J. (2011b) Withdrawal time during colonoscopy: much ado about nothing? *Gastroenterol Endosc News.* Vol.62, No.3, (March 2011) pp. 11,29. ISSN 0162-6566

Solt, J., Bajor, J., Szabó, M., Horváth, O.P. (2003) Long-term results of balloon catheter dilation for benign gastric outlet stenosis. *Endoscopy.* Vol.35, No.6, (June 2003) pp. 490-5. ISSN 0013726X

Sonoda, H, Kohnoe, S, Yamazato, T, Satoh, Y. Morizono, G., Shikata, K., Morita, M., Watanabe, A., Morita, M., Kakeji, Y., Inoue, F., Maehara, Y. Colorectal cancer screening with odour material by canine scent detection. *Gut.* (January 2011) [Epub ahead of print] ISSN 0017-5749

Stunkel, L., Benson, M., McLellan, L., Sinaii, N., Bedarida, G., Emanuel, E., Grady, C. (2010) Comprehension and informed consent: assessing the effect of a short consent form. *IRB.* Vol.32, No.4, (July-August 2010) pp. 1-9. ISSN 0193-7758

Thakkar, K., El-Serag, H.B., Mattek, N., Gilger, M.A. (2007) Complications of pediatric EGD: a 4-year experience in PEDS_CORI. *Gastrointest Endosc.* Vol.65, No. 2, (February 2007) pp. 213-21. ISSN 0016-5107

Turpie, A.G. (2008) New oral anticoagulants in atrial fibrillation. *Eur Heart J.* Vol.29, No.2. (December 2008) pp. 155-65. ISSN 0195-668X

Uraoka, T., Kato, J., Kuriyama, M., Hori, K., Ishikawa, S., Harada, K., Takemoto, K., Hiraoka, S., Fujita, H., Horii, J., Saito, Y., Yamamoto, K. (2009) CO_2 insufflation for potentially difficult colonoscopies: Efficacy when used by less experienced colonoscopists. *World J Gastroenterol.* Vol.15, No.41, (November 2009) pp. 5186-92. ISSN 1007-9327

Van den Broek, F.J., Fockens, P., van Eeden, S., Stokkers, P.C., Ponsioen, C.Y., Reitsma, J.B., Dekker, E. (2011) Narrow-band imaging versus high-definition endoscopy for the diagnosis of neoplasia in ulcerative colitis. *Endoscopy.* Vol.43, No.2, (February 2011) pp. 108-15. ISSN 0013726X

Wada, Y., Kudo, S-E., Misawa, M., Ikehara, N., Hamatani, S. (2011) Vascular pattern classification of colorectal lesions with narrow band imaging magnifying endoscopy. *Dig Endosc.* Vol.23, Suppl.1, (May 2011) pp. 106-11. ISSN 1443-1661

Ward, B., Shah, S., Kirwan, P., Mayberry, J.F. (1999) Issues of consent in colonoscopy: if a patient says 'stop' should we continue? *J R Soc Med.* Vol.92, No.3, (March 1999) pp. 132-3. ISSN 0141-0768

Warkentin T.E., Greinacher, A., Koster, A. (2008) Bivalirudin. *Thromb Haemost.* Vol.99, No.5. (May 2008) pp. 830-9. ISSN 0340-624

Waye, J.D., (2010) Improving lesion detection during colonoscopy. *Gastroenterol Hepatol.* Vol.6, No.10, (October 2010) pp. 647-52. ISSN 1554-7914

Waye, J.D., Kahn, O., Auerbach, M.E. (1996) Complications of colonoscopy and flexible sigmoidoscopy. *Gastrointest Endosc Clin North Am.* Vol.6, No.2, (April 1996) pp. 343-7. ISSN 1052-5157

Wexner, S.D., Beck, D.E., Baron, T.H., Fanelli, R.D., Hyman, N., Shen, B., Wasco, K.E.; American Society of Colon and Rectal Surgeons; American Society for Gastrointestinal Endoscopy; Society of American Gastrointestinal and Endoscopic Surgeons. (2006) A consensus document on bowel preparation before colonoscopy: prepared by a task force from the American Society of Colon and Rectal Surgeons (ASCRS), the American Society for Gastrointestinal Endoscopy (ASGE), and the Society of American Gastrointestinal and Endoscopic Surgeons (SAGES). *Gastrointest Endosc.* Vol.63, No.7. (June 2006) p. 894-909. ISSN 0016-5107

Wexner, S.D., Garbus, J.E., Singh, J.J. (2001) SAGES Colonoscopy Outcomes Study Group. A prospective analysis of 13,580 colonoscopies. Reevaluation of credentialing guidelines. *Surg Endosc.* Vol.15, No.3. (March 2001) pp. 251-61. ISSN 1432-2218

Wexner, S.D., Litwin, D., Cohen, J., Earle, D., Ferzli, G., Flaherty, J., Graham, S., Horgan, S., Katz, B.L., Kavic, M., Kilkenny, J., Meador, J., Price, R., Quebberman, B., Reed, W., Sillin, L., Vitale, G., Xenos, E.S., Eisen, G.M.,

Dominitz, J., Faigel, D., Goldstein, J., Kalloo, A., Peterson, B. Raddawi, H., Ryan, M., Vargo, J., Young, H., Simmang, C., Hyman, N., Eisenstat, T., Anthony, T., Cataldo, P., Church, J., Cohen, J., Denstman, F., Glennon, E., Kilkenny, J., McConnell, J., Nogueras, J., Orsay, C., Otchy, D., Place, R., Rakinic, J., Savoca, P., Tjandra, J.; American Society for Gastrointestinal Endoscopy, Society of American Gstrointestinal Endoscopic Surgeons, American Society of Colorectal Surgeons. (2002) Principles of privileging and credentialing for endoscopy and colonoscopy. *Gastrointest Endosc.* Vol.55, No.2, (February 2002) pp. 145-148. ISSN 0016-5107

Williams, J.E., Le, T.D., Faigel, D.O. (2011) Polypectomy rate as a quality measure for colonoscopy. *Gastrointest Endosc.* Vol.73, No.3, (March 2011) pp. 498-506. ISSN 0016-5107

Wilschut, J.A., Steyerberg, W.W., van Leerdam, M.D., Lansdorp-Vogelaar, I., Habbema, J.D., van Ballegooijen, M. (2011) How much colonoscopy screening should be recommended to individuals with various degrees of family history of colorectal cancer? *Cancer.* (March 2011) [Epub ahead of print] pp. 1-9. ISSN 1097-0142

Wilson, W., Taubet, K.A., Gewitz, M., Lockhart, P.B., Baddour, L.M., Levison, M., Bolger, A., Cabell, C.H., Takahashi, M., Baltimore, R.s., Nwburger, J.W., Strom, B.L., Tani, L.Y., Gerber, M., Bonow, R.O., Pallasch, T., Shulman, S.T., Rowley, A.H., Burns, J.C., Ferrieri, P., Gardner, T., Goff, D., Durack, D.T.; American Heart Association Rheumatic Fever, Endocarditis, and Kawasaki Disease Committee; American Heart Association Council on Cardiovascular Disease in the Young; American Heart Association Council on Clinical Cardiology; American Heart Association Council on Cardiovascular Surgery and Anesthesia; Quality of Care and Outcomes Research Interdisciplinary Working Group. (2007) Prevention of infective endocarditis: guidelines from the American Heart Association: a guideline from the American Heart Association Rheumatic Fever, Endocarditis, and Kawasaki Disease Committee, Council on Clinical Cardiology, Council on Cardiovascular Surgery and Anesthesia, and the Quality of Care and Outcomes Research Interdisciplinary Working Group. *Circulation* Vol.116, No.15, (October 2007) pp. 1736-54. ISSN 0009-7322

Winawer, S.J., Krabshuis, J., Lambert, R., O'Brien, M., Fried, M. (2011) Cascade colorectal cancer screening guidelines: A global conceptual model. *J Clin Gastroenterol*. Feb 4, 2011, [Epub ahead of print] pp. 297-300. ISSN 0192-0790

Wolff, W.I. (1989) Colonoscopy: history and development. *Am J Gastro*. Vol.84, No.9, (September 1989) pp. 1017-25. ISSN 0002-9270

Wolff, W.I., Shinya, H. (1971) Colonfiberoscopy. *JAMA.* Vol.217, No.11, (September 13, 1971) pp. 1509-12, ISSN 0098-7484

Yamano, H., Yoshikawa, K., Kimura, T., Yamamoto, E., Harada, E., Kudou, T., Katou, R., Hayashi, Y., Satour, K. (2010) Carbon dioxide insufflation for colonoscopy: evaluation of gas volume, abdominal pain, examination time and transcutaneous partial CO_2 pressure. *J Gastroenterol*. Vol.45, No.12, (December 2010) pp. 1235-40. ISSN 0944-1174

Part 1

The Technique

1

Preparing for Colonoscopy

Rosalinda S. Hulse
Jordan Hospital
Plymouth, MA,
USA

1. Introduction

Colorectal cancer is the third leading cause of cancer-related mortality in the United States and the fourth most common cancer in men and women. Colonoscopy is the best screening test done to detect and prevent colorectal cancers. Abnormal growths such as a polyp, a tumor, or a suspicious-looking lesion in the colon or rectum can be biopsied or removed preventing the initiation of the carcinogenic process and potential metastases into other areas of the body, thereby, allowing patients to obtain a more effective treatment (s) with fewer side effects. Patients whose cancers are found early and treated in a timely manner are more likely to survive than those whose cancers are not found until symptoms appear (Atreja, A., Nepal, S. & Lashner, B., 2010; American Cancer Society [ACS], n.d, 2005). Figure 1 shows a picture of a polyp. Figure 1.a shows a picture of a cancerous tumor of the colon.

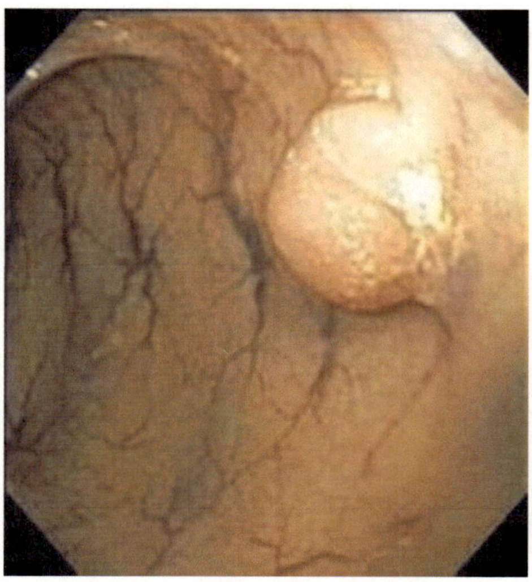

Fig. 1. Polyp in sigmoid colon

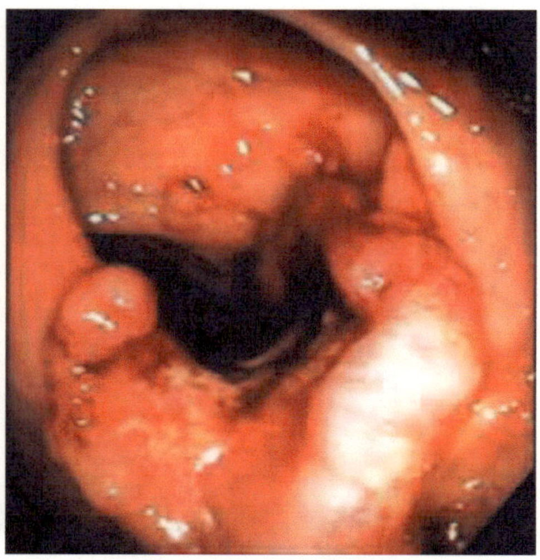

Fig. 1.a Cancerous tumor in the colon

The hardest part of the colonoscopy procedure is the preparation. It usually starts one-to-two weeks prior to the test depending on the recommendation of the physician. Careful planning and strict adherence to these instructions is crucial to the success of the test. Many individuals who have undergone this procedure will attest to the difficulty in complying with these instructions and the harshness of taking the oral prep. As a result, many are hesitant to go through with it risking the possibility of missing diagnoses of cancerous or non-cancerous lesions, tumors or polyps in the colon or rectum.

The key to a successful colonoscopy is good bowel prep, which also depends on the right choice of bowel cleansing agent. The colon needs to be totally clean for good visualization to avoid missing any abnormal or suspicious-looking areas. A small polyp or lesion can hide behind a small piece of stool. Poor or inadequate bowel prep may lead to a prolonged and costly procedure and a potentially inaccurate exam. It may also increase the chance of being aborted; to be repeated at another time which may be at an interval sooner than what is called for or suggested in the standard guidelines. A repeated colonoscopy also increases the risks and complications, such as perforation and bleeding of the colon, and infection (Lawrence, E. & Pickhardt, P., 2010; Hendry, P., Jenkins, J. & Diament, R., 2007; Froehlich, F., et al, 2005). Preparing for colonoscopy may sound complicated, uncomfortable and time-consuming, but it doesn't have to be. Following the instructions carefully and being prepared ahead of time will help the individual tolerate the procedure with minimal discomfort.

This chapter will discuss the step-by-step process in preparing for this procedure for the adult population, explaining the different types of oral preps (including the adjuncts) to take as well as diet modification that will achieve the best results, taking into consideration any medical condition the individual might have. Special conditions that might be adversely affected by the prep, such as diabetes and any heart condition that require taking blood thinners will also be discussed. Tips to alleviate the discomfort while taking the prep will be outlined as well. The goal is to explain the process in a simple, non-intimidating fashion to encourage more individuals to avail of this life-saving screening procedure minimizing any fear and anxiety they may have. A well-informed individual is better able to follow directions carefully to ensure good results. Figure 2 shows an adequately clean transverse colon.

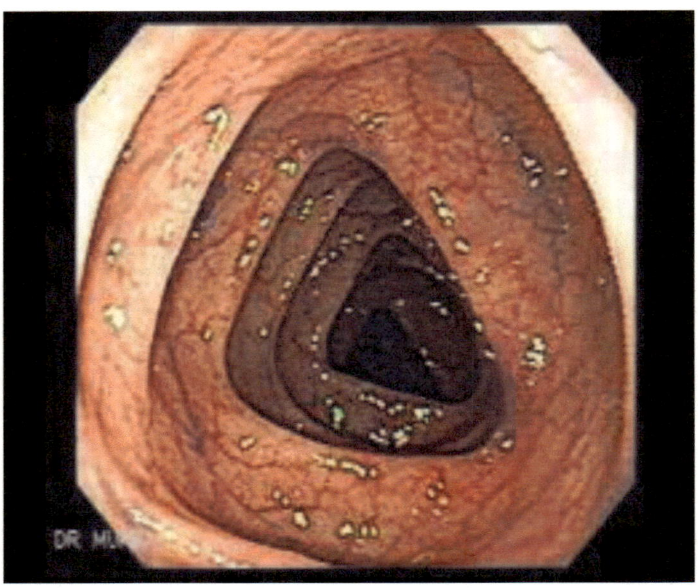

Fig. 2. Transverse Colon

2. Bowel cleansing preps

Some key questions need to be answered prior to selecting an appropriate bowel cleansing agent for the individual:

1. Does the individual have any condition (s) that is contraindicated to taking a bowel prep (i.e. bowel obstruction, perforation, and severe ileus)? If the answer is "yes," then another alternative diagnostic exam need to be considered.
2. Is the individual at risk for fluid and/or electrolyte imbalances? If the answer is "yes," then avoid the sodium phosphate group. Choose the polyethylene glycol.
3. Can the individual tolerate full volume solutions? If not at risk for fluid and electrolyte imbalance and cannot tolerate large doses, choose low-volume polyethylene glycol or sodium phosphate. Sodium picosulfate and magnesium citrate can also be another alternative to sodium phosphate. This is the choice in most European countries and is currently not available in the United States (Atreja, A., Nepal, S. & Lashner, B., 2010). Otherwise, a 4-L polyethylene glycol solution is the choice especially if the individual has a history of poor bowel prep or is worried about cost or insurance coverage.

Compliance to completing a bowel prep is also dependent on a number of factors, namely, poor palatability of the prep, concomitant medications, comorbitites affecting renal and hepatic functions, time of test i.e. early morning or late in the afternoon, sex, and cost (Atreja, A., Nepal, S. & Lashner, B., 2010 & ASGE, 2009). Colonoscopies performed in the afternoon have shown higher rates of poor bowel prep and lower rates of adenoma detection (Varughese, S., Kumar,A.,George, A., & Castro, F., 2010; Sanaka,M., Shah,N., Mullen,K. et al,2006; Ness,R., Manam, R., Hoen,H. et al, 2001). One study found males to have poorer preps than females and the authors recommended these individuals schedule their colonoscopies in the afternoon to take advantage of the split-dosage regimen. The authors also found that colonoscopies performed within 6-8 hours of the end of the bowel prep resulted in a better cleansing than those performed more than 8 hours after ingestion of the last prep dose (Marmo, R., Rotondano, G., Riccio, G. et al. 2010).

The criteria for good bowel prep include:

- Require a short period of ingestion and the ability to empty out the colon in a rapid fashion without grossly or microscopically altering the lining of the colon
- Will not cause undue shifts in fluid and electrolyte balances
- Are safe to administer in light of existing comorbidities
- Easy to complete regimen
- Reimbursed by health insurance company or is inexpensive

Unfortunately, none of the preparations currently available on the market meet all these criteria. As a result, several adjunctive methods have been added along with the main prep and are now available on the market to make it easier and tolerable for the individual to take (Lawrence, M. & Pickhardt, P., 2010).

Historically, bowel cleansing agents evolved from preparations prior to surgical and radiologic exams. These included enemas, ingestion of cathartics as well as dietary restriction of low residue diet for 2-3 days prior to the procedure (Wexner, S., et al. 2006). These were harsh regimens which were time consuming, uncomfortable and inconvenient for the patient; hence, compliance was difficult. In addition, the early preparations contained mannitol, which, when fermented by bacteria in the colon resulted in combustible methane and hydrogen, which created a high risk for gas explosion when cautery was used. This was also true for sorbitol preparations (ASGE, 2009). This led to the development of an osmotically balanced solution with minimal water absorption or secretion into the colon by Davis and his colleagues in the 1980s (Davis, 1980). The solution was polyethylene glycol, "a high-molecular weight, nonabsorbable polymer in a dilute electrolyte solution that has an osmotic effect on the colon (Atreja, A., Nepal, S. & Lashner, B., 2010)." There are several commercially prepared bowel cleansers, and the compounds used in these preps generally fall into three major groups according to their mechanism of action: isosmotic (the polyethylene glycol group), hyperosmotic (the sodium phosphate group), and bowel stimulants (Atreja, A., Nepal, S. & Lashner, B., 2010; ASGE, 2009; Barkun, A. et.al, 2006; Wexner, S., Beck, D., Baron, T., et al., 2006). Other preparations have since been introduced to improve palatability and compliance, e.g. low volume prep such as PEG and Bisacodyl (Halflytely) and PEG and ascorbic acid (MoviPrep). The most commonly used bowel preparations in the United States are the oral sodium phosphate (NaP) solutions and the polyethylene glycol (PEG) solutions (Atreja, A., Nepal, S. & Lashner, B., 2010 & ASGE, 2009; Barkun, A., Chiba, N., Enns, R., et al., 2006). A summary is shown on Table 1.

Product	Active Ingredient	Approved Bowel Prep By FDA for Adults	Approved Bowel Prep by FDA for Pediatrics	Amount
Isosmotic FV*				
Colyte (Flavored & Nonflavored)	Polyethylene Glycol (PEG)	Yes	No	4000 ml (4L)
GoLYTELY (Flavored & Nonflavored)	Polyethylene Glycol (PEG)	Yes	No	4000 ml (4L)
TriLyte (Flavored)	Sulfate-free Polyethylene Glycol	Yes	>6 months	4000 ml (4L)
NuLYTELY (Flavored & Nonflavored)	Sulfate-free Polyethylene Glycol	Yes	>6 months	4000 ml (4L)
Isosmotic LV**				
MoviPrep	PEG & Ascorbic Acid	Yes	No	2000 ml (2L)
Halflytely	PEG & Bisacodyl	Yes	No	4 Bisacodyl Delayed-Release tablets plus 2000 ml (2L) PEG
Glycolax	PEG-3350 without electrolytes	No	No	255 grams
Miralax	PEG-3350 without electrolytes	No	No	255 grams
Hyperosmotic				
Osmoprep	Sodium phosphate (oral)	Yes +	No	32 tablets

Visicol	Sodium phosphate (oral)	Yes +	No	40 tablets
Fleet Enema	Sodium phosphate (enema)	Yes +	>12 years	135 ml
Magnesium Citrate	Magnesium citrate (oral)	Yes	>6 years	300 ml
Fleet Phospho-Soda EZ-Prep	Sodium phosphate (oral)	Available as prescription only$\pm$	No	75 ml
LoSoPrepKit	Magnesium citrate plus Bisacodyl oral & suppository	Yes	No	One package
Picolax	Sodium picosulfate & magnesium citrate	No. Available only in Europe & UK	Yes	Two sachets dissolved in 300 ml solution
CitraFleet	Sodium picosulfate & magnesium citrate	No. Available only in Europe & UK	No	Two sachets dissolved in 300 ml solution
Stimulant laxatives				
Picolax #	Sodium picosulfate & magnesium citrate	No. Available only in Europe & UK	Yes	Two sachets dissolved in 300 ml solution
CitraFleet#	Sodium picosulfate & magnesium citrate	No. Available only in Europe & UK	No	Two sachets dissolved in 300 ml solution
Senna	Senna	No	No	100 tablets

*Full Volume +Black Box warning included # Classified as osmotic and stimulant laxative
**Low Volume $\pm$FDA recommends against over-the-counter use

Table 1. Commonly Used Bowel Preparation Agents

2.1 Isosmotic or the polyethylene glycol group

Polyethylene glycol solutions are nonabsorbable fluids that act as purgatives to evacuate the colon of stool. These are high volume gut lavage solutions that are osmotically balanced and do not induce a significant electrolyte and fluid shifts, hence, are more effective, better tolerated, and safer for individuals who have advanced liver or kidney disease, poorly compensated congestive heart failure, or have documented electrolyte imbalances. These also do not cause significant physiologic changes in the individual's vital signs, weight, and blood counts. However, some rare adverse events have been reported in association with polyethylene glycol ingestion. These include Mallory-Weiss tear, esophageal perforation, colitis, cardiac dysrhythmias, hyponatremia, aspiration, pancreatitis, and a syndrome of inappropriate antidiuretic hormone secretion (Lichtenstein, G., Cohen, L. & Uribarri, J., 2007). Commercially prepared polyethylene glycol solutions come in full volume: flavored and unflavored GoLYTELy, flavored and unflavored Colyte, NuLytely (sulfate-free), Trilyte flavored (sulfate-free); and low volume: Halflytely and MoviPrep (ASGE, 2009).

The standard large volume polyethylene glycol (PEG) solutions, Colyte and GoLYTELY have been studied extensively and were found to have the most evidence for safety and effectiveness. The sodium sulfate in PEG allow for a reduction in sodium absorption in the small intestine. These solutions are also inexpensive and most health insurance companies reimburse the cost. The conventional adult dose is 4L, given as 240ml of the solution every 10 minutes 12-15 hours prior to the procedure until the 4L is consumed and rectal output is clear and watery. If given through a nasogastric tube, 20 to 30ml is instilled every minute. However, because of the large volume required to cleanse the colon and its poor palatability (salty taste and smell of sulfates), about 15% of individuals do not complete the prep (Atreja, A., Nepal, S. & Lashner, B., 2010 & Wexner, S., Beck, D., Baron, T., et al., 2006). The main complaint was nausea, bloating, abdominal cramping, and vomiting. To remedy this, splitting the dose allowed for better compliance and tolerability by the patients; half the dose was ingested the night before the procedure and the other half taken 4-5 hours prior to the procedure (Marmo, R., Rotondano, G., Riccio, G. et al, 2010). This method resulted in a better cleansing of the colon. With the traditional method of single dosing, the long interval between the end of the prep and the start of the procedure allowed secretions from the small intestine to flow into the large intestine, obscuring the view of the cecum and ascending colon. A study conducted by Varughese and associates found that for colonoscopies scheduled in the afternoon, ingestion of the one gallon or 4 L solution of polyethylene glycol resulted in superior cleansing of the colon and was better tolerated by the study participants. There were fewer side effects, too. This method evacuated the contents of the large intestine in a timely manner and did not allow time for the contents of the small intestine to flow to the large intestine thereby obscuring the view (Varughese, S., Kumar,A.,George, A., & Castro, F., 2010). Stimulant laxatives or ascorbic acid were also added to low-volume PEG solutions (e.g. MoviPrep) to improve compliance and palatability (Atreja, A., Nepal, S. & Lashner, B., 2010).
Other suggestions to make ingestion of PEG solutions more tolerable are:

- Adding flavor enhancers, such as Crystal Light, Gatorade, lemon juice or lemon slices.
- Chilling the solution or adding ice cubes and drinking through a straw.
- Taking metoclopramide (Reglan) 5-10mg tablets prior, to prevent nausea.
- Adding one bottle of magnesium citrate (about 300 ml) or two to four tablets of bisacodyl 5mg/tab to decrease the volume ingested.
- Stopping ingestion of the prep once the stool is clear and watery on the day of the test.
- Administration of the prep via a nasogastic tube for individuals with altered mental status or with swallowing disability.
- Ingestion of sulfate-free or flavored PEG solutions, such as NuLytely and TriLyte (flavors come in cherry, pineapple, orange, lemon-lime, and citrus-berry).
- Ingestion of a low-volume solution (2 liters) plus a stimulant laxative, e.g. HalfLytely with two bisacodyl tablets and magnesium citrate; MoviPrep which is PEG plus ascorbic acid.

A sulfate-free PEG solution was developed by Fordtran et al in the 1990s to improve palatability and smell of PEG solutions. The improved taste is the result of a decreased amount of potassium, increased amount of chloride and no sodium sulfate. Examples of these products are NuLYTELY and TriLyte and come in different fruit flavors. Dosing is the same as the 4L PEG solution. It is comparable in terms of safety, tolerance, and effectiveness to the conventional PEG solutions (Wexner, S., Beck, D., Baron, T., et al. 2006). Low-volume

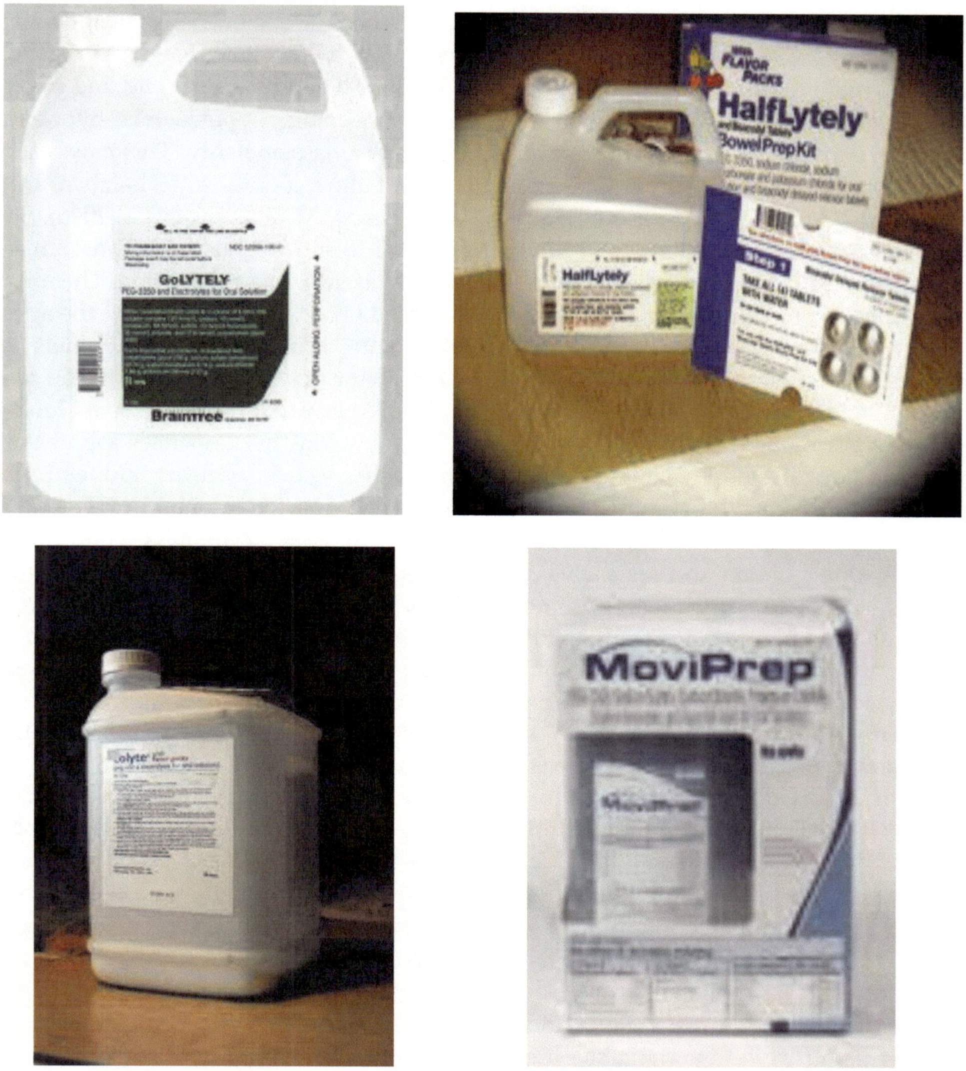

Fig. 3. Several commercially prepared polyrethylene glycol solutions:
Top left, GoLytely; top right, HalfLytely.
Bottom left, Colyte and bottom right, MoviPrep.

PEG preparations (e.g. PEG + ascorbic acid, PEG + electrolytes) were developed to improve patient tolerance by reducing the amount of solution required, and thus, reducing volume-related symptoms such as nausea, bloating, and abdominal cramping. Studies have shown equal efficacy with full volume PEG solutions but with improved compliance and tolerance by patients (Ell, C., Fischbach, W., Bronisch, H. et al. 2008; Bitoun, A., Ponchon, T., Barthet, M. et al., 2006; DiPalma, J., Wolff, B., Meagher, A. & Cleveland, M., 2003).

2.2 Hyperosmotic or the sodium phosphate solutions

Sodium phosphate is widely used worldwide and is an effective bowel cleansing agent. It is better tolerated than PEG preps due to its smaller volume (1.5 -2 liters compared with polyethylene glycol's 4 liters) and better flavor. Its hyperosmotic property draws water into the colon stimulating peristalsis and eventually affecting a bowel movement. Unfortunately, this is the main disadvantage of NaP solutions, because it causes major fluid and electrolyte shifts in the body, such as hyperphosphatemia, hypocalcemia, hypokalemia, hyponatremia and/or hypernatremia, hypovolemia and increased plasma osmolality. This may lead to an acute phosphate nephropathy in patients with renal failure (ASGE, 2009; Balaban, D., 2008; Khurana, A., McLean,L, Atkinson, S. et al., 2008; Curran, M. & Plosker, G., 2004). Sodium phosphate solutions are therefore, not recommended in individuals with congestive heart disease, bowel obstruction, hepatic and renal disease, ascites, and megacolon. The following may also be at risk of injury to the kidneys if prescribed NaP: individuals over the age of 55, patients who are already dehydrated, patients with acute colitis, individuals taking diuretics, ACE (angiotensin converting enzyme) inhibitor drugs, ARB (angiotensin receptor blockers), and non-steroidal anti-inflammatory drugs (NSAIDS) (Ker, T., 2006; Hookey, L., Depew, W. & Vanner, S., 2002). A study done by Yakut and his associates found that in a selected group of elderly patients without comorbidities such as heart, kidney and liver failure, and diabetes, the administration of NaP preparation for colonoscopy was safe and well tolerated, with a low frequency of side effects (Yakut, M., Kubilay, C., Gülseren, S. et al., 2010). Dong Choon and associates conducted a retrospective study between August of 2005 and May of 2008 in patients with normal kidney function, undergoing colonoscopy at a health center in Korea using NaP solution as the bowel cleansing agent and found that it was safe and effective and no untoward renal injury was noted (Dong Choon, S., Sung Noh, H., Jeong Hwan, K. et al. 2010). Abaskharoun and colleagues also corroborated this findings with their own retrospective study in a Canadian health center (Abaskharoun, R., Depew, W. & Vanner, S., 2007). A prospective study by Casais et al. found that hyperphosphatemia in low-risk individuals was related to low weight and can be minimized with adequate hydration. It was their recommendation to prescribe an appropriate NaP dose according to the individual's weight (Casais, M., Guillermo, R-D., Perez, S, et al., 2009). In December 2008, the Federal Drug Administration (FDA) has recommended NaP preparations be removed as an over-the-counter bowel prep to avoid inappropriate use or overdosing, and a black box warning be included in the labels of prescription products warning consumers of the risk of acute phosphate nephropathy. C.B. Fleet Company voluntarily recalled its oral NaP products, Fleets Phospho-Soda and Fleet EZ-PREP. Sodium phosphate comes in tablet form or aqueous solution. The tablet form, Visicol and OsmoPrep, are the only two sodium phosphate prep available in the United States. The aqueous solution is no longer available (US FDA, 2008; Ainley, E., Winwood, P. & Begley, J., 2005). Figure 4 shows examples of sodium phosphate products available in the market.

The differences in efficacy and safety of PEG and NaP solutions in cleansing the bowel prior to colonoscopy have been studied extensively, and, in general, the histology of the normal colon has been shown to be preserved with PEG solutions.

Sodium phosphate solutions can alter the macroscopic as well as the microscopic appearance of the mucosa of the colon mimicking inflammatory bowel diseases. Thus, these preps are to be avoided in individuals with or suspected with colitis or inflammatory bowel diseases (Bucher, P., Gervaz, P., Egger, J., et al., 2006; Rejchrt, S., Bures, J., Siroky, M. et al. 2004).

Magnesium Citrate is a saline laxative and also a hyperosmotic, and like sodium phosphate, acts by drawing water into the colon. Since it contains magnesium, and elimination is

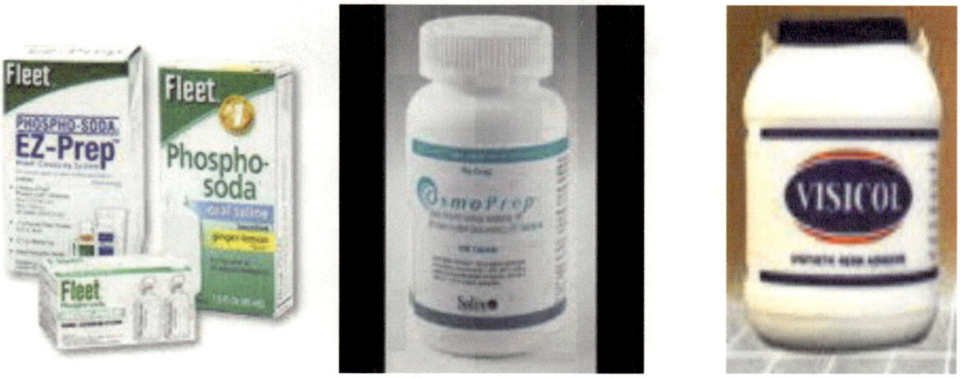

Fig. 4. Sodium phosphate products available in the US: OsmoPrep and Visicol. The aqueous formula is available only as a prescription.

through the kidneys, administer with extreme caution in individuals with renal insufficiency or failure (Atreja, A., Nepal, S. & Lashner, B., 2010). Magnesium citrate is often used as an adjunct to bowel prep. In addition to the PEG solution, adding magnesium citrate to the prep reduces the amount of PEG solution required to 2L. Taken the night before the procedure (one 300 ml bottle of magnesium citrate) plus two bisacodyl tablets and 2L of PEG solution, has shown to be just as effective as taking the full dose of PEG solution. Used alone, magnesium citrate is not an effective bowel cleansing agent prior to colonoscopy procedures. Magnesium citrate is often used as an adjunct to bowel prep (Atreja, A., Nepal, S. & Lashner, B., 2010; Wexner, S., Beck, D., Baron, T., et al., 2006).

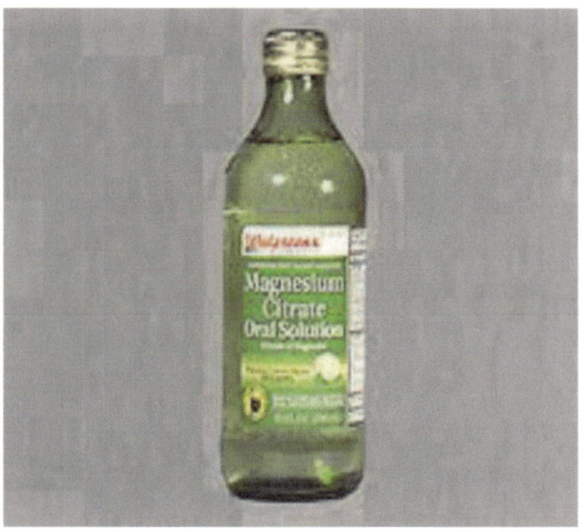

Fig. 5. Magnesium Citrate bottle

2.3 Stimulant preparations

Stimulant laxatives such as bisacodyl (Dulcolax) have been added to low volume PEG solutions and have achieved comparable results to those given the standard dose of PEG solutions (Atreja, A., Nepal, S. & Lashner, B., 2010). It is poorly absorbed in the small intestine and its active ingredients stimulate colon motility, with an onset of action between 6-10 hours (ASGE, 2009).

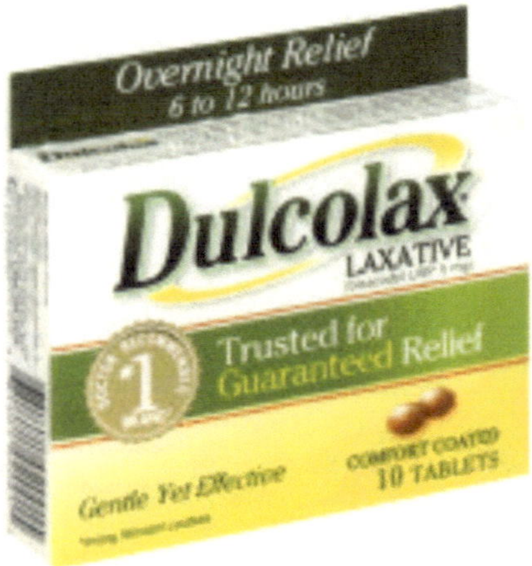

Fig. 6. Dulcolax tablets

Sodium picosulfate is another cathartic with osmotic action on the bowel similar to NaP. It is a saline laxative used in combination with magnesium citrate. An observational study done in Canada by Love and his colleagues found that administration of sodium picosulfate and magnesium citrate yielded a high percentage positive rate for efficacy (Yakut, M., Kubilay, Ç., Gülseren, S. et al., 2010). This preparation is mostly used in Europe and Canada and is not available in the United States (ASGE, 2009).

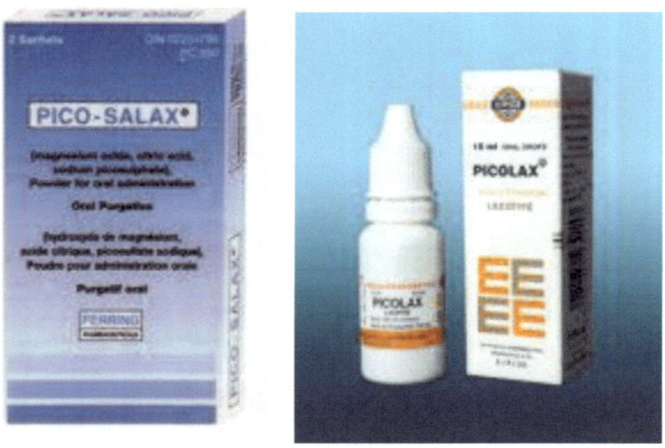

Fig. 7. Sodium picosulfate products. Not available in the US

Senna, an anthracene derivative also helps stimulate colon peristalsis by increasing smooth muscle wall activity. A low dose senna (four 8.6 mg tablets of Sennakot) added to a low-volume solution of polyethylene glycol have been found to be just as effective as taking the full-volume PEG solution. It is usually taken within 2 to 6 hours of starting the PEG solution. A study found that there was better visualization of the right colon when senna was added to the magnesium citrate prep and was also better tolerated by the subjects (Vradelis, S., Kalaitzakis, E., Sharifi, Y. et al 2009).

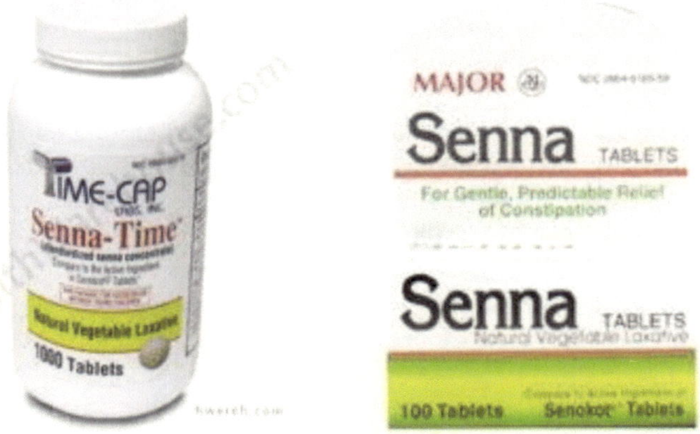

Fig. 8. Senna products

2.4 Adjunct bowel preparation agents

Enemas are useful in cleansing the distal colon in preparation for a sigmoidoscopy, but not recommended as prep for a full colonoscopy. They are used as adjuncts when patients come poorly prepped. The common types are: tap water enemas, soap suds enemas, sodium biphosphate (Fleet), and oil-based enemas such as, cottonseed oil plus docusate (Colace) and diatrizoate sodium (Hypaque). The last one is an iodinated water-soluble contrast agent used in radiographic exams that has a cathartic property. It slows absorption of water from the bowel so that the stool is softer. One study found that combining diatrizoate sodium with a low-volume saline laxative prep (preferably magnesium citrate) was just as effective as, if not better, than the other regularly prescribed preps. It consistently outperformed the standard high-volume PEG solutions in terms of effectiveness as a bowel cleanser and patient compliance and tolerance (Lawrence, E. & Pickhardt, P., 2010). One disadvantage to using this prep was that some individuals developed severe allergic reactions such as anaphylaxis and angioedema. Others have experienced muscle cramps and intermittent leakage of stool in their undergarments for up to 24 hours after the test (Atreja, A., Nepal, S. & Lashner, B., 2010; Lawrence, E. & Pickhardt, P., 2010 & Sohn, N. & Weinstein, M., 2008; Wexner, S., Beck, D., Baron, T., et al., 2006).

Dietary modifications alone are inadequate prep for colonoscopy, but are a beneficial adjunct, by decreasing the formation of solid residue. Drinking clear liquids is recommended in **ALL** bowel preps and helps maintain adequate hydration (Atreja, A., Nepal, S. & Lashner, B., 2010; ASGE, 2009; Dykes, C. & Cash, B., 2007; National Guideline Clearinghouse, 2006).

Carbohydrate-electrolyte solutions such as Gatorade and E-Lyte have been added to both PEG and NaP solutions to improve palatability and to avoid severe fluid and electrolyte shifts (Wexner, S., Beck, D., Baron, T., et al., 2006).

Antiemetic agents such as metoclopramide (Reglan 5-10mg) are commonly used to prevent nausea and vomiting associated with taking bowel preparations.

Antifoaming agents, such as Simethicone (three 80 mg tablets), an anti-gas, anti-flatulent agent, has been added to the prep to reduce the bubbles and improve visibility during colonoscopy (Tongprasert, S., Sobhonslidsuk, A. & Rattansiri, S., 2009).

Nasogastric or orogastric tube installation is usually reserved for inpatients that are unable to drink the polyethylene glycol solutions, for patients who are unresponsive or those on mechanical ventilators.

Rectal Pulsed Irrigation administered immediately prior to the colonoscopy preceded by intake of magnesium citrate the night before is also another alternative, though this is time consuming, expensive and requires expert nursing skill to be efficiently performed (Wexner, S., Beck, D., Baron, T., et al., 2006).

Clebopride is another adjunct that has gained some interest among endoscopists. It is a D-2 dopamine antagonist with antiemetic and prokinetic properties which can improve the efficacy of bowel cleansing. A study was done to evaluate the efficacy, safety, tolerability, and acceptance of Clebopride as an adjunct to PEG solution as prep for colonoscopy. The authors found that Clebopride was better accepted by patients and was better tolerated as well. It diminished the symptom of nausea, abdominal distention, and borborygmus (Abdullah, M., Aziz Rani, A., Fauzi, A. et al., 2010).

3. Special considerations

Diabetes Mellitus. Diabetic patients need to follow certain pre- and post- colonoscopy instructions to prevent hyper- or hypoglycemia episodes. The individual needs to discuss his/her medications with the physician at least two weeks prior to the test. Individuals taking insulin may need to have their regular dosages adjusted the day before and the day of the procedure. See tables 2 and 3 for general guidelines.

Cardiac conditions. Individuals taking blood thinners will need to consult their physician as to when to stop taking these medications prior to colonoscopy. A blood test to check the PT/INR will need to be drawn in the morning the day before the exam. He or she **should not** stop taking his or her other cardiac medications without consulting his or her physician. Blood pressure medications are generally allowed to be taken even on the day of the procedure.

The elderly. The elderly often have poorer bowel preps which may be attributed to a decrease or alteration in intestinal motility secondary to the aging process or other comorbidities. Constipation contributes to the poor quality of the colonoscopy which may be associated with the elderly's sedentary lifestyle, inadequate intake of fiber, depression, and dementia (Yakut, M., Kubilay, Ç., Gülseren, S. et al., 2010). They are also at risk for fluid and electrolyte imbalance, especially phosphate intoxication, due to concomitant medication use, comorbidities, poor kidney function or other gastrointestinal disorders. Adequate hydration without compromising cardiac function is of utmost importance with this population.

Pregnancy. The need for colonoscopy during pregnancy is rare, hence the safety and efficacy of the bowel preps have not been studied. If it is deemed that the potential benefit of colonoscopy outweigh the small, but possible risks, then the pregnant woman may be cleansed with PEG solutions. NaP preps may be used with caution in select patients (ASGE, 2009; National Guideline Clearing House, 2006).

The *pediatric* population will be discussed in another chapter.

4. Colonoscopy bowel preparations: general patient instruction guidelines

Two weeks prior to your procedure:

- You need to speak with or see the physician who will be performing your colonoscopy to go over your medical and surgical history, medications you take on a regular basis, allergies, any other pertinent information relevant to your procedure or concerns you may have. For women, please let the physician know if you are pregnant or maybe pregnant. If you have kidney or liver disease and are on fluid restriction, your prep and diet may need to be adjusted.

- Your physician will advise you what medications you need to discontinue and when to discontinue these prior to the test. These include all types of blood thinners or antiplatelet medications, anti-inflammatory drugs, multivitamin with iron and any other medication containing iron preparation, and bulk-forming agents.
- If you have diabetes, it is advisable to schedule an appointment early in the day so that you can eat after and take your medications as close to your usual time as possible. You will be asked to bring your blood glucose meter and test strips and any treatment you use when you experience low blood sugar levels on the day of the exam.
- For asthma sufferers, you need to bring your inhaler (s) the day of the exam.
- For individuals using a CPAP or BiPAP machines, you will be asked to bring these on the day of the exam as well.
- You will be asked to arrange for a ride to your colonoscopy as you will not be allowed to drive a car, take the bus or taxi home after the procedure. You will be given sedation medications for the procedure and the effects usually linger for a few hours after the test is completed. You will spend about 1-2 hours in the endoscopy suite, which includes the pre-procedure prep, the colonoscopy itself, and post-procedure recovery time. You will go home after to rest and allow the rest of the sedatives to wear off. If you arrive without an escort, your test will be cancelled or rescheduled.

Seven days prior to your procedure:

- Stop taking the following medications:
  - Iron, vitamin E and medications containing either component
  - Garlic, Ginko Biloba, ginger
  - Blood thinners (anticoagulant) such as warfarin (Coumadin), Fondaparinux (Arixta), enoxaparin (Lovenox)
  - Antiplatelets such as prasugrel (Effient), clopidogrel (Plavix), cilostazol (Pletal), anagrelide (Agrylin), pentoxifyline (Trental), dipyridamole (Persantine), dipyridamole with aspirin (Aggrenox), aspirin and any other products containing aspirin (Anacin, Alka Seltzer, Bufferin).

Note: You must have your PT/INR checked in the morning the day before your test if you are on Coumadin or Warfarin, Plavix or Jantovan.

Five to three days prior to your test:

- Confirm your ride.
- If you need to cancel or reschedule your appointment, this is the time to do so. Call the office where you booked your appointment.
- Review the diet you need to follow as well as medication schedule if you are a diabetic. Most heart medications such as ones for high blood pressure are generally allowed to be taken even on the day of the exam. Diuretic medications are usually asked to be taken after the procedure is completed.
- Purchase your prescription bowel prep, but **DO NOT MIX or PREPARE** the solution until the day before the exam, if not taking the pill form.
- Stop taking bulk-forming agents such as Metamucil or Citrucel.

Two days before the procedure:

- Stop taking **ALL** anti-inflammatory drugs such as ibuprofen and ibuprofen products (Advil, Motrin, Nuprin), Voltaren, naproxen (Aleve, Anaprox, Midol Extended Relief, Naprelan, Naprosyn), Indocin, Relafen, Voltaren. Acetaminophen (Tylenol) is okay to take for any headache or discomfort you might be experiencing.
- Stop eating seeds, nuts, corn, popcorn, whole grains.
- Drink a minimum of eight glasses of water throughout the day.
- Do not eat any solid food after midnight.

Day before the procedure:

- Beginning at breakfast, **DO NOT EAT ANY SOLID FOOD**. Instead, start a clear liquid diet which means drinking liquids that you can see through, e.g. apple juice, white grape juice, ginger ale, lemon-lime soda, Gatorade, Kool-Aid, Jello, coffee (without the creamer), tea, Seltzer, broth, bouillon or consommé. **Do not drink liquid that is red, blue, or purple (cherry, purple grape, or berry flavors).** Also avoid milk, milk products, non-dairy creamers, or alcohol.
- For diabetics, the following are suggested clear food choices:
  - Apple juice (4 oz.) 15 Gm carbohydrate
  - Plain Jello without fruit (regular sweetened, ½ C.) 15 Gm carbohydrate
  - Grape juice (white, 4 oz.) 20 Gm carbohydrate
  - Any sports drink such as Gatorade (8 oz.) 15 GM carbohydrate
  - Italian Ice 3 0 Gm carbohydrate
  - Ice pops, orange or yellow popsicles 15 Gm carbohydrate
  - Coffee or tea with 1 tsp. sugar (one packet) 4 Gm carbohydrate
  - Fat-free beef or chicken broth, bouillon or consomme´ no carbohydrate
  - Clear diet soda, such as ginger ale no carbohydrate
  - Seltzer (flavored or nonflavored) no carbohydrate
  - Flavored water no carbohydrate
  - Tea with slice of lemon

*Note: Aim for 45 grams of carbohydrate during mealtimes and 15-30 grams for snacks. Read the label of commercially prepared drink items for carbohydrate measurement per serving. Refer to Table 2 for diabetic medication guidelines.

- In addition to water, drink a variety of liquid throughout the day (recommended every hour while awake). Your body needs a combination of water, sugar, and electrolytes. It will keep you from being dehydrated, weak, and hungry and you will be better able to tolerate the bowel prep. A new product on the market, called Colonoscopy Prep Assistant, helps individuals keep track of their hydration status. It is a web application that tracks the number of glasses of fluid the patient has taken, the time interval between drinks, and notifies the patient when it's time to take the next glass of fluid. This application is available for free in the Android market and iTunes and can also be downloaded at www.wellapps.com.
- For individuals taking polyethylene glycol (PEG) prep, do the following:
  - In the morning, mix the PEG solution as directed and refrigerate.
  - Around 1:30 PM, take one tablet of metoclopramide (Reglan), if prescribed, to prevent or relieve the nausea that accompanies ingestion of the PEG solution.

Medications	Morning	Lunch	Dinner/Supper	Bedtime
Actos, Actoplus Met, Avandamet, Avandia, Metformin, Janumet, and Januvia	Take your usual dose	Take your usual dose	Take your usual dose	
Amaryl, Avandaryl, Duetact, Glipizide, Glucovance, Glyburide, Metaglip, Prandin, and Starlix	**Do not take**	**Do not take**		
Humalog, Regular or Novolog Insulin	If prescribed a fixed dose, take ½ the regular amount OR cover your carbs with usual carb ratio	If prescribed a fixed dose, take ½ the regular amount OR cover your carbs with usual carb ratio		
Lantus or NPH Insulin	Take your usual dose			Take your usual dose
Novolog Mix 70/30, Novolin 70/30, Premixed insulin75/25	Take half the usual dose at breakfast		Take half the usual dose at dinner time	

Table 2. General guidelines for diabetic medications the **day before** colonoscopy

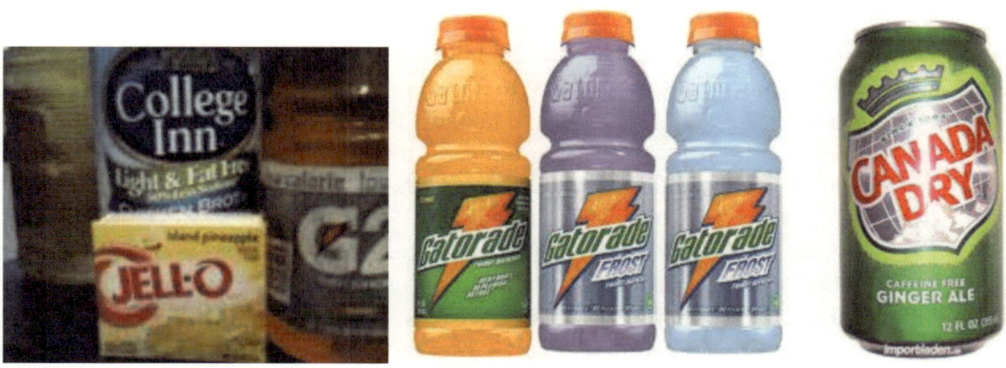

Fig. 9. Varieties of clear liquid: broth, Jello, apple juice or white grape juice, Gatorade, and ginger ale

    - If prescribed the 4-L GoLytely, take one glass (8 oz) every 15-20 minutes half-an-hour after taking the metoclopramide tablet, until half gallon is gone. Remember to drink clear liquids or water in between until you go to bed. Be sure to stay close to the bathroom. The rest of the half gallon will be taken the next day, about 3-4 hours prior to the scheduled procedure. If you have a morning appointment, you may need to get up in the middle of the night to complete your prep. If your test is in the afternoon, you may start taking the rest of the prep at 6 AM, one glassful every 15-20 minutes until the half gallon is consumed.
    - If nausea continues, take a second tablet of metoclopramide around 5 or 6 PM. Let your physician know if you are having difficulty completing the prep or uncomfortable side effects such as nausea, vomiting continues.
    - Another approach would be to take 3L the night before and 1L the day of the procedure.
- For low-volume PEG preparations plus bisacodyl tablets, the clear liquid diet the day before is also followed.
    - Around noon time, take four (5mg) bisacodyl delayed-release tablets.
- Start taking the PEG solution after a bowel movement occurs following taking the bisacodyl tablets. Keep drinking a glassful of the prep every 10-15 minutes until the 2 liters is consumed. You may take a break in-between dose if bloating, nausea, or vomiting ensues. Resume after the symptom (s) subsides.
- For low-volume PEG prep (MoviPrep) with magnesium citrate, do the following:
- Upon waking up the day before the exam, prepare the solution by mixing pouches 1 & 2 into the disposable container provided. Add lukewarm to the top line and mix until completely dissolved. Refrigerate. At around 5 PM, start drinking a cupful of the solution (about 8 oz.) down to the first mark on the container. Make sure you follow this with clear liquid of your choice. Keep drinking the solution down to the next line and so forth every 15 minutes until the liter is consumed.
    - The process will be repeated again for dose #2, but will not be taken until around 7:30 PM the same evening.
- For individuals taking the sodium phosphate (NaP) prep, do the following:
    - Only clear liquids are consumed the day before the procedure.
    - For the aqueous NaP prep, take a 30 to 45 ml solution with at least 8 oz. of water (or any other preferred clear liquid) 10-12 hours prior to your scheduled exam. The second dose will be ingested at least 3-4 hours prior to your test the next day.
    - Continue to drink clear fluids until you go to bed.
    - Another recommended approach is to take the two doses of NaP, three hours apart in-between dose, starting at 4 PM or 5 PM for the first dose followed by the second dose around 9 PM, and supplemented around 10 PM by four bisacodyl (5mg) tablets.
    - For individuals prescribed the pill form (Osmo-Prep or Visicol: The recommended dose is 3 tablets every 15 minutes for 6 doses and then 2 tablets for a total of 20 tablets, the day before the procedure. This is again repeated the next day, 3 to 5 hours before the scheduled test. Osmo-Prep uses only 32 tablets in divided doses similar to Visicol. Again, these are taken with water or clear liquid. Dulcolax or magnesium citrate may also be added as an adjunct to ensure clear bowel return.

Tips: Do not be surprised if you do not have a bowel movement soon after ingesting your prep. It usually takes about 2-4 hours before you have your first bowel movement. Stay close to the bathroom as you will spend most of your day on the toilet. Try to use moistened wipes or a water spray instead of toilet paper to clean yourself to minimize irritation of the anal area. If you have a colostomy, be prepared to empty out your pouch often and liquid stool may leak around your pouch as well. Remember to keep drinking plenty of clear liquids to prevent dehydration. Follow your instructions for the prep as you do not want to repeat this procedure all over again because you did not get it right the first time.

Day of the procedure:

- Take your regular medications allowed by the physician with a small sip of water. You may have clear liquids three hours before your test. Refer to Table 3 for medication guidelines if you are a diabetic and remember to check your blood sugar in the morning before coming to the colonoscopy. Also bring your glucometer, extra test strips and your treatment for any hypoglycemic (low blood sugar) episodes.
- Have your driver drive you to the colonoscopy place half-an-hour before your scheduled procedure or whatever time you were instructed to arrive. Remember to bring your paper work, medications, inhalers, CPAP or BiPAP machine, and health insurance card.
- Make sure you wear comfortable clothing and bring extra clothes, underwear or peri-pads in case you have an accident and soil your clothes or underwear.

Medications	Morning	Lunch	Dinner/Supper	Bedtime
Actos, Actoplus Met, Avandamet, Avandia, Metformin, Janumet, and Januvia	Take your usual dose	Take your usual dose	Take your usual dose	
Amaryl, Avandaryl, Duetact, Glipizide, Glucovance, Glyburide, Metaglip, Prandin, Starlix	**Do not take**	Resume regularly prescribed dose if allowed to eat		
Humalog, Regular or Novolog Insulin	**Do not Take**	Resume regularly prescribed dose if allowed to eat	Resume regularly prescribed dose if allowed to eat	
Lantus or NPH Insulin	Take **half** of your regularly prescribed dose			Take your regularly prescribed dose
Novolog Mix 70/30, Novolin 70/30, Premixed insulin 75/25	**Do not Take**	Resume regularly prescribed dose if allowed to eat	Resume regularly prescribed dose if allowed to eat	

Table 3. General guidelines for diabetic medications **day of** the colonoscopy

Post procedure recovery:

- You will be cared for by a nurse or a nurse's aide and your vital signs monitored for about half-an-hour to an hour immediately after the procedure in the recovery area. This will also allow for most of the effects of the sedatives to wear off.
  - During this time, your doctor will talk to you about the results of your colonoscopy. If a biopsy was performed, the results are usually not available until a few days later as the sample (s) will be sent to the lab for analysis. He will also provide you with any pertinent additional information or instructions for follow-up.
- You will be discharged home with your designated driver once you are feeling okay and are able to tolerate oral fluids without being nauseous or vomiting. If you are diabetic, it is a good idea to check your blood sugar before going home.
- Plan to rest for the remainder of the day.
- Eat foods that are easy to digest to minimize or avoid nausea and vomiting which is mostly due to the lingering side effects of the sedatives received. Examples are, toast, soup, light sandwich (e.g. grilled cheese), tea, and coffee.
- You may occasionally feel some bloating or be flatulent. This is normal and should disappear within 24 hours. If you had a biopsy done, it is not uncommon to see some flecks of blood in your stool for a couple of days following your colonoscopy. This is usually dark in color. Call your physician if you have bright red blood in your stool, experiencing persistent nausea, vomiting, and abdominal pain or bloating.

5. Safety and efficacy

All colonoscopy bowel preparations are generally considered safe when properly dosed in individuals without contraindications to the specific product, but are not completely immune to the adverse reactions, and on occasion, severe negative outcomes. The safety of the bowel cleansing agent is related to the safety profile of the base agent, i.e, polyethylene glycol or sodium phosphate. The most commonly encountered side effects are bloating, abdominal pain, borborygmus, nausea, vomiting, dizziness, and fluid and electrolyte imbalance. Often the symptoms of nausea, vomiting and abdominal pain disappear once bowel movement commences. These symptoms have also been minimized and safety improved by splitting the dosages, adding adjuncts, administering low-volume preps, and increasing the interval time in-between dosages to 10-12 hours (ASGE, 2009; NGCH, 2006).

Generally, the administration of isotonic polyethylene glycol solutions do not cause significant physiologic changes in vital signs, individual's weight, laboratory results (complete blood count, blood chemistries, and serum electrolytes). It has been safely administered in individuals with advanced liver and kidney failure, congestive heart failure, and fluid and electrolyte imbalances. Some concerns were raised with the use of some PEG solutions, HalfLytely, in particular, in patients taking angiotensin converting enzyme drugs (ACE) or potassium-sparing drugs such as aldactone, because of the small amount of potassium found in the solution. However, there were no clinical reports noted to date (ASGE, 2009; NGCH, 2006).

Sodium phosphate, on the other hand, has been shown to alter both the macroscopic and microscopic (aphthoid erosions) mucosal lining of the intestine, which may mimic inflammatory bowel disease. This prep should then be avoided in individuals with or suspected to have inflammatory bowel disease. Serum electrolyte and fluid imbalances have also been reported with sodium phosphate use. Hyperphosphatemia was seen in 40% of healthy individuals taking NaP. This could be significant for patients with renal failure. About 20% of individuals taking NaP preps have developed hypokalemia, elevated blood urea nitrogen, increased plasma osmolality, decreased exercise endurance, significant hyponatremia, hypocalcemia, and seizures. A rare adverse event, nephrocalcinosis, has been reported in patients with acute renal failure (Balaban, D., 2008; Gonlusen, G., Akgun, H., Ertan, A., et al., 2006; NGCH, 2006). As a result, the Federal Drug Administration (FDA) has recommended that over-the-counter use of sodium phosphate solutions be discontinued and a black box warning be included in prescription products. Manufacturers of sodium phosphate products were also required to perform a "risk evaluation and mitigation strategy, including a post marketing trial," to further assess occurrence of renal injury (ASGE, 2009).

All bowel preps are contraindicated in individuals with known or suspected bowel obstruction, perforation or ileus. Bowel cleansing agents containing magnesium and phosphate should be used with caution or avoided in individuals with kidney failure. To minimize or avoid fluid and electrolyte imbalance, it is necessary to screen patients carefully and to instruct them to hydrate themselves, pre- and post-procedure. Intravenous fluids are usually given during the procedure.

6. Conclusion

Colonoscopy remains the gold standard in the screening and evaluation of the colon for colorectal disorders and diseases. For maximum visualization of the colon, it is imperative that the bowel is thoroughly cleaned. Several commercially prepared agents are available on the market, but the most commonly used ones are the polyethylene glycol and sodium phosphate preps. Adjuncts have also been recommended in addition to the main prep to make it easier to administer. The choice of an appropriate bowel cleansing agent is influenced by its safety, ease of administration and completion, cleansing effectiveness, patient tolerance, adverse effects, palatability, reimbursed by health insurance, will not interact with regularly prescribed medications, and cost. It should be tailored to every individual based on his or her state of health, comorbidities, and medications taken on a regular basis. Kidney function should be evaluated prior to choosing a bowel cleansing agent particularly in the elderly. Thus, careful screening of the patients prior to colonoscopy, prescribing the appropriate dose and bowel cleansing agent, patient education and adequate hydration before and after colonoscopy will help ensure the safety and efficacy of the procedure.

7. Acknowledgement

The author wishes to thank Kira Hulse, BS for her review of the article, Dr. Jonathan Russo, Chief of Endoscopy, for his expert advice regarding colonoscopy, and to my good friend, Marian de la Cour, BSN, MLS, for all her efforts in obtaining most of the literature referred to in this chapter.

8. References

Abaskharoun, R., Depew, W. & Vanner, S. (2007, April). Changes in renal function following administration of oral sodium phosphate or polyethylene glycol for colon cleansing before colonoscopy. *Canadian Journal of Gastroenterology,* 21(4), 227-231. ISSN 0835-7900

Abdullah, M., Aziz Rani, A., Fauzi, A., et al. (2010, January). A randomized, controlled, double-bind trial of the adjunct use of clebopride in polyethylene glycol electrolyte (PEG) solution for colonoscopy preparation. *Acta Med Indones-Indonesian Journal of Internal medicine*, 42(1), 27-30.ISSN 0125-9326

Ainley, E., Winwood, P. & Begley, J. (2005, July). Measurement of serum electrolytes and phosphate after sodium phosphate colonoscopy bowel preparation: An evaluation. *Digestive Diseases and Sciences*, 50(7), 1319-1323. ISSN 0163-2116

American Cancer Society. Colon and rectal cancer. Retrieved Feb. 14, 2011 from http://www.cancer.gov/cancertopics/types/colon-and-rectal

American Cancer Society. Cancer trends progress report-2005 update. Retrieved Feb. 14, 2011 from http://progressreport.cancer.gov/doc.asp?pid=1&did=2005&mid=vcol&chid=22

American Society for Gastrointestinal Endoscopy (ASGE) (2009, June) . Technology status evaluation report. Colonoscopy preparation. *Gastrointestinal Endoscopy*, 69(7), 1201-1209. ISSN 0016-5107

Atreja, A., Nepal, S. & Lashner, B. (2010, May). Making the most of currently available bowel preparations for colonoscopy. *Cleveland Clinic Journal of Medicine*, 77(5), 317-326. ISSN 0891-1150

Balaban, D. (2008, September/October). Guidelines for the safe and effective use of sodium phosphate solution for bowel cleansing prior to colonoscopy. *Gastroenterology Nursing*, 31(5),327-334. ISSN 1042-895x

Barkun, A., Chiba, N., Enns, R., et al. (2006, November). Commonly used preparations for colonoscopy: Efficacy, tolerability and safety – A Canadian Association of Gastroenterology position paper. *Canadian Journal of Gastroenterology*, 20(11), 699-710. ISSN 0835-7900

Bitoun, A., Ponchon, T., Barther, M. et al. on behalf of the Norcol Group (2006, December). Results of a prospective randomized multicenter controlled trial comparing a new 2-L ascorbic acid plus polyethylene glycol and electrolyte solution vs. sodium phosphate solution in patients undergoing elective colonoscopy. *Alimentary Pharmacology & Therapeutics*, 24 (11-12),1631-1642. ISSN 1365-2036

Bucher, P., Gervaz, P., Egger, J., et al., (2006 January). Morphologic alterations associated with mechanical bowel preparation before elective colorectal surgery: A randomized trial. *Diseases of the Colon and Rectum*, 49(1), 109-112.ISSN 0012-3706

Casais, M., Guillermo, R-D., Perez, S. et al. (2009, December). Hyperphosphatemia after sodium phosphate laxatives in low risk patients: Prospective study. *World Journal of Gastroenterology*, 15(47), 5960-5965. ISSN 1007-9327

Curran, M. & Plosker, G. (2004,). Oral phosphate solution: A review of its use as a colorectal cleanser. *Drugs*, 64(15), 1697-1714. ISSN 0012-6667

Davis, G., Santa Ana, C., Morawski, S. & Fordtran, J. (1980, May). Development of a Lavage solution associated with minimal water and electrolyte absorption or secretion. *Gastroenterology*, 78, 991-995. ISSN 0016-5085

DiPalma, J., Wolff, B., Meagher, A. & Cleveland, M., (2003, October). Comparison of reduced volume versus four liters sulfate-free electrolyte lavage solutions for colonoscopy colon cleansing. *American Journal of Gastroenterology*, 98(10), 2187-2191. ISSN 0002-9270

Dong Choon, S., Sung Noh, H., Jeong Hwan, K. et al. (2010, April). Change in renal function after sodium phosphate preparation for screening colonoscopy. *World Journal of Gastroenterology*, 16(16), 2010-2016.ISSN 1007-9327

Dykes, C. & Cash, B. (2007, January). Key safety issues of bowel preparations for colonoscopy and importance of adequate hydration. *Gastroenterology Nursing*, 31(1), 30-37. ISSN 1042-895x

Ell, C., Fischbach, W., Bronisch, H. et al. (2008, April). Randomized trial of low-volume PEG solution versus standard PEG + electrolytes for bowel cleansing before colonoscopy. *American Journal of Gastroenterology*, 103(4), 883-893. ISSN 0002-9270

Froelich, F., Wietlisbach, V., Gonvers, F., et al. (2005,March). Impact of colonic cleansing on quality and diagnostic yield of colonoscopy: The European Panel of Appropriateness of Gastrointestinal Endoscopy European multicenter study. *Gastrointestinal Endoscopy*, 61(3), 378-384. ISSN 0016-5107

Gonlusen, G., Akgun, H., Ertan, A. et al. (2006, January). Renal failure and nephrocalcinosis associated with oral sodium phosphate bowel cleansing: Clinical patterns and renal biopsy findings. *Archives of Pathology and Laboratory Medicine*, 130(1) 101-106. ISSN 0003-9985

Hendry, P., Jenkins, J. & Diament, R. (2007, October). The impact of poor bowel preparation on colonoscopy: a prospective single centre study of 10,571 colonoscopies. *Colorectal Diseases*, 9(8), 745-748. ISSN 1463-1318

Hookey, L., Depew, W. & Vanner, S. (2002,December). The safety profile of oral sodium phosphate for colonic cleansing before colonoscopy in adults. *Gastrointestinal Endoscopy*, 56(12), 895-902. ISSN 0016-5107

Khashab, M & Rex, D. (2005,February). Efficacy and tolerability of a new formulation of sodium phosphate tablets and a reduced sodium phosphate dose, in colon cleansing: A single center open-label pilot trial. *Alimentary Pharmacology & Therapeutics*, 21(4), 465-468. ISSN 1365-2036

Ker, T. (2006, October). Comparison of reduced volume versus four-liter electrolyte lavage solutions for colon cleansing. *American Surgeon*, 72(10), 909-911. ISSN 0003-1348

Khurana, A., McLean, L., Atkinson, S. et al. (2008, March 24). The effect of oral sodium phosphate drug products on renal function in adults undergoing bowel endoscopy. *Archives of Internal Medicine*, 168(6) 593-597.ISSN0003-9926

Lawrence, E. & Pickhardt, P. (2010, August).Low volume hybrid bowel preparation combining saline laxatives with oral contrast agents versus standard polyethylene glycol lavage for colonoscopy. *Diseases of the Colon & Rectum*, 53(8), 1176-1181. ISSN 0012-3706

Lichtenstein, G., Cohen, L. & Uribarri, J. (2007,September). Review article: Bowel preparation for colonoscopy-the importance of adequate hydration. *Alimentary Pharmacology & Therapeutics*, 26(5), 633-641. ISSN 1365-2036

Marmo, R., Rotondano, G., Riccio, G. et al. (2010,August). Effective bowel cleansing before colonoscopy: A randomized study of split-dosage versus non-split dosage regimens of high-volume versus low-volume polyethylene glycol solutions. *Gastrointestinal Endoscopy*, 72(2), 313-320. ISSN 0016-5107

Makkar, R. & Shen, B. (2008, March). What are the caveats to using sodium phosphate agents for bowel preparation? *Cleveland Clinic Journal of Medicine*, 75(3), 173-176. ISSN 0891-1150

National Guideline Clearinghouse (NGCH), (2006). A consensus document on bowel preparation before colonoscopy. Retrieved on Feb. 24, 2011 from http://www.guideline.gov/content.aspx?id=9619&search=colonoscopy.

Ness ,R., Manam, R., Hoen,H. et al (2001, June). Predictors of inadequate bowel preparation for colonoscopy. *American Journal of Gastroenterology,* 96(6), 1797-1802. ISSN 0002-9270

Rejchrt, S., Bures, J., Siroky, M. et al. (2004,May). A prospective, observational study of colonic mucosal abnormalities associated with orally administered sodium phosphate for colon cleansing before colonoscopy. *Gastrointestinal Endoscopy,* 59(5), 651-654. ISSN 0016-5107

Rex,D., Di Palma, J.,Rodriguez, R. et al. (2010, August). A randomized clinical study comparing reduced-volume oral sulfate solution with standard 4-liter sulfate-free electrolyte lavage solution as preparation for colonoscopy. *Gastrointestinal Endoscopy,* 72(2), 328-336. ISSN 0016-5107

Rex, D. (2007, September). Dosing considerations in the use of sodium phosphate bowel preparations for colonoscopy. *Annals of Pharmacotherpy,* 41(9), 1466-1475. ISSN 1060-0280

Sanaka, M., Shah,N., Mullen,K. et al (2006 December). Afternoon colonoscopies have higher failure rates than morning colonoscopies. *American Journal of Gastroenterology,* 101(12), 2726-2730. ISSN 0002-9270

Sohn, N. & Weinstein, M. (2008,April). Management of the poorly prepared colonoscopy patient: Colonoscopic colon enemas as a preparation for colonoscopy. *Diseases of the Colon & Rectum,* 51(4), 462-466. ISSN 0012-3706

The Harvard Medical School Family Health Guide (2006). Retrieved February 14, 2010 from http://www.health.harvard.edu/fhg/updates/preparing-for-a-colonoscopy.shtml

Tongprasert, S., Sobhonslidsuk, A. & Rattanasiri, S. (2009, June 28). Improving quality of colonoscopy by adding simethicone to sodium phosphate bowel preparation. *World Journal of Gastroenterology,* 15(24), 3032-3037.ISSN 1007-9327

US Food and Drug Administration (FDA) (2008, December 11). Oral sodium phosphate (OSP) products for bowel cleansing (marketed as Visicol and OsmoPrep, and oral sodium phosphate products available without a prescription. *FDA Alert.* Retrieved March 01, 2011 from http://www.fda.gov/Safety/MedWatch/SafetyInformation/SafetyAlertsforHumanMedicalProducts/ucm094900.htm.

Varughese, S., Kumar,A.,George, A., & Castro, F., (2010,November). Morning-only one-gallon polyethylene glycol improves bowel cleansing for afternoon colonoscopies: A randomized endoscopist-blinded prospective study. *The American Journal of Gastroenterology,* 105(11), 2368-2374. ISSN 0002-9270

Vradelis, S., Kalaitzakis, E., Sharifi, Y. et al (2009,April 14). Addition of senna improves quality of colonoscopy preparation with magnesium citrate. *World Journal of Gastroenterology,* 15(14), 1759-1763. ISSN 1007-9327

Wexner, S., Beck, D., Baron, T., et al. (2006,June). A consensus document on bowel preparation before colonoscopy : Prepared by a task force from the American Society of Colon and Rectal Surgeons (ASCRS), the American Society for Gastrointestinal Endoscopy (ASGE), and the Society of American Gastrointesinal and Endoscopic Surgeons (SAGES). *Diseases of the Colon and Rectum,* 49(6), 792-809. ISSN 0012-3706

Yakut, M., Kubilay, Ç., Gülseren, S. et al. (2010,June). The efficacy and safety of colonoscopy with oral sodium phosphate in elderly patients. *Turkish Journal of Gastroenterology.* 21(2), 140-145. ISSN 1300-4948

2

Sedation and General Anaesthesia for Colonoscopy in Childhood

Alicja Bartkowska-Śniatkowska[1], Jowita Rosada-Kurasińska[1] and Małgorzata Grześkowiak[2]
University of Medical Sciences,
[1]Department of Paediatric Anaesthesiology and Intensive Therapy
[2]Department of Teaching Anaesthesiology and Intensive Therapy
Poznań,
Poland

1. Introduction

Fiberoptic colonoscopy was successfully introduced into paediatric practice several decades ago and has improved the detection and management of gastrointestinal diseases in children worldwide (El Mouzan et al, 2005). Since the early 1970's colonoscopy has become more useful and more advanced method for diagnosis and treatment in many large-bowel diseases in paediatric population (Steiner et al, 2006). This expansive development has also been possible thanks to the rapid development of anaesthetic techniques and new drugs. There are many indications for colonoscopy in children: diarrhea, hematochezia, unexplained rectal bleeding, abdominal pain, inflammatory bowel disease, polyposis syndrome, polypectomy, vascular ablation, dilation of stricture, foreign body removal, decompression. All reports have shown that this procedure could be safe and useful tool in children of all age groups only if it is based on good practice standards and experienced management, provided by both paediatric gastroenterologist and paediatric anaesthesiologist (Dillon et al, 1998).

Children are often difficult and non-cooperative patients. Due to the anatomical differences, when compare with adults, they need diagnostic specificity and ability to be examined by the paediatric endoscopist. His opinion and comfort during the procedure is a key for effective and satisfactory diagnostic or therapeutic procedure. On the other hand children are completely different group of patients with the higher risk of unpredictable events during invasive procedures being associated with the younger child is. Therefore they need paediatric anaesthesiologist to provide deep sedation or general anaesthesia. In some cases, conscious sedation should be also provided by anaesthesiologist if the child is extremely ill. Although paediatric colonoscopy is performed routinely in hospitals still the most important thing to remember to perform this procedure at least safely, reasonably quickly, and comfortably for the children (Strauss & Giest, 2003). They feel pain and discomfort connected with the overinsuflation of the bowel and heavy-handed instrumental technique. They are more sensitive to dehydration as a consequence of preoperative and preanaesthetic management and this could be reflected in cardiovascular and respiratory complications.

Finally, they can present different responses to the administered drugs that could complicate procedural and post-procedural course (Groot & Mulder, 2010).
Thus, conscious sedation, deep sedation, and general anaesthesia have been widely adopted in paediatric gastroenterological practice because the number of noninvasive and minimally invasive procedures performed in pediatric population has grown exponentially.
Evidenced Base Medicine (EBM) does not allow to answer which method is the best and could be recommended as a standard. To optimize the choice one should be considered three main aspects:

1. Ideal and excellent conditions for instrumental technique
2. Short recovery time
3. High level of satisfaction

The first point is assessed by the endoscopist and his opinion is the most important. Reduced total time for sedation and recovery of patients undergoing colonoscopy plays a special role as large number of procedures are undertaken as day-cases. The last aspect, the patients' satisfaction, is the most difficult to assess because of the age of child and the child is sleeping during the procedure. Additionally discomfort and pain is more with instrumental procedure than sedation or anaesthesia. When child is not able to give an answer, parents' or relatives' opinion will be important but also somewhat subjective.

2. Preanaesthetic management

Children should be routinely assessed by anaesthesiologist in connection with the plan for anaesthesia at least one day before sedation or general anaesthesia. In childrens' hospitals there should be a special room - a preoperative assessment clinic - where children and parents can get answers and explanations to their questions and where good conditions exist for comfortable examination of the child (Cavill & Kerr, 2009a). Equally important is getting the consent for anesthesia during this visit signed by each patient (in Poland over 16 years old) and/or parents or the legal representatives (Steiner et al, 2006, Malviya S, 2011).
Babies and younger children are not very often interested in this visit. They don't understand what happens nor the purpose of this interest. They may be running around the room, not accepting the examination and sometimes crying upon seeing doctor or nurse wearing an white. The person responsible for this first contact (in different countries are different systems e.g. doctors, register nurses) should be strongly experienced in the paediatric field.

2.1 Assessment of child's state of health

Children differ significantly from adults depending on their anatomy, physiology and pathophysiology the greater the difference the smaller child is. Therefore the ratio of complications in the perioperative period is higher than in adults, especially the risk of cardiac arrest. In paediatric anaesthetic cases the incidence of cardiac arrest is assessed to be approximately 1,4 in 10,000. Moreover, an overall mortality of 26% was reported following cardiac arrest (from current database of Paediatric Perioperative Cardiac Arrest (POCA) Registry (Bharti et al, 2009). Compared to adults, two predictors of mortality are the same: ASA physical status 3–5 and emergency surgery. Despite this, 33% of paediatric patients who suffered a cardiac arrest were ASA physical status 1–2. The most important causes are cardiovascular (37%), medication related (32%), respiratory (20%), equipment related (7%) and other (4%).

2.1.1 American Society of Anesthesiologists (ASA) scoring system

The ASA scoring system is helpful in the description of physical status of a patient and is routinely used by the anaesthesiologists all over the world (Saklad, 1941). Even though there is a correlation between ASA score and perioperative mortality it was never intended for risk mortality prediction (Table 1).

Code - ASA	Description
I	A normal healthy patient
II	A patient with mild systemic disease
II	A patient with severe systemic disease
IV	A patient with severe systemic disease that is a constant threat to life
V	A moribund patient who is not expected to survive without the operation
VI	A declared brain-dead patient whose organs are being removed for donor purpose

Table 1. ASA classification (modified)

Neonates are classified as ASA III and infants as ASA II due to their immature organs and significantly unpredictable responses to the drugs. When the endoscopist desires to perform both the colonoscopy and the sedation only by himself he should remember the statistics about the high risk found for paediatric patients even though ASA physical status was assessed for I or II.

2.1.2 Airway associated problems in children

Inadequate ventilation and difficult intubation are everyday hazards in paediatric anaesthesia and can cause higher morbidity and mortality in this group of patients. During the preoperative visit the ability to recognize "difficult to ventilate patient" is essential. Neonates, and smaller children have a unique anatomy of the larynx with the shape of funnel. Other important differences are a large tongue, a long epiglottis, and short and narrow trachea and bronchi which result in increased resistance. Intercostal muscles are very poorly developed and ventilation is therefore diaphragmatic and rate dependent, abdominal distension may cause splinting of the diaphragm (Berg, 2006). Some congenital defects of upper airways disturb normal ventilation (e.g. Pierre-Robin syndrome, Marfan's syndrome, mucopolysaccharidosis) (Inal, 2010).

Assessment should be based on the search for predictors of the difficult airways. A number of useful tests are available for clinical practice. The modified Mallampati scoring system can be applied among older children, who are able to open the mouths and protrude the tongues (Table 2)

Class	Comment
Class 1	Faucial pillars, soft palate, visible uvula
Class 2	Faucial pillars and soft palate visible, uvula masked by base of tongue
Class 3	Only soft palate visible
Class 4	Soft palate not visible

Table 2. Mallampati Scoring Scale

When the child is classified as class 3 or 4 the child should be assessed further using laryngoscopy to obtain a better view of things capable of causing higher risk of respiratory disturbances during deep sedation or general anaesthesia. (Cormack & Lehane, 1984)

Grade	Comment
Grade 1	Whole of glottis visible
Grade 2	Glottis incompletely visible
Grade 3	Epiglottis but not glottis visible
Grade 4	Epiglottis not visible

Table 3. Laryngoscopy Scoring

The most important thing to remember is that combination of sedatives and opioid analgesics decrease the ability to sustain sufficient ventilation, as worse as concomitant defects.

Airway obstruction (another adverse event) should be distinguished from the respiratory depression. Upper airway obstruction in paediatric patients arises from both anatomical structures and laryngospasm. The latter one results from the closure or spasm of the glottic muscles including the false and true vocal cords. This state could be very dangerous during procedural and deep sedation in young children when secretions from upper airway and a impaired cough irritate the larynx and triggered the spasm (Becker & Haas, 2007).

2.2 Requirement laboratory tests

There are many different opinions about the necessity of the laboratory tests among the children before medical procedures. The range of these tests depends on the invasiveness of medical or diagnostic procedure on the one hand and comorbidity of chronic diseases on the other. Healthy children (ASA I and II) should be able to be sedated or receive anaesthesia without any lab tests if the gastroenterologist doesn't see any unusual risk factors from the bowel disease e.g. unexplained bowel bleeding, diarrhea or inflammation. If he does, it is necessary to collect venous blood and check at least blood type, CBC, electrolytes, coagulation parameters before the procedure. For those children with congenital defects or diseases and coexisting severe systemic diseases it is necessary to consider additional laboratory tests and/or to send the child to proper consultant.

2.3 Exclusion criteria

Contraindications for sedation or anaesthesia for elective procedures include the presence of or contact with patients with contagious diseases (postpone procedure for the intubation period, usually 2 to 3 weeks), abnormalities in the physical examination or laboratory tests e.g. productive cough, purulent chest or nasal secretions, pyrexia or signs of viraemia. Anaesthesia in the presence of upper respiratory tracts infection is associated with a higher risk of excess secretions, airway obstruction, laryngospasm and bronchospasm. Children just inoculated (before 3rd day after vaccination containing killed and 3rd week after vaccines with live, attenuated microorganisms) should not be electively sedated or anaesthetized. Vaccines often stimulate the immune system to react as if there were a real infection. A child found to be post viral infection, afebrile, and with no chest signs is probably fit for the procedure even if he has a runny nose (Berg, 2006).

2.4 Feeding before the procedure

Before having a colonoscopy, the bowel needs to be completely empty. This requirement is helpful for anaesthesia because every patient before sedation or general anaesthesia needs to be fasting to perform anaesthesia safely and comfortably. In the last decade the idea of a shorter fasting is preferred among the paediatric and adult anaesthesiologist. Prolong fasting doesn't decrease the risk of gastric aspiration even though it helps to minimize the volume of gastric fluid up to 0.4 ml/kg but there is no reduction in gastric pH which is closed to 2.5 (Royal College of Nursing, 2005). In small children the rate of gastric emptying after feeding breast milk is about 25 minutes while that after the administration of formula compound is 50 minutes. For this reason minimally safe time from the breast milk feeding is 4 hours and for artificial feeding mixtures and solid foods - 6 hours. If the child needs hydration, up to 2 hours before procedure is possible to give clear fluids including water, apple juice, weak tea. Children stratified to a high-risk group of regurgitation are not allowed to be fed 6 (or even 8 hours) regardless of the type of the food (Table 4).
Children with diagnosed chronic disease could continue the most of their medications as usual.

	No risk of gastric aspiration	High risk of gastric aspiration
Clear fluid	2 hours	6 (8) hours
Breast milk	4 hours	6 (8) hours
Formula/cow's milk, solid food	6 hours	6 (8) hours

Table 4. Restrictions of feeding before sedation or anaesthesia in children

2.5 Premedication

The aim of premedication is to achieve state of controlled perioperative emotions and behaviors among the child. For children, any medical procedure can be very distressing and may lead to a lack of cooperation and refusal (Machotta, 2010). Knowledge about the reasons of this behavior is important to develop strategies and techniques to minimize preoperative stress and fear. Another desired effect of premedication is to cause amnesia, especially in the group of patients undergoing colonoscopic procedure, often repeatedly. Additionally, premedication could be helpful in inhibiting unwanted vegetative reflexes and reduction of the secretion of saliva and mucus in the airways, so typical and characteristic for pediatric population under 5-7 years old. The last indication for specific premedication is the elimination of pain accompanying the disease to minimize child's discomfort. Considering all these aspects, adequate preparation and the use of anxiolytic premedication are important modalities. Non-pharmacological interventions are interesting and could be an alternative to the use of sedative drugs in the future (Vagnoli et al, 2010)
In many cases parental presence could be helpful, even during the initiation of sedation or the induction of general anesthesia. The enthusiasts of the use of psychological methods try to introduce completely modern methods including even the presence of a clown in the preoperative room (Vagnoli et al., 2010). They achieved a significantly better effect when compared to parental presence or the influence of midazolam. In many hospitals this practice is not common for not only medical but also organizational and administrative reasons.

The best-documented practice for premedication of children for minor procedures seems to be the pharmacological method with midazolam (Kentrup et al, 1994, Isik et al, 2010).

2.5.1 Midazolam

Midazolam (described in 3.1.1) is indicated for premedication because it produces amnesia, anxiolysis and sedation. Oral administration is a favorite choice for premedication in children with the dose of 0.5 - 0.75 mg/kg given 30 minutes before the procedure but the effect is not always predictable (Robinson, 2000). Recently for smaller children (up to 30 kg of body weight) a syrup can be prepared for use by the hospital pharmacy department to avoid the use of intravenous route. The total volume of this mixture is limited to the 6 ml. Older children willingly use tablets. Oral midazolam is useful prior to planned intravenous sedation and general anaesthesia but does not give the prolonged depression of consciousness (Baygin et al, 2010, Kazak et al, 2010, Kulikov et al, 2010)

2.5.2 Clonidine

Clonidine is a partial agonist of central and peripheral alfa-2 adrenoreceptors and is a central imidazole receptor agonist. It also effects alfa-1 receptors (alfa1:alfa2 > 200:1). It is a known antihypertensive agent but with its sedative and analgesic effects potentiates volatile anaesthetic agents and decreases intraoperative requiments for propofol, although recovery time may be prolonged. It has a synergistic analgesic effect with opioids (Thompson, 2007). Oral clonidine premedication in dose of 4 - 5 mcg/kg has been shown to reduce the incidence of sevoflurane induced emergence agitation. (Tazeroualti et al, 2007). It also attenuates reflex sympathetic responses and may improve cardiovascular stability during anaesthesia (Cao et al, 2011).

2.5.3 Dexmedetomidine

Dexmedetomidine, an imidazole compound, is the pharmacologically active dextroisomer of medetomidyne and is the most selective central alfa-2 adenoreceptor agonist available clinically. This agonist has eight times higher affinity for the alfa-2 adenoreceptor than clonidine. It offers beneficial pharmacological properties, provides dose-dependent sedation, analgesia, sympatholysis and anxiolysis without significant respiratory depression (Goksu et al., 2008). Like clonidine, dexmedetomidine reduces occurrence of sevoflurane emergence agitation in a dose of 2.5 mcg/kg (Ozcengis, 2011). Both agents also can be administered intranasally for premedication in doses of 0.5-1 mcg/kg for dexmedetomidine and 2-4 mcg/kg for clonidine(Yuen, 2008; Basker, 2009).

Clonidine and dexmedetomidine preoperatively have similar levels of anxiety and sedation postoperatively as midazolam. However, children given alpha-2 agonists had less perioperative sympathetic stimulation and less postoperative pain than those given midazolam (Ali & El Ghoneimy, 2010, Al-Zaben, 2010, Dere et al, 2010, Schmidt, 2007).

3. Procedural sedation

Procedural sedation and analgesia (PSA) is intended to result in a depressed level of consciousness that allows the patient to maintain oxygenation and airway control independently. It is divided into two types: minimal sedation and conscious sedation.

3.1 Minimal sedation (anxiolysis)

Minimal sedation could be accurate and sufficient type of sedation for gastrointestinal procedures performed in older children. They are able to respond to verbal stimulation normally, but cognitive function and coordination may be impaired. What is most important is that ventilatory and cardiovascular functions are unaffected.

3.2 Conscious sedation (moderate sedation)

This type of sedation is usually performed for smaller and for older children and the depression of consciousness is drug-induced. Conscious sedation also commonly known as "moderate sedation" means that patient retains the ability to respond to vocal and light touch commands at any time during the sedation. Usually the circulatory system is not disturbed. Additionally patients have to be able to breathe spontaneously and protect their own airway. This last condition is extremely difficult to achieve in babies and smaller children because of specific anatomy and unpredictable response to drugs. In this group of patients intravenous administration of hypnotic drugs could provoke depression of spontaneous breathing and result in the need for manual or automatic ventilation via facial mask. This type of sedation could very often change from "moderate" to "deep" without clear symptoms and therefore requires the presence and expertise of an experienced pediatric anesthesiologist.

Some authors suggest that intravenous procedural sedation can be administered by the endoscopist, who both administers the sedation drug and performs the procedure. Of course this can only be done when qualified nurse helps the doctor monitor the patient's state of consciousness and vital signs. This method seems to be safe in the endoscopist's hands when restricted to ASA I and ASA II patients. Children relegated to ASA III and more status should have anaesthesia performed by a pediatric anaesthesiologist even if only minimal procedural sedation is planned (Hansen et al, 2003, Heuss et al, 2003, Lee et al, 2003). Other authors, highly experienced in paediatric anaesthesiology are opposed to idea "sedationist-operator". They claim the best and the safest method of sedation for children is to have it performed by an anesthesiologist who is highly experienced and understands the differences of paediatric population.

3.3 Drug regimens

Pharmacologic regimens that ensure safe, effective and efficient sedation for all paediatric patients would be ideal but are not always achievable. Those used should act predictably and rapidly and allow the anaesthesiologist to induce the desired level of sedation necessary for the procedure being performed. After the procedure, the drugs should allow the child to awaken quickly and they should not prolong the recovery time.

Various drugs are available to provide procedural sedation. Midazolam either alone or in combination with an opioid analgesic is commonly selected for procedural sedation. Combining use of a benzodiazepine and an opiate may be preferable for longer procedures but increases the risk respiratory and circulatory depression. Specific reversal agents for opioids (naloxone) and benzodiazepines (flumazenil) must be available during the procedure.

3.3.1 Midazolam

The effect of midazolam as a short acting benzodiazepine (in children half-life 2.5-4 hours) is controlled, reversible and produces light sedation, anxiolysis, and amnesia. Midazolam is characterized by a relatively high volume of distribution (V_d) compared with other benzodiazepines because of its lipophilicity. In obese patients the activity could be increased from 2.7 hours to 8.4 hours. Midazolam is cleared by hepatic hydroxylation to 1-hydroxymidazolam (which has about 10% of the pharmacologic activity as parent compound).

Age	Administration route			Comment
	Intravenous	Rectal	Oral	
Up to 6 month	0.04 - 0.1 mg/kg b.w.	-	-	-
6 month–5 year	0.05 - 0.1 mg/kg	0.35 - 0.45 mg/kg	0.5 mg/kg	Total dose 6 mg/kg/d
5 - 12 year	0.025 - 0.05 mg/kg	0.35 - 0.45 mg/kg	0.5 mg/kg	Total dose 0.4 mg/kg/d; max 10 mg/d
5 - 12 year	0.025 - 0.05 mg/kg	0.35 - 0.45 mg/kg	0.5 mg/kg	Total dose 0.4 mg/kg/d; max 10 mg/d
12 -18 year	2.5 mg	0.35 - 0.45 mg/kg	0.5 mg/kg	i.v. bolus 1 mg; Total dose 10 mg
	1 - 1.5 mg			i.v. bolus 1 mg; Total dose 3.5 mg

Table 5. Midazolam dosing for procedural sedation in children.

Intravenous administration is the best way in this group of patients but sometimes oral, rectal and possibly nasal method might be equally as good for colonoscopy as well as other procedures (Wood, 2011). The most important thing to consider is the route of the administration of the drug to the child. Dosing of midazolam depends very strictly on the age and body weight of patient.

Intravenous doses of midazolam should be titrated to effect, especially in neonates and small babies, to achieve a desirable level of sedation and prevent inadvertent and deeper sedation (Robinson, 2000).

3.3.2 Other benzodiazepines

Diazepam has an extremely long half-life (0.8-2.25 day) especially in neonates and babies but also in obese patients (3.9 day and 3.29 day). Additionally, its active metabolites have long half-lives (*N*-desmethyldiazepam, nordiazepam). Lorazepam is another benzodiazepine that may be used for mild-to-moderate sedation; its limitation is onset of action up to 15-20 minutes after administration. The duration of action of lorazepam is longer (6-8 hours) than that of midazolam (30-60 min).

3.3.3 Other sedative drugs

In the literature there are also proposals for the use of other sedatives (e.g. etomidate, propofol or ketamine) for procedural sedation. These drugs are registered as anaesthetic drugs, not sedative, so according to the strict recommendations of the Food and Drug Administration (FDA) and The Helsinki Declaration on Patient Safety in Anaesthesiology 2010 are not allowed for procedural "sedation". (Mellin-Olsen et al, 2010)

Given the above specific conditions midazolam is the only single drug that can be used by the non-anaesthesiologists for procedural sedation.

3.3.4 Analgesic opioids

Analgesic opioids (described in 4.1.4) should be added when more painful colonoscopy is planned. Reducing the dose of opioids of about 50% is recommended because of the accumulation of side effects, especially depression of spontaneous ventilation.

3.4 Indications and contraindications for procedural sedation in children

Children are sometimes a major challenge for doctors and nurses. On the other side is necessary to understand their immaturity and lack of experience to accept fear, pain or disconnection from parents.

3.4.1 Indications for conscious sedation in children

Indications in the paediatric population differ from those among adults. They could be divided into two groups depending on the side of interest: patient and doctor.

Indication of the patient	Indication of the doctor
Unexplained fear Unaccepted discomfort Claustrophobia Prolonged and repeated procedures	Babies and small children Non-cooperative children Diagnostic and therapeutic procedures associated with pain

Table 6. Indications for conscious sedation during colonoscopy in children

3.4.2 Contraindications for procedural sedation in children

Contraindications for procedural sedation, whether performed by an anaesthesiologist or by non-anaesthesiologist are following:

- Congenital defects of respiratory system
- Acute respiratory insufficiency
- Persistent respiratory insufficiency
- Congenital Central Hypoventilation Syndrome (CCHS)
- Important circulatory insufficiency
- Neuromuscular diseases
- Impaired or loss of consciousness in the history
- Child too excitable, even after the earlier application sedatives
- Child with behavioral disorders
- Lack of agreement of child and/or parents and/or legal representatives

Additionally special conditions for performing conscious sedation should be met in the following general situations:

- Neonates, particularly preterm birth neonates, especially with regard to individual susceptibility to depressive influence of sedatives on respiratory depression
- Children below 1 year and 5 year, with regard to higher risk complications and adverse events after overdosing of drugs and/or insufficient sedation
- Renal insufficiency
- Liver insufficiency

3.5 Complications of procedural sedation

Factors that increase the risk of complications during conscious sedation in children are: age below 12 months and coexisting congenital and/or chronic diseases.
The most important adverse events after conscious sedation among children are:

- Loss of protective reflexes of the upper respiratory tract
- Closure and upper airway obstruction
- Allergic reaction
- Breathing disturbances
- Cardiac arrest

3.6 Equipment and supplies

The place use to perform colonoscopy under procedural sedation should be equipped with an oxygen supply, a suction system, airway management equipment, resuscitation medications and equipment, intravenous accesses equipment, cardiac monitor equipment and a defibrillator.
Monitoring. All the time of performing procedure should be monitored ECG, pulse oximeter, respiratory rate, systemic blood pressure and other clinical sign such skin color.
The state of unconsciousness should be regularly assessed from the beginning to the end of sedation and this data be documented in the chart. In paediatric practice the most common used scale is Ramsay sedation scale.

Score	Response
1	Anxious or restless or both
2	Cooperative, orientated and tranquil
3	Responding to commands
4	Brisk response to stimulus
5	Sluggish response to stimulus
6	No response to stimulus

Table 7. Ramsay Sedation Scale

3.7 Recovery of the child after procedural sedation

Procedural sedation can be successfully performed for many interventional or diagnostic colonoscopy procedures in children. It should be provided by well-trained and credentialed professionals at all the times.
After successfully completing procedural sedation the child should breathe spontaneously, have throat reflexes present, be able to cough, and to adequately maintain an airway. Depending on the age of the child, child should sit and talk, and in this state may be given to parents.

4. Deep sedation

Deep sedation is a very good alternative for painful colonoscopy. Depression of consciousness is drug-induced but much deeper than in procedural sedation. The patient is not easily arousable but can respond following repeated or painful stimulation. Spontaneous ventilation may be inadequate and the patient may require assistance in maintaining a patent airway. Independent ventilatory function is rather impaired while cardiovascular hemostasis is usually properly maintained.

Deep sedation is indicated for possibly painful colonoscopies, therapeutic examinations and those more invasive examinations, especially when it is essential to immobilize the patient. The most discussed dilemma is how to provide deep sedation. The first method is based rather on deeper sedation rather than analgesia and to limit adverse events by using high doses of opioid analgesic. The second method involves analgesia even at the expense of less hypnosis. The truth is that the compilation of sedative and analgesic agents varies slightly when these agents are used in children, especially younger than 1 year, but much existing data suggest more variability in choices when the child is older than 7 years (Patel et al, 2009).

4.1 Drug regimens

Drugs should be administered intravenously. It is important to use small loading doses and to titrate the dosage because of the narrow margin of their safety. For this reason they should not be used by the non-anaesthesiologist according to the restrictions imposed by the FDA and The Helsinki Declaration on Patient Safety. If they are, the provider should be skilled in airway management and resuscitation, and usage should depend upon regional statutes. The most important anaesthetic for this type of procedure such colonoscopy is propofol.

4.1.1 Propofol

Propofol (alkyl phenol) is a short-acting anaesthetic characterized by both rapid onset of action (within one arm-brain circulation time) and short recovery time. Propofol causes dose-dependent cortical depression within 30 seconds from the beginning of administration, mostly without epileptiform activity, although larger doses could provoke excitatory movements (Eer et al, 2009). The incidence of excitation, cough and hiccup are similar to those of thiopental. In contrast to barbiturates, propofol attenuates laryngeal reflexes, facilitating laryngeal mask insertion or intubation. By the way of decreased responsiveness to $CO2$, propofol is respiratory depressant, especially when used in conjunction with opioid analgesics (when more than 50-70% of children will need ventilatory support). Its influence on the vascular system and heart is variable but often there is a mild cardiodepressant effect. Propofol is metabolized by the pathway of glucuronidation in the liver and removed by the kidney (88%) and the digestive system (2%).

Te newest lipid formulations of this agent limit the pain sometimes experienced during intravenous administration making propofol closed to the "ideal drug" for paediatric sedation.

One important difference from other intravenous and inhaled anaesthetics is its antiemetic effect, a desired effect in gastroenterological group of patients (Leon et al, 2011).

Effective deep sedation could be achieved by a single dose method as well as continuous infusion with recovery time independent to the duration of sedation (10-20 minutes after discontinuation).

The disadvantage of propofol is its narrow therapeutic range (high rates of hypoxia and hypotension) and risk of inadvertent general anesthesia and that is the reason why it should be routinely administered by anesthesiologists. Only this strategy allow to properly control of the level of sedation and reduced recovery time (Lightdale, 2004).

The usual standard dose of propofol used for sedation for older children is 0,5-1,5 mg/kg while children younger than 8 years should be sedated with higher doses e.g. 1,5 - 3,0 mg/kg. The best effect is achieved when continuous infusion is planned, of course keeping in mind age differences in dosing.

4.1.2 Other anaesthetic drugs

The choice of anaesthetic drug is in the hands of anaesthesiologist based on the status of patient and predictive duration of and type of colonoscopy.

4.1.2.1 Benzodiazepines

Benzodiazepines are highly lipid-soluble agents and can cross the blood-brain barrier readily. When used intravenously the onset of their effect usually takes longer than one arm-brain circulation time. Depending on their lipophilicity they have long a long persistence. These characteristics limit the usage of this group of drugs for deep sedation.

4.1.2.2 Barbiturates

Sodium thiopental is the most commonly used thiobarbiturate that induces anaesthesia rapidly within one arm-brain circulation and maintain longer than propofol. Its main limitation is its cardiodepressant effect with decreased cardiac output and blood pressure. Respiratory depression as a result of reduced $CO2$ response is deteriorated by laryngeal spasm and bronchoconstriction. The other limitation is its prolonged half-life depending on the total dosage which influences recovery time.

4.1.2.3 Ketamine

Ketamine is a derivative of phencyclidine and cyclohexamine and as a non-competitive antagonist of the NMDA receptors it is responsible for dissociative anaesthesia and analgesia. This last advantage allows one to not have to use opioids and in thus decreases the risk of respiratory depression while maintaining analgesia.
Ketamine is slow-onset anaesthetic with an effect within 1 minute after intravenous administration and a duration of action much longer than other newer agents. In addition the dissociative influence of this agent on the brain possibly bringing about hallucinations, diplopia, and temporary blindness limits its usefulness in short procedures (less than 1 hour) such as colonoscopy even these symptoms are not that prevalent among children (Gilger et al., 2004)

4.1.2.4 Etomidate

Etomidate is an imidazole characterized by rapid induction with one arm-brain circulation time and simultaneously long duration of action. In children the main contraindication of this agent is excitatory phenomenon, epileptic activity, respiratory depression, a relatively higher risk of emesis and commonly, pain at the injection site (Evered, 2003).

4.1.3 Inhaled anesthetic

Sevoflurane halogenated ether has been available for clinical use since 1990. This volatile anaesthetic agent remains popular both for induction and maintenance of anaesthesia and sedation. It has low blood/gas and oil/gas solubility. This produces a more rapid response to changes in inhaled concentration, and speedier induction and recovery. Intracranial pressure is increased but minimally at less than 1 MAC (minimal alveolar concentration). Sevoflurane produces anaesthesia and sedation without analgesia and epileptogenic spikes, decreases arterial pressure by reducing systemic vascular resistance with little effect on cardiac output until higher doses are used, and it lowers the heart rate and therefore helps to reduce myocardial oxygen consumption. This agent reduces tidal volume, respiratory rate and smooth muscle tone of the bronchi, and it is not irritant to the upper respiratory tract. Most sevoflurane is eliminated via the lungs, with 5% of the absorbed dose being metabolized by the liver. It can have toxic effect on the kidneys, liver and brain (Mushambi & Smith, 2007, Smith, 2008). The use of sevoflurane in paediatric patients which would enable rapid recovery is complicated by the frequent occurrence of emergence agitation, particularly with high concentration over 6 vol% with spontaneous breathing and over 5 vol% when ventilated mechanically (Ganzberg et al, 1999, Khattab, 2010)

4.1.4 Opiods

The following opioids (remifentanil, alfentanil and fentanil) are commonly used for induction and the maintenance of anaesthesia for endoscopic procedures (Colvin, 2007). Morphine is used additionally to maintain analgesia in the postoperative period.

4.1.4.1 Remifentanil

Remifentanil hydrochloride is a mu-receptor opioid agonist and is currently the shortest-acting opioid. The onset and peak effect is rapid and the duration of action is short (5 – 10 minutes). Therefore for longer action remifentanil should be administered continuously. There is a lack of drug accumulation even after prolonged infusions.

Remifentanil is indicated for intravenous administration during induction of anaesthesia with the infusion rate of 0.5 to 1 mcg/kg/min together with an intravenous or volatile agent. During the maintenance of anaesthesia the infusion rate may vary in accordance with the dosing guidelines. For paediatric patients aged 1 to 12 years continuous infusion of 0.25 mcg/kg/min (infusion dose range 0.05 – 1.3 mcg/kg/min) with sevoflurane (0.3 – 1.5 MAC) or isoflurane (0.4 – 1.5 MAC) is recommended.

Nonspecific blood and tissue esterase metabolizes remifentanil rapidly by hydrolysis.

Pseudocholinesterase plays no special role so if atypical plasma cholinesterase is present remifentanil's duration of action remains normal. The effects and side effects are dose dependent. After administration over 60 seconds a rapid and slower distribution half-life are 1 and 6 minutes respectively. A terminal elimination half-life lasts 10 - 20 minutes. Renal and liver insufficiencies do not affect remifentanil's pharmacokinetics (Toklu et al, 2009). Side effects, mostly dose-dependent are hypotension and bradycardia, respiratory depression, and skeletal muscle rigidity (including chest wall rigidity).

4.1.4.2 Alfentanil hydrochloride

Alfentanil hydrochloride is a an OP3 mu-opioid agonist which is ultra-short-acting (5 - 10 minutes). The onset of action is immediate (1 - 2 minutes). Administrated at doses of 8 - 40 mcg/kg it is excellent for procedures lasting up to 30 minutes e.g. colonoscopy. The recovery time is comparable to that observed with equipotent fentanil dosages. For children under 12 years of age it is not recommended.

Intravenous administration of a dose of 5 mcg/kg provides analgesia for the conscious but sedated patient; doses of 105 mcg/kg produce hypnosis; and induction of anesthesia requires doses 50-150 mcg/kg. Induction with alfentanil should be administered slowly (over 3 minutes) due to the danger of loss of vascular tone and hypotension. Fluid replacement prior to induction with this agent is important. Maintenance of anaesthesia (if

the procedure lasts up to 60 minutes) is carried out with a dose of 50 mcg/kg, but alternatively, continuous infusion 0.5 – 3 mcg/kg/min is acceptable. The infusion should be discontinued at least 10-15 minutes prior to the end of the procedure. In obese patients the dose of alfentanil should be determined on the basis of lean body weight.
After administration a rapid and slower distribution half-life are 1 and 14 minutes respectively. Terminal elimination half-life lasts 90 - 111 minutes. The volume of distribution is 0.4-1 L/kg, which is 4 – 10 times smaller than those for fentanil. The liver is responsible for major biotransformation. Metabolites are eliminated mostly by urinary excretion.
The important side effects consists of hypotension, secondary to vasodilation and bradycardia, respiratory depression, skeletal muscle rigidity (dose and speed dependent).

4.1.4.3 Fentanil

Fentanil is a strong mu-opioid agonist with a rapid onset (2 – 3 minutes) and short duration of action (20 – 60 minutes). Fentanil is 100 times more potent than morphine (100 mcg of fentanil approximately equals 10 mg of morphine). Because of its high lipophilicity it penetrates easily to the central nervous system causing the rapid onset of action. Due to its high lipophilicity there is a danger of possible redistribution of fentanil. Hemodynamics are stable after administration of fentanil, which makes this drug useful in cardiovascular diseases.
Fentanil could be administered orally, subcutaneously, or intravenously. For induction of anaesthesia doses of 0.5 – 1 mcg/kg (up to 5 mcg/kg) together with a intravenous or volatile agent are recommended and during maintenance of anaesthesia 1 – 4 mcg/kg according to a need.
The drug's large volume of distribution (3.5 – 5.9 L/kg) is responsible for relatively long half-life. The elimination half-life vary from 3.1 – 7.9 hours. There is a danger of possible redistribution of fentanil due to its lipophilicity (biphasic depression of ventilation). The liver is responsible for its metabolism. Side effects are as follows: respiratory depression, skeletal muscle rigidity (particularly if large doses are administered rapidly), and stimulation of parasympathetic system.

4.1.4.4. Morphine sulfate

Morphine sulfate is an important alkaloid of opium, a pure opioid agonist. It is mu-opioid agonist but at higher doses interacts with other opioid receptors. The onset of action after intravenous administration is 5 – 10 minutes, the duration of action 2 – 4 hours. The lipid solubility and degree of ionization are crucial in the onset and duration of analgesia as well as the effects of the central nervous system. The additional hydroxyl group on the molecule of morphine (pH 7.4) makes the molecule of morphine water soluble, more than other clinically used opioids. The most therapeutic action of morphine is analgesia but there are some others like euphoria and anxiolysis.
Administration intravenously requires average doses of 0.1 mg/kg and continuous infusion 20-25 mcg/kg/h, while intramusculary or subcutaneously doses of 0.15-0.2 mg/kg should be sufficient.
After intravenous administration the volume of distribution ranges from 1.0 to 4.7 L/kg. The terminal half-life vary from 1.5 – 4.5 hours. Morphine is metabolized to morphine glucuronide in the liver and eliminated by the kidneys.
Side effects are more extensive than others and include drowsiness, respiratory depression, peripheral vasodilation, decreased gastrointestinal motility, decreased biliary and pancreatic secretion, nausea, vomiting, alterations in the endocrine and autonomic nervous system, and release of histamine.

Analgesic opioid	Route of administration	Dosing
Morphine	i.v.	0.05-0.2 mg/kg b.w.
Fentanil	i.v.	0.5-1 mcg/kg b.w.
Alfentanil	i.v.	5-20 mcg/kg b.w.
Remifentanil	i.v.	0.25-1 mcg/kg b.w.

Table 8. Dosing of analgesic opioids during deep sedation in children

4.2 Advances in patient monitoring during deep sedation

Monitoring during colonoscopy in the paediatric population under deep sedation is essential for safety and effectiveness. The issue is controlling effects on the cardiovascular, respiratory and neurological systems particularly in younger children. Recent technologic advances include electronic vital-sign monitoring systems which should be useful to maintain physiologic condition in the perioperative time period. The most recent method is the proposal of advanced capnography as a method of providing early warning for preventing postoperative respiratory depression (American Society of Anesthesiologists, 1996, Hutchinson & Rodriguez, 2008). Only hospital and/or specially equipped endoscopy facilities are appropriate setting for colonoscopy under deep sedation among infants, babies and children.

5. General anesthesia

Colonoscopy under general anaesthesia in children allows endoscopist comfortably prepare the patient and perform painless procedure. These aspects are important because of the technical advantages during invasive colonoscopy and higher patient's satisfaction even the presence of reported symptoms.

The frequency of the episodes of perforation or bleeding is not described (Steiner et al, 2006). Similarly postprocedural pain is significantly lower after colonoscopy under general anesthesia probably because of mild and controlled insufflation resulted in lower gas excess and abdominal pain.

Complications connected with general anaesthesia are sometimes arguing by the oppositionists. They emphasize most often sore throat and hoarseness (after endotracheal intubation), postoperative nausea and vomiting (mainly after inhaled anesthetics) and rarely irritability and sleep disturbances. The serious adverse events such as respiratory complications and cardiodepressant effects are statistically comparable to others typical for paediatric anaesthesia (Samer Ammar et al, 2003, Stringer et al, 1999).

General anaesthesia is defined as reversible, controlled and temporary loss of consciousness, painless and/or muscle relaxation (anaesthesia & analgesia & muscle relaxation). It needs the usage of up to date anaesthesia machine and monitoring apparatus what increases indeed the cost of the colonoscopy and forces to organize the relevant endoscopy room.

5.1 Induction

General anaesthesia is induced by using one of the following techniques: inhalational or intravenous. Drugs used belong to the three classes according to the tenets of general anaesthesia: anaesthetics, analgesic opioids and muscle relaxants (the latter more for endotracheal intubation than colonoscopic technique).

5.1.1 Inhalational induction

The most common indication for inhalational induction of anaesthesia are following:

- young children
- no accessible veins
- fear of needles by the child
- upper airway obstructions e.g. epiglottis, asthma
- a predictably difficult endotracheal intubation
- acceptance of the use of a child's face mask

Contraindications include in fear of the child regarding the use of a face mask, a higher risk of aspiration of gastric content and the risk of malignant hyperthermia.

There are three main techniques of induction with inhaled anesthetics:

- single-breathe technique – for cooperative and older children
- normal breathing volumes – for children of all ages, especially infants and babies
- increasing doses of inhaled gases - for children of all ages

After consciousness is lost it is possible to introduce access into a peripheral vein and continue fluid and drug administration in this way. At the same time depending on the extent of colonoscopy and the child's ASA physical state is necessary to consider insertion of oropharyngeal airway, laryngeal mask airway or endotracheal tube. Laryngeal mask airway become a major advance in anesthetic airway management, particularly when children breathe spontaneously during colonoscopy. This method limits the adverse events that accompany endotracheal intubation.

The most important inhaled anaesthetic in paediatric anaesthesia is sevoflurane (described in 4.1.3).

5.1.2 Intravenous induction

Intravenously inducted anaesthesia is preferable for most routine procedures, including colonoscopy because of a less complicated technique used when applying inhaled anesthetics. Additionally it is very useful for rapid induction in patients with a higher risk of regurgitation of gastric contents. Many authors report higher comfort and tolerance for patients. After insertion of a cannula into the peripheral vein administration of the required drugs is started. In children cannulation is a painful procedure and local anaesthetics should be used on suitable veins in both forearms (EMLA [Eutectic Mixture of Local Anesthetic], 50% lidocaine and 50% prilocaine).

Currently the most commonly used intravenous hypnotic for colonoscopy is propofol (described in 4.1.1). Its disadvantage e.g. narrow therapeutic range and risk of hypoxia and hypotension applies to general anaesthesia as well as deep sedation.

5.2 Maintenance of anaesthesia

For complicated and prolonged colonoscopies in children the preferred method of maintenance could be Total Intravenous Anaesthesia (TIVA) conducted with a special infusion pump. After the loading dose continuous infusion is done. The profile of propofol allows the patient to recover quickly irrespectively of the time of anaesthesia (stop the infusion 10 minutes before the end of colonoscopy).

In the other cases the maintenance of anaesthesia can be combined with inhalation of oxygen, air, nitrous oxide, sevoflurane or isoflurane, depending on the available choices. For colonoscopy in children appropriate level of maintenance of anaesthesia could be achieved by the method of inhalational anaesthesia with spontaneous ventilation.

Other than the above described intravenous and inhaled anaesthetics there may be some additional agents which have a role in providing general anaesthesia, decision to use them belonging to the anaesthesiologist.

5.3 Recovery

After the completion of colonoscopy anaesthetic drugs should be withdrawn and 100% oxygen delivered. Removal of the endotracheal tube or laryngeal mask airway should be done when respiratory reflexes are fully returned. This maneuver is challenging in small children up to 4 year because half of them following laryngeal spasm. After the patient is ready he should be transported into the recovery area.

5.4 Drug regimens

Anaesthetic drugs (intravenous and inhaled) have to be combined with strong and short acting analgesic opioids. The introduction of these newer less-toxic, shorter-acting anaesthetic drugs has reduced the requirement for muscle relaxants not only for diagnostic procedures like colonoscopy but also for general surgery in the paediatric population. Moderate anaesthesia conducted with combination of sevoflurane–remifentanil or propofol–remifentanil can keep children immobile without producing hypotension and facilitate controlled ventilation once the effects of the intubating dose of a muscle relaxant have worn off (Meakin, 2007, Liao et al, 2010).

Neuromuscular blocking agents could be selected only for those indications like difficult airway, higher risk of gastric regurgitation, obesity, and difficulties with patient's position. The usage of these agents is limited by prolong muscle blocking and risk of postprocedural respiratory depression. Thus, only relatively short acting nondepolarizing blocking agents such mivacurium and rocuronium are recommended for colonoscopy in children (Eikermann, 2001).

Mivacurium produces onset of maximum block in 1-2 min and 25% recovery in 9–10 min. This type of action is faster and longer during anesthesia with sevoflurane than with propofol.

Rocuronium retains the characteristics of an intermediate-duration relaxant in the younger age group of children, longer in infants than in children (42 vs. 27 min).

The introduction of the newest selective relaxant binding agent (SRBA) – sugammadex (Bridion) - has been an important development in the last few years because of its ability to provide a rapid reversal from any depth of neuromuscular blockade. Sugammadex is a modified gamma-cyclodextrin, chemically water-soluble cyclic oligosaccharides with a lipophilic core, which encapsulates and inactivates rocuronium or vecuronium (Bom, 2007). Rapid reversal with this agent occurs respectively after less than 4 minutes from deep neuromuscular blockade (dose 4 mg/kg) and less than 3 minutes from moderate neuromuscular blockade (dose 2 mg/kg). Any effect on the cholinergic nervous system has not been observed. Currently there are no recommendations to use sugammadex in full-term neonates or young infants even though there have been good results off-label but for older children it is the most desirable (Meretoja, 2010).

6. Conclusion

Recently fiberoptic colonoscopy has become more useful and advanced method for treating a large number of large-bowel disorders in the paediatric population. All reports have shown that this procedure can be a safe and useful tool in children of all age groups only if it is based on good practice standards and experienced management, provided by both: paediatric gastroenterologists and paediatric anaesthesiologists. The most important trend among paediatric gastroenterologists is acceptance of the anaesthesiologist's performance of intravenous sedation and/or general anaesthesia based on differences between children and adults as were presented in this chapter. The choice of sedation or general anaesthesia for those paediatric gastrointestinal procedures is in the hands of anaesthesiologists who are the most experienced in this area. Only this pattern of conduct may provide not only optimal routine sedation or anaesthesia but the most standardized and the safest care for all age groups of children.

7. References

Ali, A. & El Ghoneimy, M. (2010). Dexmedetomidine versus fentanyl as adjuvant to propofol: comparative study in children undergoing extraxoroporeal shock wave lithotripsy. *Eur J Anaesthesiol.*, Vol.27, No.12, (December, 2010), pp.1058-1064, ISSN 0265-0215

Al-Zaben, KR.; Qudaisat, IY.; Al-Ghanem SM.; Massad IM.; Al-Mustafa MM.; Al-Owedi AS.; Abu-Halaweh SA. & Abu-Ali HM. (2010). Intraoperative administration of dexmedetomidine reduces the analgesic requirements for children undergoing hypospadius surgery. *Eur J Anaesthesiol.* Vol.27, No.3, (March, 2010), pp.247-252, ISSN 0265-0215

American Society of Anesthesiologists. Task force on sedation and analgesia by non-anaesthesiologists. Practice guidelines for the prevention, detection, and management of respiratory depression associated with neuraxial opioid administration. (1996). *Anesthesiology*, Vol.84, No.2, (Feb, 1996), pp.459-471, ISSN 0003-3022

Berg, S.(2006). Paediatric and neonatal anaesthesia, In: *Oxford handbook of anaesthesia*, Allman, K. & Wilson, I., (Eds.), 757-814, Oxford University Press, ISBN 0-19-856609-3, New York, United States

Bharti, N.; Batr, YK. & Kaur, H. (2009). Paediatric perioperative cardiac arrest and its mortality: Database of a 60-month from tertiary care paediatric centre. *Eur J Anaesthesiol.* Vol.26, No.6, (June, 2009), pp.490-495, ISSN 0265-0215

Becker, DE. & Haas, DA. (2007). Management of complications during moderate and deep sedation: respiratory and cardiovascular considerations. *Anesth Prog.*, Vol.54, No.2, pp.59-69, ISSN 0003-3006

Baygin, O.; Nodur, H. & Isik, B. (2010). Effectiveness of premedication agents administered prior to nitrous oxide/oxygen. *Eur J Anaesthesiol,.* Vol.27, No.4, (April, 2010), pp.341-346, ISSN 0265-0215

Bom A, Epemolu O, Hope F, Rutherford S & Thomson K. (2007). Selective relaxant binding agents for reversal of neuromuscular blockade. *Curr Opin Pharmacol.*, Vol.7, No.3, (June, 2007), pp.298-302, ISSN 1040-8703

Cavill G & Kerr K, (2009). Preoperative management, In: *Fundamentals of Anesthesia*, Smith T, Pinnock C & Lin T, 1-24, Cambridge University Press, ISBN 978-0-521-6924906, Cambridge, UK

Cao, J.; Shi, X.; Xu, H., Jiang, J., Pu, Y. & Miao X. (2011). Effects of premedication with clonidine on pre-operative anxiety and post-operative pain in children: a prospective, randomized, controlled trial. *Eur J Anaesthesiol*. Vol.28, No.4, (April, 2011), pp.311-315, ISSN 0265-0215

Colvin, L. (2007). Analgesic drugs, In: *Textbook of anaesthesia,* Aitkenhead, A. ; Smith, G. & Rowbotham, D., (Eds.), 64-79, Elsevier, ISBN 0-443-10078-0, United Kingdom

Cormack, RS. & Lehane, J. (1989). Difficult tracheal intubation in obstetrics. *Anaesthesia,* Vol.44, pp. 42-46, ISSN 0003-2409

De Groot, H. & Mulder, WM. (2010). Clinical practice: drug desensitization in children. *Eur J Pediatr.*, Vol.169, No.11, pp.1305-1309, (November, 2010), ISSN 0340-6199

Dere, K.; Sucullu, I.; Budak, ET.; Yeyen, S.; Filiz, AI.; Ozkan, S. & Dagli, G. (2010). A comparison of dexmedetomidine versus midazolam for sedation, pain and hemodynamic comtrol during colonoscopy under conscious sedation. *Eur J Anaesthesiol.* Vol.27, No.7, (July, 2010), pp.648-652, ISSN 0265-0215

Dillon, M.; Brown, S.; Casey, W.; Walsh, D., Durnin, M.; Abubake, K. & Drumm, B. (1998). Colonoscopy under general anesthesia in children. *Pediatrics,* Vol.102, No.2, (August, 1998), pp.381-383, ISSN 0031-4005

Eer, AS.; Padmanabhan, U. & Leslie, K. Propofol dose and incidence of dreaming during sedation. (2009). *Eur J Anaesthesiol.,* Vol.26, No.10, (October, 2009), pp.833-836, ISSN 0265-0215

Eikermann, M.; Renzing-Kohler, K.&Peters J. (2001). Probability of acceptable intubation conditions with low dose rocuronium during light sevoflurane anaesthesia in children. *Acta Anaesthesiol Scand.,* Vol.45, No.8, (September, 2001), pp.1036–1041, ISSN 1399-6576

El Mouzan, MI.; Al-Mofleh, IA.; Abdullah, AM.; Al Sanie, AM. & Al-Rashed, RS. (2005). Colonoscopy in children. *Saudi J Gastroenterol,* Vol.11, pp.35-39, 1319-3767

Evered, L (2003). Procedural sedation and analgesia for paediatric patients in the emergency department. *Paediatrics and Child Health,* Vol.8, No.8, (October 2003), pp.503-507, ISSN 1205-7088

Ganzberg, S.; Weaver, J.; Beck, FM. & McCaffrey, G. (1999). Use of sevoflurane sedation for outpatient third molar surgery. *Anesth Prog,* Vol.46, No.1, pp. 21-29, ISSN 0003-3006

Gilger, M.; Spearman, R.; Dietrich, C.; Spearman, G.; Wilsey, M. Jr. & Zayat, M. (2004). Safety and effectiveness of ketamine as a sedative agent for pediatric GI endoscopy. *Gastrointestinal Endoscopy,* Vol.59, No.6, (May 2004), pp.659-663, ISSN 0016-5107

Goksu, S.; Arik, H.; Demiryurek, S.; Mumbuc, S.; Oner, U. & Demiryurek A. (2008). Effects of dexmedetomidine infusion in patients undergoing functional endoscopic sinus surgery under local anaesthesia. *European Journal of Anaesthesiology,* Vol.25, No.1, (January 2008), pp. 22-28, ISSN 0265-0215

Hansen, JJ.; Ulmer, BJ. & Rex, DK. (2003). Technical performance of colonoscopy with nurse-administered propofol sedation (NAPS) versus midazolam/narcotics. *Gastrointest Endosc.,* 57 AB 79 (Poster 317), ISSN 0016-5107

Heuss, LT.; Schnieper, P.; Pfimlin, E. & Beglinger, C. (2003). Nurse-administered sedation with propofol under observation of the endoscopist: prospective observation study with more than 5000 patients. *Gastrointest Endosc.,* 57 AB 105 (Poster 1481), ISSN 0016-5107

Hutchinsosn, L. & Rodrguez, L. Capnography and respiratory depression. (2008). *Am J Nurs.,* Vol.108, No.2, (February, 2003), pp.35-39, ISSN 1538-7488

Inal, MT.; Memis, D.; Kargi, M.; Oktay, Z. & Sut, N. (2010). Comparison of TruView EVO2 with Miller Laryngoscope In paediatric patients. *Eur J Anaesthesiol.*, Vol.27, No.11, (November, 2010), pp.950-954, ISSN 0265-0215

Isik, B.; Baygin, O.; Kapci, EG. & Bodur, H. (2010). The effects of temperament and behavior problems on sedation failure and anxious children after midazolam premedication. *Eur J Anaesthesiol.*, Vol.27, No.4, (April, 2010), pp. 336-340, ISSN 0265-0215

Khattab, A.; El-Seify, Z.; Shaaban, A.; Radojevic, D. & Jankovic, I. (2008). Sevoflurane-emergence agitation: effect of supplementary low-dose oral ketamine premedication in preschool children undergoing dental surgery. *European Journal of Anaesthesiology*, Vol.27, No.4, (April 2010), pp. 353-358, ISSN 0265-0215

Kazak Z, Sezre GB, Yilmaz AA & Ates Y. (2010). Premedication with oral midazolam with or without parental presence. *Eur J Anaesthesiol.* Vol.27, No.4, (April, 2010), pp.347-352, ISSN 0265- 0215

Kentrup H, Skopnik H, Menke D, Thon HJ, Matern S & Heimann G. (1994). Midazolam and ketamine as premedication in colonoscopies: a pharmacodynamic study. *Int J Clin Pharmacol Ther.*, Vol.32, No.2, pp. 82-87, ISSN 0946-1965

Lee DW, Chan AC, Wong SK, Li AC, Sze TS & Chung SC. (2003). A prospective study in safety, feasibility and acceptability of patient-controlled sedation for colonoscopy. *Gastrointest Endosc.*, 57 AB 79 (Poster 316), ISSN 0016-5107

Leon A, Ahlstrand R, Thorn SE & Wattwli M. (2011). Effects of propofol on esophageal sphincters: study on young and elderly volunteers using high-resolution solid-state manometry. *Eur J Anaesthesiol.*, Vol.28, No.4, (April, 2011), pp.273-278, ISSN 0265-0215

Liao R, Li JY & Liu GY. (2010). Comparison of sevoflurane volatile induction/maintenance anaesthesia and propofol-remifentanyl total intravenous anaesthesia for rigid bronchoscopy under spontaneous breathing for tracheal/bronchial foreign body removal in children. *Eur J Anaesthesiol.*, Vol.27, No.11, (November, 2010), pp.930-934, ISSN 0265-0215

Lightdale JR. (2004). Sedation and analgesia inpaediatric patient. *Gastroinest Endosc Clin N Am*, Vol.14, No.2, pp. 385-399, ISSN 0016-5107

Machotta A,. (2010). Non cooperation and refusal during induction of anesthesia in children. *Anasthesiol Intensivmed Notfallmed Schmerzther.* Vol.45, No.6, pp.378-382, ISSN 0939 2661

Malviya s, Voepel-Lewis T, Chiravuri SD, Gibbokds K, Chimbira WT, Nafiu OO, Reynolds PI & Tait AR. (2011). Does an objective system-based approach improve assessment of perioperative risk in children? A preliminary evaluation of the 'NARCO'. *Br J Anaesth.*, Vol.106, No.3, pp. 352-358, ISSN 1471-6771

Meakin HG. (2007). Role of muscle relaxants in paediatric anesthesia. *Curr Opin Anaesthesiol*, 20, pp.227-231, ISSN 0952-7907

Mellin-Olsen J, Staender S, Whitkaer DK & Smith A. (2010). The Helsinki Declaration on Patient Safety in Anaesthesiology, *Eur J Anaesthesiol.*, Vol.27, No.7, pp.592-597, ISSN 0265-0215

Meretoja OA. (2010). Neuromuscular block and current treatment strategies for its reversal in children, *Pediatric Anesthesia*, Vol.20, pp.591–604, ISSN 1155-5645

Mushambi, M. & Smith, G. (2007). Inhalational anaesthetic agents, In: *Textbook of anaesthesia,* Aitkenhead, A. ; Smith, G. & Rowbotham, D., (Eds.), 13-33, Elsevier, ISBN 0-443-10078-0, United Kingdom

Ozcengiz, D.; Gunes, Y. & Ozmete, O. (2011). Oral melatonin, dexmedetomidine, and midazolam for prevention of postoperative agitation in children. *Journal of Anesthesia,* online first, (February 2011), pp. 22-28, ISSN 0913-8668

Patel KN, Simon HK, Stockwell CA, Stockwell JA, DeGuzman MA, Roerig PL & Rigby MR. (2009). Paediatric procedural sedation by a dedicated non anaesthesiology pediatric sedation service using propofol. *Pediatr Emerg Care.,* Vol.25, No.3, pp.133-138, ISSN 0749-5161

Robinson DN. (2000). Paediatric sedation techniques. *Current Anaesthesia & Critical Care,* Vol.11, pp.250-254, ISSN 0953-7112

Royal College of Nursing (RCN). Perioperative fasting in adults and children: an RCN guideline for the multidisciplinary team. 2005, RCN, London, www.rcn.org.uk.

Saklad M. (1941). Grading of patients for surgical procedures. *Anesthesiology,* Vol.2, pp.281-284, ISSN 0003-3022

Samer Ammar M, Pffefferkorn MD, Croffie JM, Gupta SK, Corkins MR & Fitzgerald JF. (2003). Complications following outpatient upper gastrointestinal endoscopy in children: 30-day follow-up. *Am J Gastroenterol,* Vol.98, pp.1508-1511, ISSN 0002-9270

Schmidt, A.; Valinetti, E.; Bandeira, D.; Bertacchi, M., Simões, C. Auler &J. Jr. (2007). Effects of preanesthetic administration of midazolam, clonidine, or dexmedetomidine on postoperative pain and anxiety in children. *Pediatric Anaesthesia* , Vol.17, No.7, (July 2007), pp. 667-674, ISSN 1155-5645

Smith, T. (2008). Anaesthetic gases and vapours, In: *Fundamentals of anaesthesia,* Smith, T.; Pinnock, C. & Lin, T., (Eds.), 110-146, Cambridge University Press, ISBN 978-0-521-69249-6, New York, United States

Steiner, SJ. ; Pfefferkorm, MD. & Fitzegerald, JF. (2006). Patient-reported symptoms after pediatric outpatient colonoscopy or flexible sigmoidoscopy under general anesthesia. *J Pediatr Gastroenterol Nutr.,* Vol.52, No.4, pp. 483-486, ISSN 0277-2166

Strauss, JM.& Giest, J. (2003). Total intra venous anesthesia. On the way standard practise in pediatrics. *Anaesthetist,* Vol.52, No.9, (September, 2003), pp. 763-767, ISSN 0003-2417

Stringer, MD.; Pinfield, A.; Revell, L.; McClean, P. & Puntis, JW. (1998). A prospective audit of paediatric colonoscopy under general anaesthesia. *Acta Paediatr.,* Vol.88, No.2, (February, 1998), pp.199-202, ISSN 0803-5253

Tazeroualti, N.; De Groote, F.; De Hert, S.; De Ville, A.; Dierick, A. &Van der Linden P. (2007). Oral clonidine vs midazolam in the prevention of sevoflurane-induced agitation in children. A prospective, randomized, controlled trial. *British Journal of Anaesthesia,* Vol.98, No.5, (May 2007), pp. 667-671, ISSN 1471-6771

Thompson, J.(2007). Drugs acting on the cardiovascular system, In: *Textbook of anaesthesia,* Aitkenhead, A. ; Smith, G. & Rowbotham, D., (Eds.), 110-146, Elsevier, ISBN 0-443-10078-0, United Kingdom

Toklu, S.; Yyilikci, L.; Gonen, C.; Siffci, L.; Gunenc, F.; Sahin, E. & Gokel, E. (2009). Comparison of etomidate-remifentanil and propofol-remifentanil sedation in patients scheduled for colonoscopy. *Eur J Anaesthesiol.,*May Vol.26, No.5, (May, 2009), pp.370-376, ISSN 0265-0215

Vagnoli, L.; Caprilli, S. & Messeri, A. (2010). Parental presence, clowns or sedative premedication to treat preoperative anxiety in children: what could be the most promising option? *Paediatr Anaesth.*, Vol.20, No.10, (October, 2010), pp.937-943, ISSN 1155-5645

Wood, M. (2011). The safety and efficacy of using a concentrated intranasal midazolam formulation for paediatric dental sedation. *SAAD Dig*, Vol.27, (January, 2011), pp.16-23

Yuen, V.; Hui, T.; Irvin M. & Yuen, M. (2008). A Comparison of Intranasal dexmedetomidine and Oral Midazolam for Premedication in Pediatric Anesthesia: A Double-Blinded Randomized Controlled Trial. *Anesthesia &Analgesia* , Vol.106, No.6, (June 2008), pp. 1715-1721, ISSN 1526-7598

3

Quality of Screening Colonoscopy: Learning Technical Skills and Evaluating Competence

Marco Bustamante
Department of Gastroenterology
Dr. Peset University Hospital, Valencia
Spain

1. Introduction

Colonoscopy is an essential part of colorectal cancer (CRC) screening programs since it can diagnose CRC as well as identify and excise precursor lesions before the carcinoma fully develops (Winawer et al., 1993). Although colonoscopy has shown to be effective in decreasing the incidence and mortality of CRC (Kahi et al., 2009), it does not provide total protection against cancer since, in daily practice, a clinically significant number of CRCs and adenomas still go undetected. For example, the proportion of undiagnosed CRC in patients having previously undergone colonoscopy ranges from 2.1%, when the cancer is located in the left colon and the splenic angle, to 5.9% when located in the right colon (Bressler et al., 2007). The proportion of undetected adenomas ranges from 2% for polyps ≥10 mm to 26% for polyps of between 1 and 5 mm (van Rijn, 2006). Consequently, an incidence of interval cancers has been described which ranges from 1.7 to 2.4/1000 person-years of follow-up in patients included in a control program following the excision of one or more adenomas (Pabby et al., 2005).

One of the factors which seem to have the most bearing on the number of lesions diagnosed by colonoscopy is the endoscopist him/herself. A difference of up to 20% has been described in the proportion of colonoscopies with at least one adenoma (Chen & Rex, 2007) and of up to 9 times in the proportion of patients with advanced adenomas (Barclay et al., 2006). Other studies confirm these results and suggest that some endoscopists could leave up to half of the adenomas undiagnosed (Rex, 2006b). A number of technical aspects could be responsible for these differences, in particular the ability to reach the cecum and the withdrawal technique (longer explorations, better examination of the proximal mucosa in folds and angles, better management of colon distension and better cleaning of the remains and fluids in the colon) (Rex, 2000).

Screening colonoscopy is a special situation which involves an invasive exploration of an asymptomatic subject with the theoretical promise of detecting CRC before it produces symptoms, or of reducing the individual risk of suffering CRC by detecting and excising colorectal adenomas. In this context, where the detection of lesions is crucial, it appears to be essential to have endoscopists with the necessary technical skills. A study carried out recently in the setting of a CRC screening program based on the detection of fecal occult blood showed that the endoscopist was an independent predictive factor in the detection of

adenomas (Bretagne et al., 2010). In fact, the rate of adenoma detection per endoscopist is the factor most associated with the risk of interval cancer (Karniski et al., 2010).
In conclusion, for a CRC screening program to be truly effective, it must be based on high-quality colonoscopies in such a way that the protective effect against CRC of this procedure approaches the theoretical maximum possible. For these programs it would therefore appear logical to have endoscopists who are experts in colonoscopy in order to reduce to a minimum the degree of variability in the detection of lesions attributable to the examiner. However, at the present time, with screening programs still in their infancy, the basic characteristics of Endoscopy Departments and of those endoscopists who will be in charge of such programs have yet to be defined. The training of endoscopists to carry out screening colonoscopies and their evaluation in terms of seeking possible accreditation have not yet been regulated either. In this review, we will go over the current situation of the training in colonoscopy for gastroenterology specialists, the possibility of evaluating their skills and we will make some recommendations for the future.

2. Quality parameters in screening colonoscopies

Over the past few years, much attention has been given to the definition of auditable parameters to measure the quality of colonoscopies. Systematic monitoring of certain variables allows for the quality of colonoscopies to be controlled and may be used as a tool for improvement (Lin et al., 2010; Barclay et al., 2008). This review does not intend to make a comprehensive review of the parameters used to measure the quality of colonoscopy, for which there are very recent guides and revisions, including the clinical practice guidelines on the quality of screening colonoscopies produced by the Spanish Association of Gastroenterology (Jover, J. ed., 2011). (Table 1).
However, it is worth commenting on the adenoma detection rate (ADR), the variable which has become the most important, since it is directly related to the preventive capacity of colonoscopies in terms of CRC. This rate is equal to the proportion of patients undergoing colonoscopy in which at least one adenoma has been detected. The ADR is associated with a better technique for carrying out the colonoscopy, for example, a thorough exploration of folds and angles, adequate management of distension-aspiration, control of the remains of filth and the time dedicated to the exploration (Rex, 2006b). Since it is necessary to wait for the pathology result in order to measure this parameter, other authors have suggested using the number of polypectomies as an auditable parameter, which is associated with the above, but which is more directly measurable (Williams et al., 2011). Other frequently used quality parameters are associated with the ADR. Several studies have shown that the time of withdrawal is associated with the frequency of polyp detection (Barclay et al., 2006; Rex 2000; Imperiale et al., 2009). A recent study found a significant association between the proportion of adenoma detection and the "cecal intubation time/withdrawal time" ratio < 1 for those endoscopists with higher detection rates (Benson et al., 2010). Almost all recommendations consider a minimum withdrawal time of 6 minutes for a normal colonoscopy as the threshold for a quality endoscopy (Rex et al., 2006b). The proportion of colonoscopies in which the cecum is reached is also associated with the ADR, and is a parameter which must be controlled, since in several studies, most interval CRCs were diagnosed in proximal parts of the colon (Pabby et al., 2005; Singh et al., 2006). For example, the American Society for Gastrointestinal endoscopy (ASGE)/American College of Gastroenterology (ACG) Task Force on quality in endoscopy recommends that effective

colonoscopists must be able to intubate the cecum in ≥ 90% of cases, and in ≥ 95%, when the indication for the colonoscopy is screening (Rex et al., 2006b). Other parameters may be the endoscopic resection of polyps and the control in collecting complications (Rex et al., 2006b; Romagnuolo et al., 2008; Gonzalez-Huix et al., 2010).

Indicator	Advisable level
Adenoma detection rate	> 20% (colonoscopy as a primary screening strategy) > 40% (colonoscopy as a secondary screening strategy, following a positive FOBT)
Colonoscope withdrawal time	> 6 minutes
Number of colonoscopies without supervision	400 before entering the screening program 200 anually
Cecal intubation rate	> 95% colonoscopies
Use of sedation	> 90% colonoscopies
Perforation rate	< 1/1000 colonoscopies
Post-polypectomy bleeding rate	< 1/200 polypectomies
Accurate description of polyp characteristics	100%
Endoscopic excision of pedunculated and sessile/flat polyps up to 2 cm of diameter	> 95%
Polyp retrieval rate	> 95% for polyps > 10 mm > 80% for polyps < 10 mm

Table 1. Screening colonoscopy quality indicators

However, the evaluation of these parameters may not be sufficient to increase the frequency of adenoma detection (Sawhney et al., 2008). For example, a recent study found an inverse relationship between the total duration of the exploration and the ADR. Furthermore, control of the ADR by feeding back the results to the endoscopists did not improve the ADR (Shaukat et al., 2009). This is probably due to the fact that there are other technical aspects relating to the withdrawal exploration which are essential in order to increase the lesion detection rate but which are more difficult to evaluate quantitatively. This happens, for example, with the thorough examination of the colon mucosa, especially the angles and the proximal parts of the folds, the aspiration of the liquid content and the exploration with different degrees of insufflation. In a center where a protocol for exploration on withdrawal was applied, which, in addition to time, included these technical aspects, a 10% increase in the total number of neoplasms detected was achieved, as well as a 15% increase in the number of lesions under 10 mm (Barclay et al., 2008).

Therefore, a quality colonoscopy is characterized by the combination of certain measureable parameters, as well as others which, even though they are not measurable, are essential in screening colonoscopies. These technical aspects may be responsible for the differences found between endoscopists in the frequency of lesion detection, in such a way that it seems to be of the utmost importance to ensure adequate teaching of these technical skills for all endoscopists, and especially for those who are going to be in charge of a CRC screening program. Collection and measurement of these parameters must also be the basis for control and evaluation of the endoscopist competence.

3. Current situation of learning in colonoscopy: acquisition and evaluation of competence

Competence in a procedure is the minimum level of skills, knowledge and/or expertise acquired through training and practice which is required to safely and effectively carry out a task or procedure without any help or supervision (Faigel et al., 2006). Applied to colonoscopy, competence entails the ability to confidently carry out the exploration, interpret the findings, apply the necessary treatments and manage the complications that may arise.

Clearly, the first step towards achieving competence is adequate training during the residency period in the specialty of Gastroenterology. However, specialty training programs are greatly undefined and variable, and they are mostly based on general recommendations by Scientific Societies and opinions from experts. For example, the training period necessary to acquire competence has not been clearly defined. In general terms, it appears that the training period should be no shorter than 6-12 months (Conjoint Committee for the recognition of training in Gastrointestinal Endoscopy, n.d.). In Spain, a minimum period of 6 months is recommended for basic endoscopy, with an additional 3 months for advanced endoscopy (Consejo Nacional de Especialidades Médicas, 2009), but training periods vary greatly from country to country. Generally speaking, there is no structured procedure for teaching during the residency program either, which would allow all areas of learning to be managed and for their results to be assessed. Furthermore, trainers in endoscopy are usually not trained in teaching techniques. In practice, training of endoscopists during the residency is done in a barely regulated manner, integrating teaching into the normal activities of attendance in Endoscopy Departments, and by trainers who are not specifically trained to that effect. All of this may influence the quality of the training and may be responsible for the poor quality perceived by residents in their learning in endoscopy (Wells et al., 2009).

Traditionally, two supplementary learning methods have been proposed to improve the results of standard teaching during the residency: short courses and simulators. Short courses, usually lasting two to three days, are not considered to be enough to acquire the technical skills or judgment necessary to carry out the colonoscopy, since their short duration does not allow for adequate training (Romagnuolo, 2008). In a short course, 10 supervised colonoscopies can be done at most, a long way from the Societies' recommendations and, of course, far short of the minimal number of colonoscopies required to achieve competence. The ASGE recommends that short courses be considered as training opportunities or tools for continued education but never as substitutes for a formal training program of adequate duration (ASGE Taskforce on ensuring competence in endoscopy, n.d.).

Simulators are computer-based devices which offer different degrees of difficulty, with a sense of touch through a simulated endoscope and the ability to administer sedation as well as incorporating systems which simulate pain and discomfort in the virtual patient. Moreover, data associated with the procedure, such as duration, the ability to visualize the mucosa and the ability to complete the procedure is collected. The aspect in which they have been evaluated the most is the resident's learning, with the aim of shortening the learning curve and reducing the patient's discomfort when examined by an inexperienced examiner. In general terms, it appears that the greatest benefit is obtained in the early stages of learning, in such a way that experienced endoscopists hardly obtain any benefit (Sedlack & Kolars, 2002). Moreover, it would appear that even for inexperienced endoscopists, the learning curve flattens after only 7 simulated explorations (Eversbusch & Grantcharov, 2004). A randomized study compared the skills of two groups of residents, one which had received simulator training and the other which had not, before starting the traditional training program. This study showed that if the use of the simulator was extended to 10 sessions in the residents in the first group, a benefit in competence parameters was seen, which was maintained until real exploration number 80 (Cohen et al., 2006). However, this device does not seem to be of any use to endoscopists who have already completed the standard period of practical training. In fact, this type of device is able to distinguish between the user's technical capacity and differentiate expert endoscopists from novice ones (Grantcharov et al., 2005; Koch et al., 2008). In one study, for expert endoscopists, the learning curve in the device was only two simulated explorations (Eversbusch, 2004). Residents do, however, perceive this device as being effective as a supplementary learning system (Lightdale, 2010).

As regards the evaluation of competence, until now, the most usual way has been a subjective assessment whereby at the end of the residency period the trainer states that the resident can carry out colonoscopies autonomously. A more objective attempt at evaluation is the measurement of parameters which support the fact that the individual is competent to carry out the exploration. The one which has been studied the most, perhaps because it is the easiest to measure is the minimum number of colonoscopies performed, but this also involves great variability. In the United States, the ASGE recommends carrying out a minimum of 140 colonoscopies during the training period, with at least 20 polypectomies. However, the program for the specialty of surgery is different with only a minimum of 50 explorations being required (Accreditaton Council for Graduate Medical Education, 2006). The Canadian and Australian Societies of Gastroenterology require 100 complete, totally unassisted explorations up to the cecum to have been carried out (Romagnuolo, 2006; Conjoint Committee for the recognition of training in Gastrointestinal Endoscopy, n.d.). In Spain, the minimum number of colonoscopies which must be carried out is 150 (Consejo Nacional de Especialidades Médicas, 2009). However, carrying out a specific number of colonoscopies does not guarantee competence in this exploration since learning varies greatly from individual to individual. In a recent study, it was determined that the number of colonoscopies necessary to reach the cecum in 90% of explorations was 150, and 200 in 95% (Lee et al., 2008). However, another study suggested a threshold of 500 colonoscopies for all residents to have autonomy of ≥ 90% to carry out colonoscopies (Spier et al., 2010). The first resident to become autonomous did so after carrying out 330 colonoscopies. It would therefore appear that linking the evaluation of competence to having carried out a specific number of explorations is not an adequate system. This was demonstrated by Cass et al., who designed an evaluation system with key points which should be learned in order to carry out a colonoscopy, which included, for example correct identification of any anomalies found in the exploration (Cass et al., 1993). Adequate competence in these variables was not reached with the minimum number of colonoscopies recommended by the experts (Cass et al., 1996). Another finding of this study was that the subjective assessment overestimated the resident's competence compared to objective assessments. Moreover, nowadays competence assessment cannot focus solely on variables related to diagnostic colonoscopy, such as the number of procedures carried out or the percentage that reached the cecum. These days a student cannot be considered competent if he/she is not capable of carrying out the endoscopic treatment of the lesions found.

Finally, in addition to the basic training, continued practice is necessary to maintain competence. The secondary results of a Canadian study showed that endoscopists who carried out less than 240 colonoscopies per year had significantly more incomplete colonoscopies than those who carried out 370 per year (Shah et al., 2007). A similar study in the U.S. showed that endoscopists who carried out less than 100 colonoscopies per year had a significantly lower proportion of complete colonoscopies (Wexner et al., 2001).
In conclusion, there are still no standardized or universally accepted methods to achieve and evaluate competence when autonomously carrying out colonoscopies. Carrying out a certain number of explorations does not guarantee competence, and specific tools must be developed to assess cognitive aspects and competence skills.

4. Towards a new teaching system: structured learning and training the trainers

Colonoscopy is a complex procedure at the psychomotor level which also requires a solid knowledge base allowing for clinical and therapeutic decisions to be made. Traditionally, however, the learning of endoscopy has been based on passing from watching explorations to carrying them out outside the context of an organized teaching system which ensures that learning is carried out correctly. This procedure has several limitations which affect the quality of the learning, such as the ever greater work load of endoscopy departments which reduces the time assigned to each exploration, the reduction of the residents' overall working hours, who thus have less time to dedicate to practicing colonoscopy, and the fact that every person learns in a different way and at a different pace. An alternative teaching system which allows these difficulties to be overcome is therefore necessary. In this system, the responsibility for learning would no longer lie on the student but would focus on the trainer, who must follow a structured teaching system based on communication and feedback with the student, and who must also be responsible of evaluating the student in each of the phases.

4.1 The teaching process. The role of trainers and endoscopy departments

The trainer must have broad technical knowledge and experience in diagnostic and therapeutic colonoscopy, and must be able to finalize a procedure when the student fails. This, however, is not enough. He/she must know what the resident needs to learn, know the basic concepts of the learning process and apply teaching techniques which ensure the resident's training. The learning of colonoscopy includes three areas: i) cognitive skills which include the indications and contraindications of the test, the identification and classification of lesions and clinical decision-making based on the findings; ii) technical skills, which include methods for advancing the endoscope and handling the loops that are formed, the ability to carry out the test adequately and in a reasonable time, as well as the ability to apply endoscopic treatments, and iii) procedure-related skills, such as information to the patient, informed consent, risk assessment, the safe administration of sedation-analgesia and the drafting of an adequate report of the exploration (Raman & Donnon, 2008).
The colonoscopy teaching process should go through three phases: acquisition of theoretical knowledge, observation of the procedure with comments by the tutor and tutored practice. Each of these phases will be planned beforehand and it will be the active responsibility of the trainer to ensure that the way in which students go through each one of the phases is not left to chance (Figure 1).

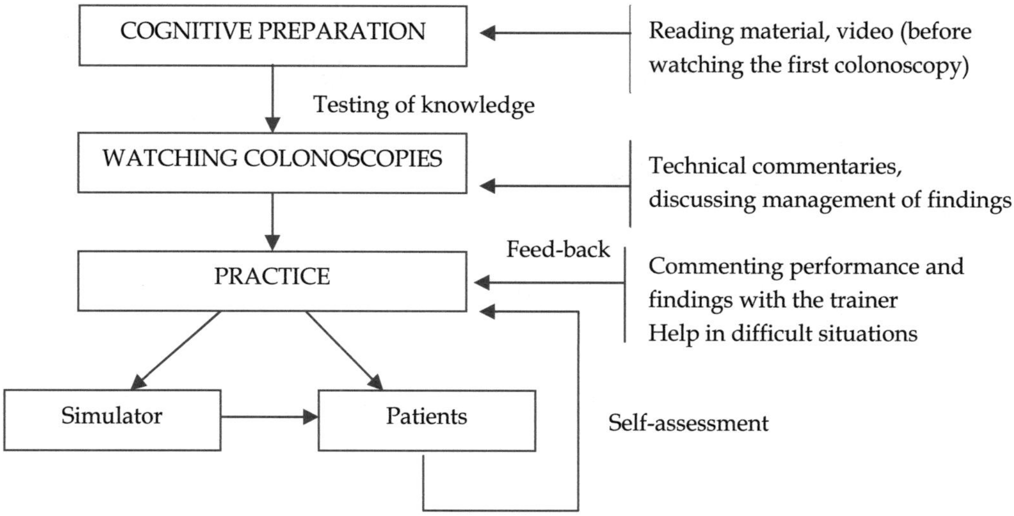

Fig. 1. Teaching phases in colonoscopy

Evaluation of the student by the trainer and the feedback between both is a fundamental part of this process and is supported by recent evidence. For example, the use of checklists which ensure the inclusion of key points in colonoscopic technique and the design of a system for evaluating trainees, with feedback to the trainers on their results, seems to improve the effectiveness of teaching certain aspects of endoscopy (Alevi, 2010).

As for the role of endoscopy departments, a working group suggested that endoscopy departments where teaching is carried out must have at least two designated trainers, each with one or two sessions dedicated to the teaching process. Furthermore, at least 300 colonoscopies should be carried out annually in the department, of which at least 100 should be carried out by the student. It would also be advisable to have audiovisual teaching material available. The department should have a record of the student's colonoscopy activity, including the parameters described above (Teague, 2002). Teaching should be student oriented (trainer-student), with dedicated time established and separated from the needs of the department.

4.2 Answer to these demands. Training the trainers and evaluation systems

The main problem behind implementing such a change in the form of teaching is the trainer's and institution's lack of knowledge of learning techniques. The solution would involve the training of trainers, which has shown to be effective in improving the results of the teaching process. For example, in the aforementioned study by Alevi et al. (Alevi, 2010), trainers attended a previous educational module on the effective practice of feedback with the student. This training is necessary because an analysis of cognitive tasks, in which 3 colonoscopists were asked to explain what they were doing and why, allowed the relevant steps and important clinical decisions that were omitted during traditional training to be identified (Sullivan, 2008).

In the United Kingdom, in 2004, a structured training program on endoscopy was put into practice. This system is based, firstly, on the training of trainers by means of a three-day course, where they learn teaching techniques. The trained trainers complete 3-day courses locally, where the technical principles of colonoscopy are taught. Finally, the students must

continue developing their technical skills in their own centers (Balfour, 2001). This centrally organized system has been shown to improve the quality of explorations, reduce complications and increase the students' satisfaction with their training (Haycock, 2010). The importance of training the trainers is included in the recent recommendations by the United European Gastroenterology Federation (UEGF), where it recommends providing trainers in gastroenterology with a standardized tool for teaching (Berberat, 2010).
As for the evaluation of the student, supervision must be done by the trainer by way of the systematic collection and evaluation of a series of technical data. In general terms, the resident should be successful in 80-90% of the technical objectives included in the training program in order to complete it successfully (ASGE standards of training committees, 1999). These parameters should coincide with the quality markers for colonoscopy and should, amongst others, include intubation in the cecum and ileum, adenoma detection rate, technical ability to carry out standard polypectomies and recover polyps for pathological analysis, an acceptable rate of complications, the number of colonoscopies carried out and a correct use of sedation (Romagnuolo, 2008; Joint Advisory Group [JAG] on Gastrointestinal Endoscopy, n.d.a; JAG, 2010). This evaluation should also include cognitive criteria and assessment of tasks related to the procedure (table 2).

Cognitive criteria	Related tasks
Identification of risk factors	Reviewing of patient chart and images
Evaluation of indications and contraindications	Obtention of informed consent
Recognizing and managing complications	Preparation of an accurate report
Planning management based on findings	Discussion of findings with the patient, family and other healthcare providers

Table 2.

The development of several tools for objectively measuring competence is currently underway. For example, the Accreditation Council for Graduate Medical Education (ACGME) developed a structured tool for evaluating residents (ACGME, 2000) which could be effective in terms of teaching colonoscopy (Spier, 2010). More recently, authors in the Mayo Clinic have developed a tool to objectively measure the quality in conducting colonoscopies longitudinally in time, which also includes parameters of endoscopic treatment (Sedlack, 2010). Other groups have proposed similar tools (Vassilou, 2008; Tang, 2006). A structured evaluation is also to be found in the English system, in which the latest component of this system is monitoring and auditing (Balfour, 2001). Although all these instruments have to be specifically validated in the evaluation of competence, it is clear that this is the path that must be taken in order to achieve a more objective assessment of the individual ability to carry out colonoscopies.

5. Credentialing of individuals and units

The final goal of healthcare systems is to provide high quality medical services. In the case of colonoscopy, local institutions and stakeholders are responsible for designing and implementing a quality assurance program able to ensure quality and safety of all phases of the colonoscopy process including pre- and post-procedural aspects. This quality control program must apply to individuals and endoscopy units in a standarized way.

5.1 Granting privileges to individuals for colonoscopy

A privilege is the authorizacion by a local institution (hospital or endoscopy unit) for a physician to perform a particular procedure (Faigel, 2009). Granting privileges is the mainstay of this process as it requires reviewing in a systematic and reproductible manner the performance of endoscopists and units involved in the colonoscopy process. Privileges must be granted only to competent individuals, and healthcare providers must stablish specific policies for granting, complying with local, regional and national regulations (fig. 2). The process for granting privileges includes a formal review of the applicant´s credentials by a physician member of the healthcare institution, including documentation of the accomplished training. The reviewer should also have privileges to perform colonoscopy. If the applicant´s credential acomplish healthcare institution criteria, a proctoring evaluation must follow. Proctoring includes direct observation of the applicant performing a pre-specified number of procedures, with evaluation of a group of criteria that should include the aforementioned technical and cognitive items (Tables 1 and 2). The proctor must be an unbiased individual, with expertise in colonoscopy to allow judgement of the applicant skills but uninvolved in teaching or active patient care (Dominitz, 2008). A written guideline of the whole competence assessment process must be included in the institution´s bylaws. Competence must be reassessed periodically through a renewal of privileges process, performed in a similar way to the initial credentialing process. Again the institution must have a written guideline for the renewal process, including timing of reevaluation and recommendations for additional training.

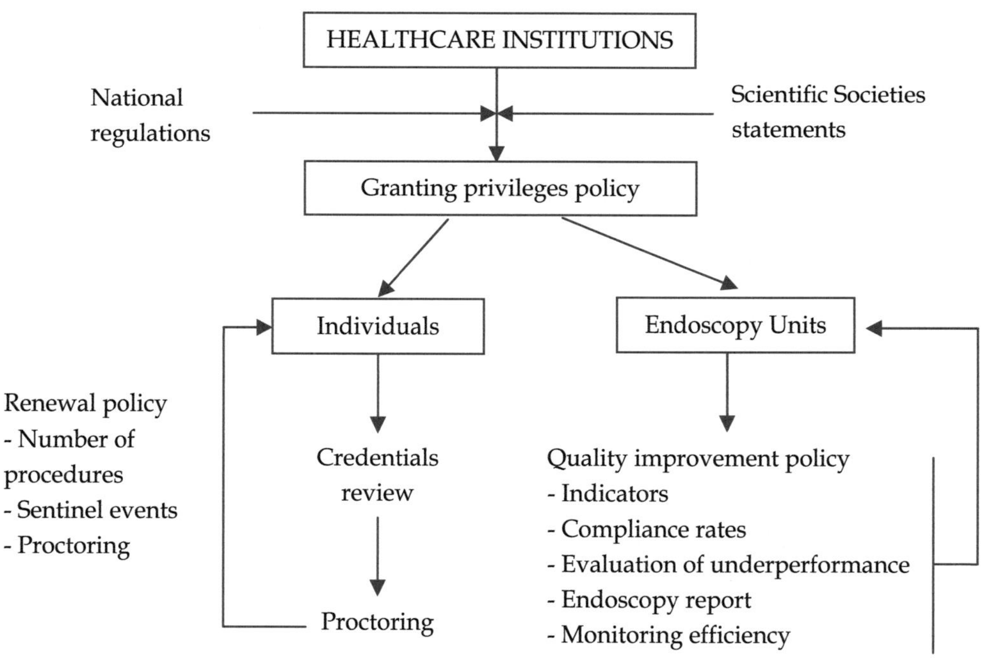

Fig. 2. Granting and renewal of privileges for individuals and endoscopy units

5.2 Credentialing for endoscopy units

Units are responsible for maintaining and enhancing the quality of endoscopic procedures, by means of an institutional policy for quality improvement (Faigel, 2009). Individual

quality indicators must be assessed periodically and improvement plans must be implemented if needed. Poor performance must be addressed offering feed-back and plans for improvement to underperformers. Each institution should have policies for reviewing and reporting sentinel events. This term is used to describe significant deviations from optimal patient care, which in the case of colonoscopy, should include adverse outcomes of sedation, bleeding, perforation and infections. Inappropriate indications, lack of informed consent and inadequate colonoscopy report should also be included and formally assessed. All the process of quality control, indicators, feed-back and consequences of repeated underperformance should be pre-specified and written-down.
Units should be evaluated and subject to a formal credentialing and re-credentialing process. The ASGE is recognizing units which adhere to ASGE guidelines on privileging and quality assurance with a Certificate of Recognition award (ASGE, n.d.a). In the UK the British Global Rating Scale is the standard of accreditation for endoscopy services (JAG, n.d.b) and in Spain the Spanish Association of Gastroenterology (AEG) has recently launched a practice guideline for quality in screening colonoscopy aimed to define auditable quality indicators for endoscopists and units (table 1) (AEG & SEED working group, 2011).

6. Conclusions and recommendations

The performance of screening colonoscopy requires high quality standards to guarantee the efficiency of the CRC screening programs. Since there is a great variability between endoscopists in the detection of colorectal lesions, only experienced examiners with adequate technical and cognitive skills should be in charge of those programs. However, there is a lack of uniformity and standardization in the evaluation of technical skills, and classical teaching programs may not be enough to meet all the quality requirements.
Recently, much attention has been given to the definition of auditable parameters to measure the quality of colonoscopies. Systematic monitoring of certain variables allows for the quality of colonoscopies to be controlled and may be used as a tool for evaluation and improvement. The identification of these variables may also point out the main issues to be taught, leading to a more structured way of teaching.
Based on the current evidence the following general recommendations may be stressed:

- The use of auditable parameters to assess quality is of paramount importance in screening colonoscopy. These parameters will be also useful to evaluate competence.
- The teaching process should be structured in different phases, and monitoring and evaluation in each phase is advisable. Teaching techniques should be learned by the trainer, preferably during training the trainers courses. Endoscopy units should be adapted to teaching activities.
- A structured and reproducible system of evaluating competence, taking into account cognitive and technical skills, should be designed and validated.
- Local institutions and stakeholders are responsible for designing and implementing a quality assurance program able to ensure quality and safety of all phases of the colonoscopy process. Granting privileges for individuals and endoscopy units is advisable.

7. References

ACGME (2006). ACGME program requirements for general sugery resident trainees in endoscopic procedures. Access on march 2011. Available from: http://www.acgme.org/acWebsite/RRC_440/440_policyArchive.asp

ACGME (2000). Toolbox of assessment methods. Access on march 2001. Available from: http://www.acgme.org/outcome/assess/toolbox.pdf

Alevi, D.; Baiocco, P.J.; Chokhavatia, S.; Kotler, D.P.; Poles, M.; Zabar, S.; Gillespie, C.; Ark, T. & Weinshel, E. (2010). Teaching the competences: using observed structured clinical examinations for faculty development. *Am J Gastroenterol*, Vol. 105, No. 5, (May 2010), pp. 973-977, ISSN 0002-9270

American Society for Gastrointestinal Endoscopy (n.d.). ASGE Endoscopy Unit Recognition Program. Access on march 2011. Available from: http://www.asge.org/ITTIndex.aspx?id=6254

ASGE Standards of Training Committees. (1999). Principles of training in gastrointestinal endoscopy. *Gastrointest Endosc*, Vol. 49, No. 6, (June 1999), pp. 845-853, ISSN 0016-5107

ASGE Taskforce on ensuring Competence in Endoscopy. (n.d.). Ensuring Competence in Endoscopy. ASGE/ACG Executive Briefing. Access on march 2011. Available from: http://www.acg.gi.org/physicians/pdfs/ExecutiveBriefing.pdf.

Balfour, TW. (2001). Training for colonoscopy. *J R Soc Med*, Vol. 94, No. 4, (April 2001), pp. 160-161, ISSN 0141-0768

Barclay, R.L.; Vicari, J.J.; Doughty, A.S.; Johanson, J.F. & Greenlaw, R.L.. (2006). Colonoscopic withdrawal times and adenoma detection during screening colonoscopy. *New Engl J Med*, Vol. 355, No. 24, (December, 2006), pp. 2533-2541, ISSN 0028-4793

Barclay, R.L.; Vicari, J.J. & Greenlaw, R.L.. (2008). Effect of a time-dependent colonoscopic withdrawal protocol on adenoma detection during screening colonoscopy. *Clin Gastroenterol Hepatol*, Vol. 6, No. 10, (October 2008), pp. 1091-1098, ISSN 1542-3565

Benson, M.E.; Reicheiderfer, M.; Said, A.; Gaumnitz, E.A. & Pfau, P.R.. (2010). Variation in colonoscopic technique and adenoma detection rates at an academic gastroenterology unit. *Dig Dis Sci*, Vol. 55, No. 1, (January 2010), pp.166-71, ISSN 0163-2116

Berberat, P.O.; de Wit, N.J.; Bockhorn, M.; Lundell, L. & Drenth, J.P.. (2010). Training innovations in gastroenterology and educational resources: a new vision of gastrointestinal education across Europe. *Eur J Gastroenterol Hepatol*, Vol. 22. No.12, (December 2010), pp. 1393-1396, ISSN 0954-691X

Bressler, B.; Paszat, L.F.; Chen, Z.; Rothwell, D.M.; Vinden, C. & Rabeneck, L.. (2007). Rates of new or missed colorectal cancers after colonoscopy and their risk factors: a population-based analysis. *Gastroenterology*, Vol. 132, No. 1, (January 2007), pp. 96-102, ISSN 0016-5085

Bretagne, J.F.; Hamonic, S.; Piette, C.; Manfredi, S.; Leray, E.; Durand, G. & Riou F..(2010). Variations between endoscopists in rates of detection of colorectal neoplasia and their impact on a regional screening program based on colonoscopy after fecal occult blood testing. *Gastrointest Endosc*, Vol. 71, No. 2, (February 2010), pp. 342-345, ISSN 0016-5107

Cass, O.W.; Freeman, M.L.; Peine, C.J.; Zera, R.T. & Onstand, G.R.. (1993). Objective evaluation of endoscopy skills during training. *Ann Intern Med*, Vol. 118, No. 1, (January 1993), pp. 40-44, ISSN 0003-4819

Cass, O.W.; Freeman, M.L.; Cohen, J., et al.. (1996). Acquisition of competency in endoscopic skills (ACES) during training: a multicenter study (abstract). *Gastrointest Endosc*, Vol. 43, No. 4, pp. 308, (April 1996), ISSN 0016-5107

Chen, S.C. & Rex, D.K.. (2007). Endoscopist can be more powerful than age and male gender in prediction adenoma detection at colonoscopy. *Am J Gastroenterol*, Vol. 102, No. 4, (April 2007), pp. 856-861, ISSN 0002-9270

Cohen, J.; Cohen, S.A.; Vora, K.C.; Xue, X.; Burdick, J.S.; Bank, S.; Bini, E.J.; Bodenheimer, H.; Cerulli, M.; Gerdes, H.; Greenwald, D.; Gress, F.; Grosman, I.; Hawes, R.; Mullen, G.; Schnoll-Sussman, F.; Starpoli, A.; Stevens, P.; Tenner, S. & Villanueva, G.. (2006). Multicenter, randomized, controlled trial of virtual- reality simulator training in acquisition of competency in colonoscopy. *Gastrointest Endosc*, Vol. 64, No. 3, (September 2006), pp. 361-368, ISSN 0016-5107

Conjoint Committee for the Recognition of Training in Gastrointestinal Endoscopy. (n.d.). Information for registrants. Access march 2010, Available from: http://conjoint.gesa.org.au/information.html

Consejo Nacional de Especialidades Médicas. Ministerios de Sanidad y Consumo y de Educación y Cultura (2009). Guia de formación de Especialistas. Aparato Digestivo. In: *BOE, Lunes 26 de Octubre de 2009*. Access on march 2011. Available from: http://www.msps.es/profesionales/formacion/docs/NPaparatoDigestivo.pdf

Dominitz, J.A.; Ikenberry, S.O.; Anderson, M.A.; Banerjee, S.; Baron, T.H.; Cash, B.D.; Fanelli, R.D.; Gan, S.I.; Harrison III, M.E.; Lichtenstein, D.; Shen, B.; Van Guilder, T. & Lee, K.K.. (2008). Renewal of and proctoring for endoscopic privileges. *Gastrointest Endosc*, Vol. 67, No. 1, (January 2008), pp. 10-16, ISSN 0016-5107

Eversbusch, A.; Grantcharov, T.P. (2004). Learning curves and impact of psychomotor training on performance in simulated colonoscopy: a randomized trial using a virtual reality endoscopy trainer. *Surg Endosc*, Vol. 18, No. 10, (October 2004) pp. 1514-1518, ISSN 0930-2794

Faigel, D.O.; Cotton, P.B.. (2009). The London OMED position statement for credentialing and quality assurance in digestive endoscopy. *Endoscopy*, Vol. 41, No. 12, (December 2009), pp. 1069-1074, ISSN 0013-726X

Faigel, D.O.; Baron, T.H.; Lewis, B., Petersen, P., Petrini, J., et al. (2006). Ensuring competence in endoscopy. Access on march 2011. Available from: http://www.asge.org/WorkArea/showcontent.aspx?id=3384.

González-Huix, F.; Figa, M. & Huertas, C.. (2010). Criterios de calidad que deben exigirse en la indicación y en la realización de la colonoscopia. *Gastroenterol Hepatol*, Vol. 33, No. 1, (January 2010), pp. 33-42, ISSN 0210-5705

Grantcharov, T.P.; Carstensen, L.; Schulze, S.. (2005). Objective assessment of gastrointestinal endoscopy skills using a virtual reality simulator. *JSLS*, Vol. 9, No. 2, (April-June 2005), pp. 130-133, ISSN 1086-8089

Haycock, A.V.; Patel, J.H.; Tekkis, P.P. & Thomas-Gibson, S.. (2010). Evaluating changes in gastrointestinal endoscopy training over 5 years: closing the audit loop. *Eur J Gastroenterol Hepatol*, Vol. 22, No. 3, (March 2010), pp. 368-373, ISSN 0954-691X

Imperiale, T.F.; Glowinski, E.A.; Juliar, B.E.; Azzouz, F. & Ransohoff, D.F.. (2009). Variation in polyp detection rates at screening colonoscopy. *Gastrointest Endosc*, Vol. 69, No. 7, (June 2009), pp. 1288-1295, ISBN 0016-5107

Joint Advisory Group on Gastrointestinal Endoscopy. (n.d.). Access on march 2011. Available from: www.thejag.org.uk

Joint Advisory Group on Gastrointestinal Endoscopy. (2010). JAG Trainee Certification, guidance for colonoscopy. Access on march 2011. Available in: http://www.thejag.org.uk/AboutUs/DownloadCentre.aspx

Joint Advisory Group on Gastrointestinal Endoscopy (JAG). (n.d.). The global rating scale. Access on march 2011. Available from: http://www.grs.nhs.uk/

Jover, J. (ed.) (2011). *Guía de práctica clínica de calidad en colonoscopia de cribado del cáncer colorrectal*, Edimsa, ISBN 978-84-7714-362-8, Madrid

Kahi, C.J.; Imperiale, T.F.; Juliar, B.E. & Rex, D.K.. (2009). Effect of screening colonoscopy on colorectal cancer incidence and mortality. *Clin Gastroenterol Hepatol*, Vol. 7, No. 7, (July 2009), pp. 770-775, ISSN 1542-3565

Kaminski, M.F.; Regula, J.; Kraszewska, E.; Polkowski, M.; Wojciechowska, U.; Didkowska, J.; Zwierko, M.; Rupinski, M.; Nowacki, M.P. & Butruk E.. (2010). Quality indicators for colonoscopy and the risk of interval cancer. *New Engl J Med*, Vol. 362, No. 19, (May 2010), pp. 1795-1803, ISSN 0028-4793

Koch, A.D.; Buznick, S.N.; Heemskerk, J.; Botden, S.M.B.I.; Veenendaal, R.; Jakimowicz, J.J. & Schoon E.J.. (2008). Expert and construct validity of the Simbionix GI Mentor II endoscopy simulator for colonoscopy. *Surg Endosc*, Vol. 22, No. 1, (January 2008), pp.158-162, ISSN 0930-2794

Lee, S.H.; Chung, H.K.; Kim, S.J.; Kim, J.O.; Ko, B.M.; Hwangho, Y.; Kim, W.H.; Park, D.H.; Lee, S.K.; Park C.H.; Baek, I.H.; Park, D.I.; Park, S.J.; Ji, J.S.; Jang, B.I.; Jeen, Y.T.; Shin, J.E.; Byeon, J.S.; Eun, C.S. & Han, D.S.. (2008). An adequate level of training for technical competence in screening and diagnostic colonoscopy: a prospective multicenter evaluation of the learning curve. *Gastrointest Endosc*, Vol. 67, No. 4, (April 2008), pp. 683-689, ISSN 0016-5107

Lightdale, J.R.; Newburg, A.R.; Mahoney, L.B.; Fredette, M.E. & Fishman L.N.. (2010). Fellow perceptions of training using computer-based endoscopy simulators. *Gastrointest Endosc*, Vol. 72, No. 1, (July 2010), pp. 13-18, ISSN 0016-5107

Lin, O.S.; Kozarek, R.A.; Arai, A.; Gluck, M.; Jiranek, G.C.; Kowdley, K.V.; McCormick, S.E.; Schembre, D.B.; Soon, M.S. & Dominitz, J.A.. (2010). The effect of periodic monitoring and feedback on screening colonoscopy withdrawal times, polyp detection rates, and patient satisfaction scores. *Gastrointest Endosc*, Vol. 71, No. 7, (June 2010), pp. 1253-1259, ISSN 0016-5107

Pabby, A.; Schoen, R.E.; Weissfeld, J.L.; Burt, R.; Kikendall, J.W. Lance, P.; Shike, M.; Lanza, E. & Schatzkin, A.. (2005). Analysis of colorectal cancer occurrence during surveillance colonoscopy in the dietary Polyp Prevention Trial. *Gastrointest Endosc*, Vol. 61, No. 3, (March 2005), pp. 385-391, ISSN 0016-5107

Raman, M. & Donnon, T.. (2008). Procedural skills education - colonoscopy as a model. *Can J Gastroenterol*, Vol. 22, No. 9, (September 2008), pp. 767-770, ISSN 0835-7900

Rex, D.K.. (2000). Colonoscopic withdrawal technique is associated with adenoma miss rates. *Gastrointest Endosc*, Vol. 51, No. 1, (January 2000), pp. 33-36, ISSN 0016-5107

Rex, D.K.; Petrini, J.L.; Baron, T.H.; Chak, A.; Coen, J.; Deal, S.E.; Hoffman, B.; Jacobson, B.C.; Mergener, K.; Petersen, B.T.; Safdi, M.A.; Faigel, D.O. & Pike, I.M.. (2006). Quality indicators for colonoscopy. *Am J Gastroenterol*, Vol. 101, No. 4, (April 2006), pp. 873-885, ISSN 0002-9270

Rex, D.K.. (2006). Maximizing detection of adenomas and cancers during colonoscopy. *Am J Gastroenterol*, Vol. 101, No.12, (December 2006), pp. 2866-2877, ISSN 0002-9270

Romagnuolo, J.; Enns, R.; Ponich, T.; Springer, J.; Armstrong, D. & Barkun, A.N.. (2008). Canadian credentialing guidelines for colonoscopy. *Can J Gastroenterol*, Vol. 22, No. 1, (January 2008), pp. 17-22, ISSN 0835-7900

Sawhney, M.S.; Cury, M.S.; Neeman, N.; Ngo, L.H.; Lewis, J.M.; Chuttani, M.; Pleskow, D.K. & Aronson, M.D.. (2008). Effect of institution-wide policy of colonoscopy withdrawal time ≥ 7 minutes on polyp detection. *Gastroenterology*, Vol. 135, No. 6, (December 2008), pp.1892-1898, ISSN 0016-5085

Sedlack, R.E. & Kolars, J.C.. (2002). Colonoscopy curriculum development and performance-based assessment criteria on a computer-based endoscopy Simulator. *Acad Med*, Vol. 77, No. 7, (July 2002), pp. 750-751, ISSN 1040-2446

Sedlack, R.E.. (2010). The Mayo Colonoscopic Skills Assessment Tool: validation of a unique instrument to assess colonoscopic skills in trainees. *Gastrointest Endosc*, Vol. 72, No. 6, (December 2010), pp. 1125-1133, ISSN 0016-5107

Shah, H.A.; Paszat, L.F.; Saskin, R.; Stukel, T.A. & Rabeneck, L.. (2007). Factors associated with incomplete colonoscopy: a population-based study. *Gastroenterology*, Vol.132, No. 7, (June 2007), pp. 2297-2303, ISSN 0016-5085

Shaukat, A.; Oancea, C.; Bond, J.H.; Church, T.R. & Allen, J.I.. (2009). Variation in detection of adenomas and polyps by colonoscopy and change over time with a performance improvement program. *Clin Gastroenterol Hepatol*, Vol. 7, No. 7, (July 2007), pp. 1335-1340, ISSN 1542-3565

Singh, H.; Turner, D.; Xue, L; Targownik, L.E.; Bernstein, C.N. (2006). Risk of developing colorectal cancer following a negative colonoscopy examination. Evidence for a 10-year interval between colonoscopies. *JAMA*, Vol. 95, No. 20, (May 2006), pp. 2366-2373, ISSN 0098-7484

Spier, B.J.; Benson, M.; Pfau, P.R.; Nelligan, G.; Lucey, M.R. & Gaumnitz, E.A.. (2010). Colonoscopy training in gastroenterology fellowships: determining competence. *Gastrointest Endosc*, Vol. 71, No. 2, (February 2010), pp. 319-324, ISSN 0016-5107

Sullivan, M.E.; Ortega, A.; Wasserberg, N; Kaufman, H.; Nyquist, J. & Clark, R.. (2008). Assessing the teaching of procedural skills: can cognitive task analysis add to our traditional teaching methods? *Am J Surg*, Vol. 195, No. 1, (January 2008), pp. 20-23, ISSN 0002-9610

Tang, B.; Hanna, G.B.; Carter, F; Adamson, G.D.; Martindale, J.P. & Cuschieri, A.. (2006). Competence assessment of laparoscopic operative and cognitive skills: objective structured clinical examination (OSCE) or observational clinical human reliability assessment (OCHRA). *World J Surg*, Vol. 30, No. 4, (April 2006), pp. 527-534, ISSN 0364-2313

Teague, R.; Soehendra, N; Carr-Locke, D.; Segal, R.; Nagy, G.; Chao, W. & Sakai, Y.. (2002). Setting standards for colonoscopic teaching and training. *J Gastroenterol Hepatol*, Vol. 17, (Suppl. s1), (February 2002), pp. S50-S53, ISSN 0815-9319

van Rijn, J.C.; Reitsma, J.B.; Stoker, J.; Bossuyt, P.M.; van Deventer, S.J. & Dekker, E.. (2006). Polyp miss rate determined by tandem colonoscopy: a systematic review. *Am J Gastroenterol*, Vol. 101, No. 2, (February 2006), pp. 343-350, ISSN 0002-9270

Vassilou, M.C.; Sroka, G.; Poulose, B.K.; Kaveva, P.A. Fayez, R., Dunkin, B.J., Fried, G.M. & Marks, J.M.. (2008). CAGES: a global assessment tool for evaluation of technical performance during gastrointestinal endoscopy [abstract]. *Gastrointest Endosc*, Vol. 67, No. 5, (April 2008), pp. AB300, ISSN 0016-5107

Wells, C.; Inglis, S. & Barton, R.. (2009). Trainees in gastroenterology views on teaching in clinical gastroenterology and endoscopy. *Medical Teacher*, Vol. 31, No. 2, (January 2009), pp. 138-144, ISSN 0142-159X

Wexner, S.D.; Garbus, J.E.; Singh, J.J. & SAGES Colonoscopy Study Outcomes Group. (2001). A prospective analysis of 13,580 colonoscopies: reevaluation of credentialing guidelines. *Surg Endosc*, Vol. 15, No. 3, (May 2001), pp. 251-261, ISSN 0930-2794

Williams, J.E.; Le, T.D. & Faigel, D.O.. (2011). Polypectomy rate as a quality measure for colonoscopy. *Gastrointest Endosc*, Vol. 73, No. 3, (March 2011), pp. 498-506, ISSN 0016-5107

Winawer, S.J.; Zauber, A.G.; Hoh, M.N.; O´Brien, M.J.; Gottlieb, L.S.; Sternberg, S.S.; Waye, J.D.; Schapiro, M.; Bond, J.H.; Panish, J.F.; Ackroyd, F.; Shike, M.; Kurtz, R.C.; Hornsby-Lewis, L.; Gerdes, H.; Stewart, E.T. & the National Polyp Study Workgroup. (1993). Prevention of colorectal cancer by colonoscopic polypectomy. *New Engl J Med*, Vol. 329, No. 27, (December 1993), pp. 1977-1981, ISSN 0028-4793

4

Maintaining Quality in Endoscopy

Anita Balakrishnan[1], Stephen Lewis[2] and Kenneth B Hosie[1]
[1]*Department of Surgery*
[2]*Department of Gastroenterology,*
Derriford Hospital, Plymouth,
United Kingdom

1. Introduction

If something is worth doing it is worth doing well.
A colonoscopy is only of value if the procedure accurately assesses the whole of the mucosa with minimal morbidity and distress to the patient. Colonoscopic examination properly performed is safe, sensitive and well-tolerated by the majority of patients. The benefits of colonoscopy are within acceptable cost-benefit rates; screening colonoscopies carry a cost of $20,000 per year of life saved(Pignone, Saha et al. 2002; Smith, Cokkinides et al. 2002; Winawer, Fletcher et al. 2003). However complications, such as the need for repeat procedures, and the use of surgical intervention for endoscopically-removable polyps, will reduce this cost-benefit ratio thereby reducing patient acceptance of this examination.
The inconsistency in the degree of technical expertise of colonoscopists as documented in the literature suggests the need for standardization of the quality of colonoscopy service provision nationally and internationally(Marshall and Barthel 1993; Rex, Cutler et al. 1997; Rex 2000; Postic, Lewin et al. 2002; Gatto, Frucht et al. 2003; Rabeneck, Souchek et al. 2003; Schoenfeld, Cash et al. 2005; Barclay, Vicari et al. 2006; Rex, Petrini et al. 2006; Simmons, Harewood et al. 2006; Shah, Paszat et al. 2007; Rabeneck, Paszat et al. 2008; Imperiale, Glowinski et al. 2009). These studies have contributed to the identification of a number of parameters that can be analysed to determine the quality of the colonoscopic procedures performed by an individual endoscopist or within an endoscopy unit(Rex, Petrini et al. 2006; Lieberman, Nadel et al. 2007) (Table 1). This chapter examines these factors which contribute to quality outcomes by review of the published evidence and expert opinion.

2. Patient experience

Pre-procedural checks are essential to identify risk factors that may contribute to an adverse outcome from colonoscopy. Such risk factors include the use of anti-coagulants that may predispose to bleeding following a therapeutic component of colonoscopy such as biopsy or polyp removal, or the existence of comorbidities such as heart failure, respiratory problems or renal failure(Sharma, Nguyen et al. 2007; Ko, Riffle et al. 2010). Indeed the commonest complications following colonoscopy are respiratory depression due to oversedation and renal failure induced by dehydration due to the effects of bowel preparation(Sharma, Nguyen et al. 2007; Ko, Riffle et al. 2010). The American Society of Anesthesiologists (ASA) score is a crude but effective parameter in the risk assessment for sedation and correlates with sedation-related complications of endoscopy(Dominitz, Eisen et al. 2003; Sharma, Nguyen et al. 2007; Vargo 2007).

Appropriate indication for procedure
Informed consent obtained, including discussion of risks of and alternatives to colonoscopy
Use of recommended post-polypectomy and post-resection surveillance intervals
Documentation of the adequacy of bowel preparation
Caecal intubation rates evidenced by photodocumentation
Adenoma detection rate in asymptomatic (screening) individuals
Withdrawal time (minimum $\geq$ 6 minutes in individuals with intact anatomy)
Biopsies taken in patients with chronic diarrhoea
Sufficient biopsies obtained in patients with inflammatory bowel disease
Endoscopic resection of polyps where possible or documentation of unresectability
Incidence of perforation or bleeding documented
Post polypectomy bleeding managed endoscopically (nonoperatively)

Adapted from Rex et al, Gastrointestinal Endoscopy 2006; 63 (4):S16-S28

Table 1. Quality indicators for colonoscopy

3. Bowel preparation

Bowel preparation is another important factor in ensuring successful colonoscopic outcomes as poor bowel preparation has been shown to not only increase procedure time but also to decrease the adenoma detection rate(Harewood, Sharma et al. 2003; Froehlich, Wietlisbach et al. 2005; Chiu, Lin et al. 2006). Common bowel preparation regimens include split dose sodium picosulphate or polyethylene glycol-electrolyte solutions. Patient related factors such as prior constipation, comorbid status and mobility may affect the regime prescribed as well as compliance thereby determining the success of bowel preparation(Athreya, Owen et al. 2011). The quality of bowel preparation and mucosal views should be documented for every case and is considered adequate if it permits the detection of polyps of 5mm or greater(Rex, Bond et al. 2002). High rates of inadequate bowel preparation should highlight the need for investigation into the method of patient information and the sufficiency of the bowel preparation regimen in use.

4. Patient information

Patients are often anxious about the impending procedure and their reassurance and subsequent tolerance of the procedure is dependent on the manner and professionalism of the doctors and nurses as well as the physical environment(Ko, Zhang et al. 2009). The use of electronic media such as information videos has been found to positively supplement the written information contained in leaflets by improving patients knowledge of colonoscopy and decreasing anxiety levels compared to information leaflets alone(Luck, Pearson et al. 1999). A consultation with either a medical professional or a nurse specialist prior to the procedure is necessary to allow detailed explanation of the procedure prior to obtaining informed consent. During the consent process, specific risks of colonoscopy should be explained including bleeding, perforation, infection, sedation adverse events, missed diagnosis, missed lesions and intravenous site complications(Rex, Petrini et al. 2006).

5. Endoscopy facilities

Appropriate waiting facilities, bathrooms and endoscopy rooms are essential in ensuring a comfortable patient experience. In addition, endoscopy departments are obliged to adhere to the published guidelines for endoscope disinfection(Banerjee, Shen et al. 2008; Beilenhoff, Neumann et al. 2008) and to have full resuscitation facilities including a cardiac defibrillator and emergency drugs tray(Working Party of the Clinical Services Committee of the British Society of Gastroenterology 1991). Procedure rooms should be equipped with pulse oximetry, piped oxygen and suction, electronic blood pressure cuffs and facilities for ECG monitoring(Working Party of the Clinical Services Committee of the British Society of Gastroenterology 1991).

6. Ensuring appropriate indications and surveillance intervals

Colonoscopy should be performed in accordance with accepted guidelines (Terraz, Wietlisbach et al. 2005; Rex, Kahi et al. 2006; Winawer, Zauber et al. 2006; U.S. Preventive Services Task Force 2008; Cairns, Scholefield et al. 2010) as previous studies have shown a higher rate of detection of pathology when endoscopies are performed for appropriate indications(Vader, Pache et al. 2000; de Bosset, Froehlich et al. 2002; Balaguer, Llach et al. 2005). The indications for colonoscopy in symptomatic patients are well described, and include evaluation of gastrointestinal bleeding of unknown origin, investigation of unexplained iron deficiency anaemia, evaluation of an abnormality (such as a filling defect, stricture or wall thickening) on barium enema or CT, assessment of chronic inflammatory bowel disease of the colon and changes in bowel habit such as diarrhoea(American Society for Gastrointestinal Endoscopy 2000). In particular, endoscopists should adhere to the recommended surveillance guidelines post-resection or post-polypectomy as well as the guidelines for surveillance in patients with Crohn's or ulcerative colitis, which make the assumption of caecal intubation, adequate bowel preparation and careful examination(Rex, Petrini et al. 2006). Overuse of surveillance colonoscopy is not cost-effective and unnecessarily exposes patients to the discomfort and risks of a colonoscopy.

7. Sedation and analgesia

Ensuring an adequate yet safe degree of sedation is of paramount importance for successful colonoscopy and increases the likelihood of the patients' willingness to have a repeat procedure if necessary. Recent studies have suggested that "moderate" sedation, in which patients continue to respond purposefully to either verbal commands alone or with light tactile stimulation without requiring intervention to maintain a patent airway or spontaneous ventilation, is sufficient for colonoscopy and safer than deep sedation, in which ventilation may be inadequate and airway protection may be required(Triebwasser and Browning 2001; American Society of Anesthesiologists 2002; Faigel, Baron et al. 2002; Brisith Society of Gastroenterology 2003; Waring, Baron et al. 2003; Rex 2006). Agents used for sedation include benzodiazepines (midazolam, diazepam), narcotics (fentanyl, meperidine), propofol, neuroleptic tranquilizers (droperidol), antihistamines (diphenhydramine), and dopaminergic receptor antagonists (promethazine). A meta-analysis showed no difference in the incidence of hypoxemia, need for supplemental oxygen, physician satisfaction with the procedure, or rates of patient pain or discomfort when either midazolam or diazepam was co-administered with a narcotic for colonoscopy (McQuaid and Laine 2008).

The use of propofol as a sole sedative agent was associated with higher rates of patient satisfaction and less memory of the procedure compared to midazolam co-administered with a narcotic, however no significant difference was noted in the incidence of bradycardia, hypotension, hypoxemia, physician satisfaction, or the number of patients reporting pain or discomfort(McQuaid and Laine 2008). Rates of propofol use are increasing in the United States, with >20% of physicians using propofol routinely for endoscopy. The narrow therapeutic window of propofol and the lack of a reversal agent can contribute to rapid depression of consciousness and cardiovascular function, necessitating additional training and monitoring when using this agent(American Society of Anesthesiologists 2002; Faigel, Baron et al. 2002; Vargo, Cohen et al. 2009). Combining propofol with midazolam and narcotics is believed to allow lower doses to be used thus improving the safety profile(Cohen, Dubovsky et al. 2003; Cohen, Hightower et al. 2004). The use of patient controlled analgesia using narcotics such as alfentanyl and fentanyl has also been associated with high patient satisfaction and willingness to undergo repeat procedure(Usta, Turkay et al. 2011).

The inhalational agent nitrous oxide is also used for sedation and analgesia in colonoscopy due to its rapid onset of action and short recovery time. Randomised trials comparing nitrous oxide to intravenous opiates with or without benzodiazepines failed to show a clear difference between the two groups in terms of pain relief, reaction times or complex psycho-motor co-ordination(Lindblom, Jansson et al. 1994; Saunders, Fukumoto et al. 1994; Notini-Gudmarsson, Dolk et al. 1996; Trojan, Saunders et al. 1997; Forbes and Collins 2000; Maslekar, Gardiner et al. 2009; Welchman, Cochrane et al. 2010). Patients given intravenous sedation had worse recall of the procedure and reduced manual dexterity compared to those given nitrous oxide(Lindblom, Jansson et al. 1994; Saunders, Fukumoto et al. 1994; Notini-Gudmarsson, Dolk et al. 1996; Trojan, Saunders et al. 1997; Forbes and Collins 2000; Maslekar, Gardiner et al. 2009; Welchman, Cochrane et al. 2010). All studies showed reduced post-procedural stay in patients given nitrous oxide compared to intravenous sedation(Lindblom, Jansson et al. 1994; Saunders, Fukumoto et al. 1994; Notini-Gudmarsson, Dolk et al. 1996; Trojan, Saunders et al. 1997; Forbes and Collins 2000; Maslekar, Gardiner et al. 2009; Welchman, Cochrane et al. 2010).

Carbon dioxide insufflation has been recommended during colonoscopy as carbon dioxide is highly soluble and can thus be passively absorbed by the colon and excreted by the lungs, thereby minimizing intra-procedural and post-procedural discomfort(Williams 1986). In addition the rapid absorbance of carbon dioxide allows double contrast CT or barium enema to be performed on the same day if necessary, while the minimal interference of carbon dioxide with colonic blood flow reduces the risk of ischaemia(Williams 1986). Studies comparing the use of carbon dioxide insufflation to the more routinely used air insufflation in colonoscopy have demonstrated decreased levels of pain and shorter examination times in the carbon dioxide insufflations group (Bretthauer, Thiis-Evensen et al. 2002; Sumanac, Zealley et al. 2002; Church and Delaney 2003; Uraoka, Kato et al. 2009; Yamano, Yoshikawa et al. 2010).

8. Measurements of technical expertise

8.1 Caecal intubation rates

Caecal intubation (passage of the colonoscope to a point proximal to the ileocaecal valve) is necessary to ensure adequate visualisation of the entire colon. A significant fraction of colonic neoplasms are located in the right colon(Imperiale, Wagner et al. 2000; Rabeneck, Souchek et al. 2003), hence successful caecal intubation should be specifically noted, ideally by photo documentation(Rex 2000). Intubation of the terminal ileum or visualization of the lips of the ileocaecal valve may be further necessary if there is any doubt as to whether the caecum has been entered. Failure to intubate the caecum is associated with decreased sensitivity of the examination as well as the need for further radiographic imaging or repeat colonoscopy, thereby reducing the cost-effectiveness of the procedure. Recommended caecal intubation rates are ≥90% for all cases(Marshall and Barthel 1993) and ≥95% of screening cases in healthy adults(Rex, Petrini et al. 2006; Rabeneck, Rumble et al. 2007; Levin, Lieberman et al. 2008; National Health Service Cancer Screening Programmes 2011). Procedures which have been aborted due to poor bowel preparation, severe colitis, equipment failure and those performed solely for the treatment of strictures or polyp removal (where complete colonic imaging has been previously performed) are not included in calculation of the caecal intubation rate(Rex, Bond et al. 2002; Rex, Petrini et al. 2006).

8.2 Adenoma detection rate in screening

The adenoma detection rate (ADR) in asymptomatic patients undergoing screening colonoscopy is an important quality indicator in colonoscopy. A recent study by Kaminski *et al* demonstrated that the ADR of the endoscopist was an independent risk factor for the subsequent development of interval cancers (cancers occurring during surveillance colonoscopy after a previous screening colonoscopy). The number of interval cancers was significantly higher in patients who had undergone colonoscopy by endoscopists with an ADR of <20% compared to those who had undergone colonoscopy by endoscopist with an ADR of ≥20% (Kaminski, Regula et al. 2010). Studies of different practice groups have shown large disparities in the rates of adenoma detection between endoscopists within the same practice for both screening and symptomatic indications(Barclay, Vicari et al. 2006; Chen and Rex 2007; Imperiale, Glowinski et al. 2009) highlighting the possibility that suboptimal colonoscopy rather than technological limitations may be a significant contributing factor to the miss rate of incident cancers(Rex, Hewett et al.; Rex, Petrini et al. 2006). The decrease in sensitivity of colonoscopy associated with missed adenomas also has implications on surveillance intervals, as guidelines for surveillance interval assume thorough examination of the colon and cannot compensate for disparities in technical expertise between colonoscopists. Tandem colonoscopy studies demonstrated adenoma miss rates ranging from 0-6% for adenomas more than 1cm in size, 12-13% for those between 6-9mm, and 15-27% for those under 5mm(Hixson, Fennerty et al. 1990; Rex, Cutler et al. 1997). CT-colonography in turn demonstrated miss rates between 12 and 17% for adenomas greater than 1cm in size, indicating that tandem colonoscopies may underestimate the true prevalence of missed lesions (Pickhardt, Nugent et al. 2004; Van Gelder, Nio et al. 2004). Colonoscopy screening studies have consistently demonstrated adenoma prevalence rates of >25% in men and >15% in women over 50 years old (Johnson, Gurney et al. 1990; Lieberman and Smith 1991; Lieberman, Weiss et al. 2000; Schoenfeld, Cash et al. 2005); hence these form the basis of the current recommended ADRs in the United States. In the United Kingdom a slightly higher ADR of 35% has been set for screening colonoscopy (performed following positive faecal occult blood tests)(National Health Service Cancer Screening Programmes 2011).

While the ADR is considered a good quality indicator for colonoscopy, this parameter cannot be determined at the time of endoscopy and requires histological confirmation before an accurate ADR can be calculated. Polypectomy rates have therefore been postulated as a suitable surrogate, as this can be calculated at the time of colonoscopy and appear to correlate with the ADR(Williams, Le et al. 2011). A disadvantage of using polypectomy rates is the potential for "gaming" -endoscopists artificially increasing their polypectomy rates by removing benign hyperplastic polyps rather than true adenomas(Rex, Hewett et al. 2010).

A recent randomized study examining the effects of the antispasmodic buscopan on polyp detection demonstrated increased polyp detection rates in only a subgroup of patients with significant colonic spasm (Lee, Cheon et al. 2010). In addition, the majority of studies to date have focused on the use of buscopan for the alleviation of colonic spasm and attendant discomfort during colonoscopy with inconsistent results (Saunders and Williams 1996; Mui, Ng et al. 2004; Yoong, Perkin et al. 2004), suggesting that further studies are necessary before buscopan can be routinely recommended for the improvement of polyp detection.

9. Withdrawal time

Measurement of colonoscope withdrawal time (the time between reaching the caecum and withdrawing the scope from the anus) has been used as a further quality indicator in units or endoscopists with low adenoma detection rates. Endoscopists who took longer than 6 minutes to withdraw the colonoscope were found to have very low miss rates and more than 2-fold higher rates of detection of both small and large adenomas(Rex 2000; Barclay, Vicari et al. 2006; Simmons, Harewood et al. 2006). It has therefore been recommended that withdrawal of the colonoscope in patients without any prior colonic surgery should last at least 6 minutes on average(Rex, Petrini et al. 2006). Mean withdrawal times are used rather than individual times as this figure is influenced by the adequacy of colon preparation as well as the length of the colon and the prominence of haustral markings. In addition a recent study has shown that the withdrawal time can be reduced safely with the use of wide angle scopes(Deenadayalu, Chadalawada et al. 2004). Despite the positive correlation between withdrawal time and ADR, Gellad *et al* showed that withdrawal times failed to correlate with 5-year interval neoplasia(Gellad, Weiss et al. 2010). In addition in their study withdrawal times beyond a threshold of 5.2 to 8.6 minutes no longer correlated with adenoma detection rates. This may be explained by the possibility that longer withdrawal times were representative of more difficult rather than more careful examinations. Additionally longer withdrawal times have been found to correlate with the detection of smaller polyps(Simmons, Harewood et al. 2006), not all of which might have been removed at colonoscopy.

10. Surrogate markers

Despite the emphasis placed on caecal intubation rates and withdrawal times as a marker of adequacy of examination, Beckly *et al* (2007) found no correlation between caecal intubation rate or withdrawal times and the detection of artificial bowel markers placed within the colon by a separate intubating colonoscopists (Beckly, Douie et al. 2007). The miss rates of these markers corroborated the findings of Postic *et al* identifying synchronous lesions in specimens of resected colon(Postic, Lewin et al. 2002) as well as the findings of tandem colonscopy studies which used a second closely sequential colonoscopy to determine the miss rate of the first colonoscopy(Hixson, Fennerty et al. 1990; Rex, Cutler et al. 1997). The higher miss rate for markers placed at the flexures highlights the fact due to the high degree of angulation required to navigate these corners lesions may be missed at these sites even with good technique. The use of surrogate markers for assessing lesion detection may therefore represent a useful addition to endoscopy training.

10.1 Colonic biopsy

The sensitivity of colonoscopy for neoplastic and other pathological processes increases when coupled with endoscopic biopsies. This is particularly relevant in patients undergoing colonoscopic surveillance for Crohn's or ulcerative colitis. The sensitivity of the examination for detecting dysplasia in this patient group is improved by quadrantic biopsies every 10cm of colon as well as biopsy of any suspicious lesions (Rubin, Haggitt et al. 1992). Panchromoscopy (dye-spray) of the colon with targeted biopsies has also been shown to increase sensitivity for dysplasia (Kiesslich, Fritsch et al. 2003; Rutter, Saunders et al. 2004).
In addition to surveillance in inflammatory bowel disease, recent guidelines also recommend the use of biopsies in patients with chronic diarrhoea(Rex, Petrini et al. 2006). Serial biopsies of macroscopically normal colon can identify microscopic (collagenous and lymphocytic) colitis in patients with normal mucosa at colonoscopy (Zins, Tremaine et al. 1995; Yusoff, Ormonde et al. 2002). Detection of collagenous colitis in particular is improved when the proximal colon is biopsied (Zins, Tremaine et al. 1995; Yusoff, Ormonde et al. 2002).

10.2 Colonoscopic polypectomy

Routine polypectomy should be performed at diagnostic colonoscopy to minimize the reduction in cost-effectiveness and increased risk associated with an additional unnecessary colonoscopy for removal of the polyp. The UK national guidelines recommend that 90% of screen-detected polyps are removed at the time of detection (National Health Service Cancer Screening Programmes 2011). Consistent referral of sessile polyps <2cm in size for surgical resection is discouraged as these polyps are frequently amenable to endoscopic removal. In cases of technically difficult polyps, referral to an endoscopist experienced in endoscopic resection may be appropriate. The need for surgical intervention, where unavoidable, should be substantiated by photo documentation of the polyp and subsequent review of images with a second endoscopist. Furthermore, correlation of the endoscopic and pathologic measurements of the polyp should be performed following surgical resection to confirm the necessity of surgical resection(Rex, Petrini et al. 2006).

11. Post-procedure quality indicators

11.1 Complication rates

All complications such as perforation or bleeding following the procedure should be monitored and documented to allow identification and correction of any systematic errors that may be contributing to the incidence of these events.
Perforations can occur during diagnostic colonoscopies, either mechanical in nature (e.g. rupture of the rectosigmoid by the instrument or perforation through a stricture) or barotrauma-related due to an excess of pneumatic pressure causing rupture of the caecum (Woltjen 2005). Therapeutic colonoscopies often run a greater risk of perforation, which can occur following polypectomy. This is most often associated with electrocautery and most

frequently occurs following attempts at removal of large polyps from the proximal colon. Submucosal saline injection prior to polypectomy has been suggested might reduce the risk, (Norton, Wang et al. 2002; Singh, Harrison et al. 2004) however randomized controlled trial evidence on this observation is lacking. Current guidelines suggest that perforation rates of greater than the rate of 1:500 overall or 1:1000 in screening patients as documented in previous studies should highlight the need for further investigation into any inappropriate practices that may be a contributory (Silvis, Nebel et al. 1976; Nivatvongs 1986; Gatto, Frucht et al. 2003; Rabeneck, Paszat et al. 2008; National Health Service Cancer Screening Programmes 2011).

Bleeding is the most common complication following colonoscopic polypectomy, and is more frequent in large polyps with a proximal colonic location. Bleeding rates of large polyps (>2cm) in the proximal colon may exceed 10% however the recommended overall acceptable rate of bleeding is 1% (National Health Service Cancer Screening Programmes 2011). The risk of bleeding (particularly immediate bleeding) may be reduced by the use of epinephrine injections (Hsieh, Lin et al. 2001; Di Giorgio, De Luca et al. 2004) or detachable snares(Iishi, Tatsuta et al. 1996; Di Giorgio, De Luca et al. 2004). Immediate bleeding can often be managed endoscopically by pressure on the stalk for up to 10-15 minutes or injection of adrenaline followed by electrocautery (Rex, Lewis et al. 1992). Delayed bleeding is rarely significant and often stops spontaneously. Exceptions are patients who continue to pass bright red blood who may be experiencing arterial bleeding; urgent repeat colonoscopy with clipping or injection and electrocautery of the bleeding site is then necessary (Rex, Lewis et al. 1992). By these means over 90% of post-polypectomy bleeding can be managed conservatively without resorting to surgical intervention(Rex, Petrini et al. 2006). Accurate assessment of the delayed complication rates of individual colonoscopists such as perforation or bleeding may be difficult as patients may present to different centres, hence regular feedback and audit systems should be in place to ensure delayed complications are recorded.

11.2 Standardised reporting

Although standardized reporting and data collection systems are currently in use for many other large scale tests such as Papanicolaou testing and mammography, these have not currently been adopted for colonoscopy. Standardization of reporting colonoscopic procedures would allow improved communication of test results to primary care providers and patients as well as standardized terms and measurement criteria. In addition this would allow the development of national databases to be interrogated for audit and research purposes. In 1997 the Quality Assurance Task Group in the United States developed a standardized colonoscopy reporting and data system (CO-RADS) in conjunction with the major national gastroenterological societies, outlining the key components of colonoscopy that should be closely monitored in every endoscopy unit(Lieberman, Nadel et al. 2007) (Table 2). The use of and adherence to this standardized reporting has not been audited and remains to be seen. No standardized national reporting system exists for symptomatic colonoscopies in many other countries including the United Kingdom. (these are however in place in the United Kingdom for screening colonoscopies). Most endoscopic units in the United Kingdom employ commonly used endoscopic data recording software such as Endosoft® or Endoscribe® which require the documentation of the major quality indicators.

Patient demographics
History of complaint and indications for colonoscopy
Assessment of patient risk and comorbid status
Technical description of procedure
Findings on colonoscopy
Assessment
Any intervention / unplanned events
Follow-up plan
Pathology

Adapted from Lieberman et al, Gastrointestinal Endoscopy 2007; 65(6): 757-766

Table 2. Key subject areas in a standardized colonoscopy report

12. Other factors

12.1 Training and accreditation

As indicated by the studies quoted above, technical competence is of paramount importance in ensuring the delivery of a high quality endoscopy service. To achieve this particular attention must be paid to the instruction of medical and surgical trainees in the necessary skills for competent colonoscopy, and in many countries including the United Kingdom endoscopists are required to be formally certified to perform independent procedures (British Society of Gastroenterology 2004). Several studies have attempted to better define the learning curve that unquestionably accompanies colonoscopic training. Lee *et al* demonstrated achievement of the basic competencies (in terms of caecal intubation rate and polyp detection rate) after 150 colonoscopies(Lee, Chung et al. 2008), however this was disputed by Spier *et al*, who showed that over 500 colonoscopies were necessary before their gastroenterological fellows could perform $\geq$ 90% of colonoscopies independently(Spier, Benson et al. 2010; Spier, Durkin et al. 2010). Simulator training has been suggested as an alternative or adjunct to colonoscopic experience on live patients; Haycock *et al* demonstrated no significant difference between the performance novice colonoscopists trained on a simulator or live patients when assessed on live cases(Haycock, Koch et al. 2010), suggesting that use of the simulator may shorten the learning curve to competency on live patients.

Once competencies are acquired continued regular colonoscopic experience is necessary to maintain the skill levels required for this procedure. A recent study from Canada revealed that patients were more likely to have an incomplete colonoscopy if the procedure was performed by a low volume endoscopist (<240 colonoscopies per year) compared to a high volume endoscopist (370 colonoscopies per year)(Shah, Paszat et al. 2007). This was corroborated by a study from the United States showing no difference in complications but significant differences in completion rates and time to completion between endoscopists that performed 100-200 colonoscopies per year and those that only performed less than 10 per year(Harewood 2005). In keeping with these findings the National Institute for Clinical Excellence (NICE) in the United Kingdom has recommended that on average colonoscopists should perform a minimum of 100 procedures per year(National Institute for Clinical Excellence 2004). while screening colonoscopists should perform at least 150 procedures per year(National Health Service Cancer Screening Programmes 2011)

12.2 Nurse endoscopists

In countries such as the United Kingdom the demand for endoscopists is rapidly outstripping the capacity for medical endoscopists to perform the service within a reasonable time-frame. This has led to the training of nurse endoscopists to meet this need. To avoid any compromise in quality, nurse endoscopists are required to train to achieve the same competencies as medical endoscopists. Two to three sessions a week are mandated to maintain competencies achieved by a closely supervised period of apprenticeship as well as attendance of national endoscopy courses(Brisith Society of Gastroenterology 2001). A recent pilot study from the Netherlands identified no difference in the caecal intubation rate and caecal intubation time between nurse endoscopists and gastrointestinal fellows in training, with 150 examinations required before independent procedures could be performed(Koornstra, Corporaal et al. 2009).

12.3 Cost effectiveness

Provision of a quality colonoscopic service should not only encompass clinical performance but also cost-effectiveness, which relies on the efficient use of resources as well as successful team-working. Challand *et al* found that colonoscopists performing >150 cases per year were more likely to achieve the recommended workload of 4 colonoscopies per 4 hour session that would be required to meet session costs, however the volume of cases of each endoscopist per year had no effect on the caecal intubation rate. In addition, endoscopists who offered $\geq$ 15% of their sessions for training were more likely to achieve the work required to meet session costs, suggesting that the most clinically effective endoscopists also offered the greatest number of training opportunities(Challand, Bullen et al. 2010).
Cost-effectiveness has also been an important factor in the development of screening and surveillance guidelines. The majority of gastroenterological societies recommend surveillance colonoscopy following adenoma detection at ten yearly frequency in low-risk groups or five yearly in groups where the miss rate for adenomas is suspected to be high(Saini, Schoenfeld et al. 2010). Three yearly surveillance is not cost-effective and the inherent risks of colonoscopy may make such frequent surveillance incrementally harmful (Saini, Schoenfeld et al. 2010). Cost-effectiveness analyses have shown that colonoscopy is not an appropriate first line screening tool but is instead often used as a further investigation in patients with positive faecal occult blood tests(Pignone 2005).

13. Conclusion/ summary

The effectiveness and safety of colonoscopy is dependent on the quality of the procedure performed. The identification of specific quality indicators for colonoscopy as described above (outlined in Table 3) has contributed to the development of recommendations for improving the quality of colonoscopy internationally. Adherence to these recommendations will ensure a thorough examination that achieves the expected sensitivity of the procedure while avoiding complications that would offset the cost-benefit ratio of the process. Ensuring quality in colonoscopy is therefore of paramount importance in ensuring the delivery of a safe, accurate, effective and acceptable service for the diagnosis and management of colonic pathology.

Disclosures: est.

Abbreviations:

ADR - adenoma detection rate
ASA - American Society of Anaesthesiologists

14. References

American Society for Gastrointestinal Endoscopy (2000). "Appropriate use of gastrointestinal endoscopy." Gastrointest Endosc 52(6): 831-7.

American Society of Anesthesiologists (2002). "Practice guidelines for sedation and analgesia by non-anesthesiologists." Anesthesiology 96(4): 1004-17.

Athreya, P. J., G. N. Owen, et al. (2011). "Achieving quality in colonoscopy: bowel preparation timing and colon cleanliness." ANZ J Surg 81(4): 261-5.

Balaguer, F., J. Llach, et al. (2005). "The European panel on the appropriateness of gastrointestinal endoscopy guidelines colonoscopy in an open-access endoscopy unit: a prospective study." Aliment Pharmacol Ther 21(5): 609-13.

Banerjee, S., B. Shen, et al. (2008). "Infection control during GI endoscopy." Gastrointest Endosc 67(6): 781-90.

Barclay, R. L., J. J. Vicari, et al. (2006). "Colonoscopic withdrawal times and adenoma detection during screening colonoscopy." N Engl J Med 355(24): 2533-41.

Beckly, J. B., W. J. Douie, et al. (2007). "Artificial bowel markers: a novel method for measuring the accuracy of colonoscopy." Dis Colon Rectum 50(7): 1047-52.

Beilenhoff, U., C. S. Neumann, et al. (2008). "ESGE-ESGENA Guideline: cleaning and disinfection in gastrointestinal endoscopy." Endoscopy 40(11): 939-57.

Bretthauer, M., E. Thiis-Evensen, et al. (2002). "NORCCAP (Norwegian colorectal cancer prevention): a randomised trial to assess the safety and efficacy of carbon dioxide versus air insufflation in colonoscopy." Gut 50(5): 604-7.

Brisith Society of Gastroenterology. (2001). "Provision of Endoscopy Related Services in District General Hospitals." Retrieved 18/02/2011, from http://www.bsg.org.uk/images/stories/docs/clinical/guidelines/endoscopy/endo_related_services.pdf

Brisith Society of Gastroenterology. (2003). "BSG Guidelines on Safety and Sedation during Endoscopic Procedures." Retrieved 18/02/2011, from http://www.bsg.org.uk.

British Society of Gastroenterology. (2004). "Guidelines for training in GI endoscopy." Retrieved 18/02/2011, from http://www.bsg.org.uk/pdf_word_docs/jag_recommendations_2004.pdf.

Cairns, S. R., J. H. Scholefield, et al. (2010). "Guidelines for colorectal cancer screening and surveillance in moderate and high risk groups (update from 2002)." Gut 59(5): 666-89.

Challand, C. P., N. Bullen, et al. (2010). "How Do You Measure Performance as a Colonoscopist?" Colorectal Dis.

Chen, S. C. and D. K. Rex (2007). "Endoscopist can be more powerful than age and male gender in predicting adenoma detection at colonoscopy." Am J Gastroenterol 102(4): 856-61.

Chiu, H. M., J. T. Lin, et al. (2006). "The impact of colon preparation timing on colonoscopic detection of colorectal neoplasms--a prospective endoscopist-blinded randomized trial." Am J Gastroenterol 101(12): 2719-25.

Church, J. and C. Delaney (2003). "Randomized, controlled trial of carbon dioxide insufflation during colonoscopy." Dis Colon Rectum 46(3): 322-6.

Cohen, L. B., A. N. Dubovsky, et al. (2003). "Propofol for endoscopic sedation: A protocol for safe and effective administration by the gastroenterologist." Gastrointest Endosc 58(5): 725-32.

Cohen, L. B., C. D. Hightower, et al. (2004). "Moderate level sedation during endoscopy: a prospective study using low-dose propofol, meperidine/fentanyl, and midazolam." Gastrointest Endosc 59(7): 795-803.

de Bosset, V., F. Froehlich, et al. (2002). "Do explicit appropriateness criteria enhance the diagnostic yield of colonoscopy?" Endoscopy 34(5): 360-8.

Deenadayalu, V. P., V. Chadalawada, et al. (2004). "170 degrees wide-angle colonoscope: effect on efficiency and miss rates." Am J Gastroenterol 99(11): 2138-42.

Di Giorgio, P., L. De Luca, et al. (2004). "Detachable snare versus epinephrine injection in the prevention of postpolypectomy bleeding: a randomized and controlled study." Endoscopy 36(10): 860-3.

Dominitz, J. A., G. M. Eisen, et al. (2003). "Complications of colonoscopy." Gastrointest Endosc 57(4): 441-5.

Faigel, D. O., T. H. Baron, et al. (2002). "Guidelines for the use of deep sedation and anesthesia for GI endoscopy." Gastrointest Endosc 56(5): 613-7.

Forbes, G. M. and B. J. Collins (2000). "Nitrous oxide for colonoscopy: a randomized controlled study." Gastrointest Endosc 51(3): 271-7.

Froehlich, F., V. Wietlisbach, et al. (2005). "Impact of colonic cleansing on quality and diagnostic yield of colonoscopy: the European Panel of Appropriateness of Gastrointestinal Endoscopy European multicenter study." Gastrointest Endosc 61(3): 378-84.

Gatto, N. M., H. Frucht, et al. (2003). "Risk of perforation after colonoscopy and sigmoidoscopy: a population-based study." J Natl Cancer Inst 95(3): 230-6.

Gellad, Z. F., D. G. Weiss, et al. (2010). "Colonoscopy withdrawal time and risk of neoplasia at 5 years: results from VA Cooperative Studies Program 380." Am J Gastroenterol 105(8): 1746-52.

Harewood, G. C. (2005). "Relationship of colonoscopy completion rates and endoscopist features." Dig Dis Sci 50(1): 47-51.

Harewood, G. C., V. K. Sharma, et al. (2003). "Impact of colonoscopy preparation quality on detection of suspected colonic neoplasia." Gastrointest Endosc 58(1): 76-9.

Haycock, A., A. D. Koch, et al. (2010). "Training and transfer of colonoscopy skills: a multinational, randomized, blinded, controlled trial of simulator versus bedside training." Gastrointest Endosc 71(2): 298-307.

Hixson, L. J., M. B. Fennerty, et al. (1990). "Prospective study of the frequency and size distribution of polyps missed by colonoscopy." J Natl Cancer Inst 82(22): 1769-72.

Hsieh, Y. H., H. J. Lin, et al. (2001). "Is submucosal epinephrine injection necessary before polypectomy? A prospective, comparative study." Hepatogastroenterology 48(41): 1379-82.

Iishi, H., M. Tatsuta, et al. (1996). "Endoscopic resection of large pedunculated colorectal polyps using a detachable snare." Gastrointest Endosc 44(5): 594-7.

Imperiale, T. F., E. A. Glowinski, et al. (2009). "Variation in polyp detection rates at screening colonoscopy." Gastrointest Endosc 69(7): 1288-95.

Imperiale, T. F., D. R. Wagner, et al. (2000). "Risk of advanced proximal neoplasms in asymptomatic adults according to the distal colorectal findings." N Engl J Med 343(3): 169-74.

Johnson, D. A., M. S. Gurney, et al. (1990). "A prospective study of the prevalence of colonic neoplasms in asymptomatic patients with an age-related risk." Am J Gastroenterol 85(8): 969-74.

Kaminski, M. F., J. Regula, et al. (2010). "Quality indicators for colonoscopy and the risk of interval cancer." N Engl J Med 362(19): 1795-803.

Kiesslich, R., J. Fritsch, et al. (2003). "Methylene blue-aided chromoendoscopy for the detection of intraepithelial neoplasia and colon cancer in ulcerative colitis." Gastroenterology 124(4): 880-8.

Ko, C. W., S. Riffle, et al. (2010). "Serious complications within 30 days of screening and surveillance colonoscopy are uncommon." Clin Gastroenterol Hepatol 8(2): 166-73.

Ko, H. H., H. Zhang, et al. (2009). "Factors influencing patient satisfaction when undergoing endoscopic procedures." Gastrointest Endosc 69(4): 883-91, quiz 891 e1.

Koornstra, J. J., S. Corporaal, et al. (2009). "Colonoscopy training for nurse endoscopists: a feasibility study." Gastrointest Endosc 69(3 Pt 2): 688-95.

Lee, J. M., J. H. Cheon, et al. (2010). "Effects of Hyosine N-butyl bromide on the detection of polyps during colonoscopy." Hepatogastroenterology 57(97): 90-4.

Lee, S. H., I. K. Chung, et al. (2008). "An adequate level of training for technical competence in screening and diagnostic colonoscopy: a prospective multicenter evaluation of the learning curve." Gastrointest Endosc 67(4): 683-9.

Levin, B., D. A. Lieberman, et al. (2008). "Screening and surveillance for the early detection of colorectal cancer and adenomatous polyps, 2008: a joint guideline from the American Cancer Society, the US Multi-Society Task Force on Colorectal Cancer, and the American College of Radiology." Gastroenterology 134(5): 1570-95.

Lieberman, D., M. Nadel, et al. (2007). "Standardized colonoscopy reporting and data system: report of the Quality Assurance Task Group of the National Colorectal Cancer Roundtable." Gastrointest Endosc 65(6): 757-66.

Lieberman, D. A. and F. W. Smith (1991). "Screening for colon malignancy with colonoscopy." Am J Gastroenterol 86(8): 946-51.

Lieberman, D. A., D. G. Weiss, et al. (2000). "Use of colonoscopy to screen asymptomatic adults for colorectal cancer. Veterans Affairs Cooperative Study Group 380." N Engl J Med 343(3): 162-8.

Lindblom, A., O. Jansson, et al. (1994). "Nitrous oxide for colonoscopy discomfort: a randomized double-blind study." Endoscopy 26(3): 283-6.

Luck, A., S. Pearson, et al. (1999). "Effects of video information on precolonoscopy anxiety and knowledge: a randomised trial." Lancet 354(9195): 2032-5.

Marshall, J. B. and J. S. Barthel (1993). "The frequency of total colonoscopy and terminal ileal intubation in the 1990s." Gastrointest Endosc 39(4): 518-20.

Maslekar, S., A. Gardiner, et al. (2009). "Randomized clinical trial of Entonox versus midazolam-fentanyl sedation for colonoscopy." Br J Surg 96(4): 361-8.

McQuaid, K. R. and L. Laine (2008). "A systematic review and meta-analysis of randomized, controlled trials of moderate sedation for routine endoscopic procedures." Gastrointest Endosc 67(6): 910-23.

Mui, L. M., E. K. Ng, et al. (2004). "Randomized, double-blinded, placebo-controlled trial of intravenously administered hyoscine N-butyl bromide in patients undergoing colonoscopy with patient-controlled sedation." Gastrointest Endosc 59(1): 22-7.

National Health Service Cancer Screening Programmes. (2011). "Quality assurance guidelines in colonoscopy." Retrieved 18/02/2011, from http://www.cancerscreening.nhs.uk/bowel/publications/nhsbcsp06.pdf

National Institute for Clinical Excellence. (2004). "Improving outcomes in colorectal cancer." Retrieved 18/02/2011, from http://www.nice.org.uk/nicemedia/live/10895/28832/28832.pdf

Nivatvongs, S. (1986). "Complications in colonoscopic polypectomy. An experience with 1,555 polypectomies." Dis Colon Rectum 29(12): 825-30.

Norton, I. D., L. Wang, et al. (2002). "Efficacy of colonic submucosal saline solution injection for the reduction of iatrogenic thermal injury." Gastrointest Endosc 56(1): 95-9.

Notini-Gudmarsson, A. K., A. Dolk, et al. (1996). "Nitrous oxide: a valuable alternative for pain relief and sedation during routine colonoscopy." Endoscopy 28(3): 283-7.

Pickhardt, P. J., P. A. Nugent, et al. (2004). "Location of adenomas missed by optical colonoscopy." Ann Intern Med 141(5): 352-9.

Pignone, M. (2005). "Is population screening for colorectal cancer cost-effective?" Nat Clin Pract Gastroenterol Hepatol 2(7): 288-9.

Pignone, M., S. Saha, et al. (2002). "Cost-effectiveness analyses of colorectal cancer screening: a systematic review for the U.S. Preventive Services Task Force." Ann Intern Med 137(2): 96-104.

Postic, G., D. Lewin, et al. (2002). "Colonoscopic miss rates determined by direct comparison of colonoscopy with colon resection specimens." Am J Gastroenterol 97(12): 3182-5.

Rabeneck, L., L. F. Paszat, et al. (2008). "Bleeding and perforation after outpatient colonoscopy and their risk factors in usual clinical practice." Gastroenterology 135(6): 1899-1906, 1906 e1.

Rabeneck, L., R. B. Rumble, et al. (2007). "Cancer Care Ontario Colonoscopy Standards: standards and evidentiary base." Can J Gastroenterol 21 Suppl D: 5D-24D.

Rabeneck, L., J. Souchek, et al. (2003). "Survival of colorectal cancer patients hospitalized in the Veterans Affairs Health Care System." Am J Gastroenterol 98(5): 1186-92.

Rex, D. K. (2000). "Colonoscopic withdrawal technique is associated with adenoma miss rates." Gastrointest Endosc 51(1): 33-6.

Rex, D. K. (2000). "Still photography versus videotaping for documentation of cecal intubation: a prospective study." Gastrointest Endosc 51(4 Pt 1): 451-9.

Rex, D. K. (2006). "Review article: moderate sedation for endoscopy: sedation regimens for non-anaesthesiologists." Aliment Pharmacol Ther 24(2): 163-71.

Rex, D. K., J. H. Bond, et al. (2002). "Quality in the technical performance of colonoscopy and the continuous quality improvement process for colonoscopy: recommendations of the U.S. Multi-Society Task Force on Colorectal Cancer." Am J Gastroenterol 97(6): 1296-308.

Rex, D. K., C. S. Cutler, et al. (1997). "Colonoscopic miss rates of adenomas determined by back-to-back colonoscopies." Gastroenterology 112(1): 24-8.

Rex, D. K., D. G. Hewett, et al. "Editorial: Detection targets for colonoscopy: from variable detection to validation." Am J Gastroenterol 105(12): 2665-9.

Rex, D. K., D. G. Hewett, et al. (2010). "Editorial: Detection targets for colonoscopy: from variable detection to validation." Am J Gastroenterol 105(12): 2665-9.

Rex, D. K., C. J. Kahi, et al. (2006). "Guidelines for colonoscopy surveillance after cancer resection: a consensus update by the American Cancer Society and US Multi-Society Task Force on Colorectal Cancer." CA Cancer J Clin 56(3): 160-7; quiz 185-6.

Rex, D. K., B. S. Lewis, et al. (1992). "Colonoscopy and endoscopic therapy for delayed post-polypectomy hemorrhage." Gastrointest Endosc 38(2): 127-9.
Rex, D. K., J. L. Petrini, et al. (2006). "Quality indicators for colonoscopy." Am J Gastroenterol 101(4): 873-85.
Rubin, C. E., R. C. Haggitt, et al. (1992). "DNA aneuploidy in colonic biopsies predicts future development of dysplasia in ulcerative colitis." Gastroenterology 103(5): 1611-20.
Rutter, M. D., B. P. Saunders, et al. (2004). "Pancolonic indigo carmine dye spraying for the detection of dysplasia in ulcerative colitis." Gut 53(2): 256-60.
Saini, S. D., P. Schoenfeld, et al. (2010). "Surveillance colonoscopy is cost-effective for patients with adenomas who are at high risk of colorectal cancer." Gastroenterology 138(7): 2292-9, 2299 e1.
Saunders, B. P., M. Fukumoto, et al. (1994). "Patient-administered nitrous oxide/oxygen inhalation provides effective sedation and analgesia for colonoscopy." Gastrointest Endosc 40(4): 418-21.
Saunders, B. P. and C. B. Williams (1996). "Premedication with intravenous antispasmodic speeds colonoscope insertion." Gastrointest Endosc 43(3): 209-11.
Schoenfeld, P., B. Cash, et al. (2005). "Colonoscopic screening of average-risk women for colorectal neoplasia." N Engl J Med 352(20): 2061-8.
Shah, H. A., L. F. Paszat, et al. (2007). "Factors associated with incomplete colonoscopy: a population-based study." Gastroenterology 132(7): 2297-303.
Sharma, V. K., C. C. Nguyen, et al. (2007). "A national study of cardiopulmonary unplanned events after GI endoscopy." Gastrointest Endosc 66(1): 27-34.
Silvis, S. E., O. Nebel, et al. (1976). "Endoscopic complications. Results of the 1974 American Society for Gastrointestinal Endoscopy Survey." Jama 235(9): 928-30.
Simmons, D. T., G. C. Harewood, et al. (2006). "Impact of endoscopist withdrawal speed on polyp yield: implications for optimal colonoscopy withdrawal time." Aliment Pharmacol Ther 24(6): 965-71.
Singh, N., M. Harrison, et al. (2004). "A survey of colonoscopic polypectomy practices among clinical gastroenterologists." Gastrointest Endosc 60(3): 414-8.
Smith, R. A., V. Cokkinides, et al. (2002). "American Cancer Society guidelines for the early detection of cancer." CA Cancer J Clin 52(1): 8-22.
Spier, B. J., M. Benson, et al. (2010). "Colonoscopy training in gastroenterology fellowships: determining competence." Gastrointest Endosc 71(2): 319-24.
Spier, B. J., E. T. Durkin, et al. (2010). "Surgical resident's training in colonoscopy: numbers, competency, and perceptions." Surg Endosc 24(10): 2556-61.
Sumanac, K., I. Zealley, et al. (2002). "Minimizing postcolonoscopy abdominal pain by using CO(2) insufflation: a prospective, randomized, double blind, controlled trial evaluating a new commercially available CO(2) delivery system." Gastrointest Endosc 56(2): 190-4.
Terraz, O., V. Wietlisbach, et al. (2005). "The EPAGE internet guideline as a decision support tool for determining the appropriateness of colonoscopy." Digestion 71(2): 72-7.
Triebwasser, A. and R. A. Browning (2001). "Sedation and analgesia by non-anesthesiologists." Med Health R I 84(10): 317-20.
Trojan, J., B. P. Saunders, et al. (1997). "Immediate recovery of psychomotor function after patient-administered nitrous oxide/oxygen inhalation for colonoscopy." Endoscopy 29(1): 17-22.
U.S. Preventive Services Task Force (2008). "Screening for colorectal cancer: U.S. Preventive Services Task Force recommendation statement." Ann Intern Med 149(9): 627-37.

Uraoka, T., J. Kato, et al. (2009). "CO(2) insufflation for potentially difficult colonoscopies: efficacy when used by less experienced colonoscopists." World J Gastroenterol 15(41): 5186-92.
Usta, B., C. Turkay, et al. (2011). "Patient-controlled Analgesia and Sedation With Alfentanyl Versus Fentanyl for Colonoscopy: A Randomized Double Blind Study." J Clin Gastroenterol.
Vader, J. P., I. Pache, et al. (2000). "Overuse and underuse of colonoscopy in a European primary care setting." Gastrointest Endosc 52(5): 593-99.
Van Gelder, R. E., C. Y. Nio, et al. (2004). "Computed tomographic colonography compared with colonoscopy in patients at increased risk for colorectal cancer." Gastroenterology 127(1): 41-8.
Vargo, J. J. (2007). "Minimizing complications: sedation and monitoring." Gastrointest Endosc Clin N Am 17(1): 11-28, v-vi.
Vargo, J. J., L. B. Cohen, et al. (2009). "Position statement: Nonanesthesiologist administration of propofol for GI endoscopy." Gastroenterology 137(6): 2161-7.
Waring, J. P., T. H. Baron, et al. (2003). "Guidelines for conscious sedation and monitoring during gastrointestinal endoscopy." Gastrointest Endosc 58(3): 317-22.
Welchman, S., S. Cochrane, et al. (2010). "Systematic review: the use of nitrous oxide gas for lower gastrointestinal endoscopy." Aliment Pharmacol Ther 32(3): 324-33.
Williams, C. B. (1986). "Who's for CO2?" Gastrointest Endosc 32(5): 365-7.
Williams, J. E., T. D. Le, et al. (2011). "Polypectomy rate as a quality measure for colonoscopy." Gastrointest Endosc.
Winawer, S., R. Fletcher, et al. (2003). "Colorectal cancer screening and surveillance: clinical guidelines and rationale-Update based on new evidence." Gastroenterology 124(2): 544-60.
Winawer, S. J., A. G. Zauber, et al. (2006). "Guidelines for colonoscopy surveillance after polypectomy: a consensus update by the US Multi-Society Task Force on Colorectal Cancer and the American Cancer Society." CA Cancer J Clin 56(3): 143-59; quiz 184-5.
Woltjen, J. A. (2005). "A retrospective analysis of cecal barotrauma caused by colonoscope air flow and pressure." Gastrointest Endosc 61(1): 37-45.
Working Party of the Clinical Services Committee of the British Society of Gastroenterology (1991). "Provision of gastrointestinal endoscopy and related services for a district general hospital. ." Gut 32(1): 95-105.
Yamano, H. O., K. Yoshikawa, et al. (2010). "Carbon dioxide insufflation for colonoscopy: evaluation of gas volume, abdominal pain, examination time and transcutaneous partial CO2 pressure." J Gastroenterol 45(12): 1235-40.
Yoong, K. Y., D. Perkin, et al. (2004). "Intravenous hyoscine as a premedication for colonoscopy: a randomized double-blind controlled trial." Endoscopy 36(8): 720-2.
Yusoff, I. F., D. G. Ormonde, et al. (2002). "Routine colonic mucosal biopsy and ileoscopy increases diagnostic yield in patients undergoing colonoscopy for diarrhea." J Gastroenterol Hepatol 17(3): 276-80.
Zins, B. J., W. J. Tremaine, et al. (1995). "Collagenous colitis: mucosal biopsies and association with fecal leukocytes." Mayo Clin Proc 70(5): 430-3.

Part 2

Applications

5

The Impact of Colonoscopy on Colorectal Cancer Incidence and Mortality

Minhhuyen T. Nguyen and David S. Weinberg
Fox Chase Cancer Center
United States of America

1. Introduction

In the United States, periodic colorectal cancer (CRC) screening rates increased from 45% of the eligible population in 2002 to 63% in 2008 (Richardson et al., 2010). Over a similar time period, colonoscopy has become the most widely utilized colorectal cancer screening tool in the United States. In other countries, colonoscopy is the most commonly recommended screening test, particularly in Europe. However, in many locales in which other screening tests such as fecal occult blood tests (FOBT) are preferred due to cost or availability, colonoscopy is used to follow up on patients screening positive (Brenner et al., 2001; Hoff & Dominitz, 2010; Classen & Lambert, 2008).

The ascendance of colonoscopy in the US corresponds with a significant reduction in colorectal cancer incidence and mortality. In the Annual Report to the Nation on the Status of Cancer from 1975-2006, microsimulation modeling demonstrated the relatively large contributions of screening, along with risk factor modifications and improved cancer treatments, to this decline (Edwards et al., 2010).

The focus of this chapter is the effectiveness of colonoscopy, as a means to decrease CRC incidence and mortality. In addition, we identify factors including tumor biology, instrumental, patient-related issues and endoscopist characteristics that may influence the impact of colonoscopy on these rates.

2. Randomized controlled trials in CRC screening using endoscopy

Currently, there are no published randomized controlled trials examining the impact of colonoscopy on CRC incidence and mortality. Before we review the published studies involving the colonoscopy, we will first examine two randomized, controlled trials of sufficient size and duration using screening flexible sigmoidoscopy to address the same questions. The results of these studies are often extrapolated to support the efficacy of colonoscopy, which is often thought to be an extended sigmoidoscopy. In the first study, Atkin and colleagues randomized more than 170,000 people in 14 United Kingdom medical centers to either once-only flexible sigmoidoscopy or no screening, with 71% included in the exam arm. The median follow-up was 11.2 years. The incidence and mortality of colorectal cancer were measured in both intention-to-treat and per-protocol analyses. Overall CRC incidence reduction was 23%-33%. Overall CRC mortality reduction was 31%-43% and distal CRC mortality reduction was 50% (Atkin et al., 2010). The protective effect appears persistent, with reduction of left-sided CRC incidence continuing at the rate of 0.02% to 0.04% per year after year 5.

In the second study with similar design, Hoff and colleagues in the NORCAP trial randomized more than 55,000 men and women between 55 to 64 years of age in Norway to once-only screening flexible sigmoidoscopy or no screening. The planned duration of follow-up was 15 years. The published study reported cumulative incidence after 7 years of follow-up. Interestingly, by intention-to-treat analysis, there was an insignificant (P= 0.16) reduction in overall CRC mortality by 27% and in rectosigmoid cancer mortality by 37%. Per-protocol analysis with its inherent risk of selection bias yielded a significant 59% reduction in overall CRC incidence and a significant 76% reduction in distal CRC incidence. The authors suggested that these findings might be the results of a short timeframe for the follow-up period (Hoff et al., 2009).

Two other randomized controlled trials using screening flexible sigmoidoscopy, namely, the SCORE trial in Italy and the PLCO trial (US National Cancer Institute-led Prostate, Lung, Colorectal and Ovarian cancer screening trial) are expected to report on their results within the next few years (Segnan et al., 2002; PLCO NCI web page).

In addition, researchers in Europe and the US are currently conducting a randomized controlled trial examining the efficacy of screening colonoscopy on CRC incidence and mortality. The Northern-European Initiative on Colorectal Cancer (NordICC) trial will randomly draw 66,000 individuals from population registries to compare screening colonoscopy with a control group of unscreened individuals for a planned follow-up period of 15 years. Final data collections and analyses are not expected until 2026 (Baxter & Rabeneck, 2010).

3. CRC incidence and mortality after colonoscopy with adenomatous polypectomy

Muto et al first proposed the adenoma-carcinoma sequence of colorectal cancer in 1975 (Muto et al., 1975). Endoscopic polypectomy interrupts the carcinogenic sequence by preventing the transformation of adenomas, thereby inhibiting cancer development. The seminal National Polyp Study (NPS) in 1993 provided primary evidence in support of this theory as well as the rationale for colonoscopy with polypectomy as the major method to prevent colorectal cancer (Winawer et al., 1993). In this study, 1418 patients were randomized post-adenoma removal to frequent (follow-up exams in years 1 and 3) and less frequent (exams in year 3) colonoscopies. Outcomes in each group were compared with three historical reference groups, two where polyps were simply observed and one general-population cohort (the Surveillance, Epidemiology, and End Results or SEER). After an average follow-up of 5.9 years, the interventional groups showed a 76% to 90% reduction in CRC incidence compared with the observed incidence in the reference groups (standardized incidence ratios (SIRs), 0.10, 0.12 and 0.24, respectively). The cancer incidence rate was 0.6 cancers per 1000 person-years.

Subsequent studies based on NPS demonstrated the persistent reduction in CRC mortality associated with the initial polypectomy. Zauber and colleagues used mathematical modeling to show that at 20 years, the cumulative mortality rate was 2.5% for patients who had an initial polypectomy, compared to 5.5% for patients who did not (Zauber et al., 2007). Colonoscopic polypectomy could reduce CRC deaths by about 90% among patients with adenomas and by about 50% in the general population. Furthermore, these significant reductions in CRC mortality were mainly associated with the index clearing colonoscopy, not with the subsequent surveillance examinations.

Similar strong reduction in CRC incidence was also reported in two other studies involving patients with adenoma removal. The Italian Multicentre Study Group, a retrospective, observational study of 1693 men and women who had polypectomy with a mean follow-up of 10.5 years, reported SIR of 0.34 and cancer incidence rate of 0.4 cancers per 1000 person-years (Citarda et al., 2001). The Telemark Polyp Study, a prospective cohort study of 799 men and women with a mean follow-up of 10 years, showed SIR of 0.2, and cancer incidence rate of 0.5 cancers per 1000 person-years, although the trend toward CRC mortality reduction was not significant (Thiis-Evensen et al., 1999).

However, other studies examining the adenoma cohorts have demonstrated much less dramatic impact of colonoscopy with polypectomy. The Polyp Prevention Trial, the Wheat Bran Fiber Trial, the Funen Adenoma Follow-Up Trial, the Australian Polyp Study and the Combined Chemoprevention Trial have all shown cancer incidence rates 2 to 4 times higher than that of the NPS, actually approaching or exceeding the expected rate in the SEER data (1.7 cancers per 1000 person-years).

The Polyp Prevention Trial was a randomized, double blind study of 2079 men and women with history of adenoma removal examining the effects of a low-fat, high-fiber diet on the adenoma incidence. Patients had surveillance colonoscopy at years 1 and 4 post-randomization. The study found no benefits of nutritional intervention on incident adenomas. In addition, the cancer incidence rate was 2.2 cancers per 1000 person-years and more than 50% of prevalent cancers could be prevented or detected earlier if the quality of colonoscopy had been improved (Schatzkin et al., 2000; Pabby et al., 2005).

The Wheat Bran Fiber Trial using a similar design studied the effects of high fiber on adenoma recurrence in 1429 men and women with adenomas. It found 41-48% recurrent adenomas located in the proximal colon and cancer incidence rate of 2.4 cancers per 1000 person-years (Alberts et al., 2000).

The Funen Adenoma Follow-Up Trial by Jorgensen et al randomized 1056 men and women with adenomas to surveillance colonoscopy at varying intervals between 6 and 48 months after the index colonoscopy with polypectomy. Its cancer incidence rate was 2.2 cancers per 1000 person-years. It found a significant six-fold reduction in CRC incidence in the post-polypectomy group if all carcinomas were assumed to develop from large (> or = 10 mm) adenomas or adenomas with severe dysplasia according to the adenoma-carcinoma sequence (Jorgensen et al., 1993). It also found a significant reduction in CRC mortality when compared with the normal population.

The Australian Polyp Study by a single surgeon studied 645 patients with adenoma removal for a mean follow-up period of 4.4 years. The cancer incidence rate was 1.05 cancers per 1000 person-years, which was at first glance indistinguishable from that of the general population. However, based on analysis of previously published data, the authors found that the risk of developing colorectal cancer in patients with adenomas was approximately 2.5 times higher than that of the general population (3.3 cancers per 1000 person-years). Therefore, the authors concluded that colonoscopy did reduce CRC incidence (Meagher & Stuart, 1994).

The Combined Chemoprevention Trial consisted of 2915 patients drawn from three previous chemoprevention trials using calcium, aspirin and antioxidant vitamins in an effort to reduce polyp recurrence. It involved a large number of endoscopists from across North America, in both university and private practices. Its cancer incidence rate was 1.74 cancers per 1000 person-years, with 84% in the early stage and approximately half found in the proximal colon (Robertson et al., 2005). The lowered cancer incidence rate, compared with the other studies, was partially attributed to the chemopreventive properties of aspirin and calcium.

4. Why these differences?

Although all of these studies include participants who had an adenoma removed, methodological differences make comparisons of results difficult. First, criteria for patient enrollment differed in these studies. For instance, the NPS patients underwent rigorous baseline colonoscopic clearance of adenomas, with some (13%) receiving at least 2 examinations, before randomization. The NPS also excluded patients with polyps larger than 3 cm in size, or with prior history of adenomas, while other trials included patients with history of adenomas and any-sized polyps (Rex & Eid, 2008). Second, colonoscopic follow-up periods varied among the studies (Table 1). The NPS, Italian Multicentre Study and the Telemark Polyp Study had a mean follow-up of 6 to 13 years, whereas the others had much shorter follow-up periods, 3-4 years at most. As discussed below, cancers detected during the shorter follow-up periods were possibly due to lesions missed initially, not true incident cancers seen in longer follow-up (Robertson et al., 2007). Third, the expected cancer incidence rates in the various cohorts are difficult to measure due to differences in the type and size of adenomas removed at study entry (Kahi et al., 2009). Fourth, differences in the rate and the timing of the follow-up colonoscopy might also lead to variable outcomes. For example, one-fifth of the NPS and one-fourth of the Italian Trial subjects did not have follow-up colonoscopic surveillance, while most of the subjects in the chemoprevention trials did. Fifth, other confounding factors such as the use of chemopreventive agents such as aspirin, family history of CRC, cigarette smoking history were not fully accounted for and might not be comparable in these studies.

Study	Number of patients	Cancer incidence rate (per 1000 pr-yrs)	Number of cancer in follow-up	Mean follow-up (years)	SIR
SEER		1.7			
NPS--Winawer 1993	1481	0.6	5	5.9	0.1-0.24
Italian Polyp Study--Citarda 2001	1693	0.4	6	10.5	0.34
Telemark Polyp Study--Thiis-Evensen 1999	799	0.5	1	10	0.2
Polyp Prevention Study--Schatzkin 2000	2079	2.2	13	3.1	
Wheat Bran Trial Alberts 2000	1429	2.4	9	3.0	
Funen Adenoma Trial--Jorgensen 1993	1056	2.2	10	4.3	
Combined Chemoprevention Trial--Robertson 2005	2915	1.74	19	3.7	
Australian Polyp Study – Meagher 1994	645	1.05	3	4.4	

Table 1. Adenoma Cohorts and Interval Cancers

5. CRC incidence in screening cohorts

Despite the significant, although variable, reduction in CRC incidence risk for patients with prior adenoma removal, these higher risk populations may not have direct applicability to screening settings where only a proportion of participants have adenomas.

The incidence of CRC has been examined in a number of screening cohorts. Lieberman et al in 2000 studied 3121 individuals, 97% of who were men, for the Veterans Affairs Cooperative Study 380. They found that 37.5% of patients had neoplastic lesions. The presence of distal lesions increased the risk of proximal lesions (OR 3.4). However, 52% of proximal advanced neoplasms had no distal lesions (Lieberman et al., 2000). When 1193 previously screened patients had a follow-up colonoscopy within 5.5 years, 22 cancers and high-grade dysplastic lesions (1.8%) were identified. Most of these lesions (15/22) were found within 36 months of the initial colonoscopy and 6 out of 9 cancers were located in the proximal colon (Lieberman et al., 2007).

In 2005, Schoenfeld et al investigated the prevalence and location of advanced colonic neoplasia in women of average and high risk (15.7% had a family history of colon cancer). Among 1463 asymptomatic women who underwent screening colonoscopy, 72 had advanced neoplasia (4.9%). Had flexible sigmoidoscopy, which visualizes only the distal colon, been the screening tool, only 35.2% of women with advanced neoplasia would have been identified, compared to 66.3% of men from the VA Cooperative Study 380 ($P<0.001$) (Schoenfeld et al., 2005). The Schoenfeld study provided support for the concept that screening needs of women may differ from those of men.

In a similar vein, the use of the screening colonoscopy in high-risk families was further advocated by the prospective, observational study with a long follow-up period of 16 years by Dove-Edwin et al. In this study, 1678 individuals from high-risk families with hereditary non-polyposis colorectal cancer (HNPCC) and moderate-risk families with up to 3 affected first-degree relatives had screening colonoscopy. Significant reduction of CRC incidence in these screening cohorts were 80% and 43% in the moderate-risk and high-risk groups, respectively, when compared to the expected incidence in similar families lacking surveillance (Dove-Edwin et al., 2005).

Brenner and colleagues studied two different patient populations in Germany, one in the state of Saarland and the other in the Rhine-Neckar region, by two different methods to assess the question of CRC protection from previous screening colonoscopy. In the study from Saarland, the prevalence of advanced neoplasms including CRC in 586 participants following colonoscopy within the previous 10 years was compared to that in 2701 participants with no previous colonoscopy. Adjusted prevalence ratios were 0.52 for overall CRC, 0.33 for combined left colon and rectum, and 1.05 for right-sided colon (cecum to transverse colon) (Brenner et al., 2010a). Thus, this study showed that in the community setting with experienced endoscopists (completing at least 200 colonoscopies and 50 polypectomies), screening colonoscopy reduced the CRC incidence strongly in the distal, but not in the proximal, colon.

In contrast, a second study by Brenner and colleagues suggested that colonoscopy protected against proximal CRC in average risk populations. This population-based, case-control study based in the Rhine-Neckar region of Germany, examined 1688 CRC cases and 1932 controls and their history of previous colonoscopy within 1 to 10 years. The adjusted odds ratios were 0.23 for overall CRC, 0.16 for left-sided CRC and 0.44 for right-sided CRC. Significant risk reduction increased over the years in both right and left colon, in both sexes, and among those with and without family history of CRC, with the exception of moderate, non-significant risk reduction for right-sided CRC in persons aged 50-59 years (Brenner et al., 2011).

Two main factors are likely explanations for the different results in these two studies. The first report included participants with advanced adenomas and CRC, while the second included only CRC patients. The development of advanced adenomas may take less time that that of CRC. In addition, the 10-year cumulative risk of progressing from advanced adenoma to CRC is estimated to be less than 50% in individuals 55 years or older (Brenner et al., 2007). Second, the frequency of patients with right-sided CRC in the second study was much higher compared to the number of patients with right-sided advanced neoplasms in the first study, resulting in better statistics.

6. CRC mortality associated with colonoscopy

Prospectively demonstrating the beneficial effect of any intervention on CRC mortality is difficult given the disease's relatively long latency, and methodological needs for many participants with long follow-up. Disease latency also contributes to a possible underestimate of CRC prevalence. In addition, prevalent and incident cancer rates are often indistinguishable in the reference groups such as SEER data. If colonoscopy reduces the incidence of CRC in different screening populations, then could we logically deduct that it has to reduce CRC mortality as well?

In a population-based, observational cohort study, Kahi et al reported on 10,492 asymptomatic average-risk patients with screening colonoscopy in a university hospital setting. Median post-colonoscopy follow-up was 8 years (range 3-16 years). Compared to expected rates from the SEER data, the SIR was 0.33 (a relative risk reduction of 67%). Likewise, the standardized mortality rate was 0.35 (a relative risk reduction of 65%) (Kahi et al, 2009).

Another study by Singh et al used Manitoba's billing claims database to follow, until 2008, a large cohort of 24,342 men and 30,461 women, who had their first colonoscopy between 1987 and 2007. CRC mortality after the index colonoscopy was compared with that of the general population. Standardized mortality ratios (SMRs) were 0.71 (29% reduction) in overall mortality, 0.53 (47% reduction) in distal CRC mortality and 0.94 (no reduction) in proximal CRC mortality (Singh et al., 2010a).

Baxter et al using a different administrative claims database from Ontario selected 719 case patients with a CRC diagnosis between 1996 and 2001, all of whom died of CRC by 2003. They were matched against 5031 controls. Colonoscopy was strongly associated with fewer deaths from left-sided CRC (adjusted OR 0.33 [95% CI, 0.28-0.39]), but not from right-sided CRC (adjusted OR 0.99 [95% CI, 0.86-1.14]) (Baxter et al., 2009). In this study, screening colonoscopy could not be differentiated from diagnostic procedures and completeness of exams could not be verified.

Because of the methodological challenges associated with the studies of CRC mortality, other investigators have turned to mathematical models in an attempt to answer the same questions. As mentioned above, Edwards and colleagues have shown by micro-simulation modeling that declines in CRC mortality rates are consistent with a relatively large contribution from screening. These declines could be accelerated further with favorable trends in higher utilization of screening (Edwards et al., 2010). Similar findings were also found by other studies (Zauber et al., 2007; Vogelaar et al., 2006). Vogelaar et al also applied a microsimulation model to the 2000 US population to study CRC risk factor prevalence, screening use and treatment use. They concluded that without many changes to the current trends (e.g., CRC screening in the eligible population rates are 43% and 47% in women and men, respectively), CRC mortality would be reduced by 17% by 2020. However, if screening use were increased to 70% of the target population, in tandem with improvement of CRC risk factors and chemotherapy effectiveness, then the reduction in CRC mortality could reach almost 50% by 2020. Screening and surveillance methods in this study included both sigmoidoscopy and colonoscopy with FOBT.

7. CRC protection in patients after a negative colonoscopy

A number of studies have demonstrated that CRC protection after a negative colonoscopy is durable, perhaps as long as 10-15 years. In two prospective cohort studies of average-risk subjects, Rex and Imperiale showed that no CRC was detected at re-screening 5 years after the negative baseline colonoscopy. In the first, the investigators re-screened 154 persons with initial negative colonoscopy at a mean of 66 months. None had cancer while 27% had at least one adenoma, only one of which was advanced. The presence of hyperplastic polyps in the baseline colonoscopy did not predict incident adenomas at re-screening. However, confounding factors including the use of non-steroidal anti-inflammatory agents might have reduced the rate of incident adenomas (Rex et al., 1996). The second study had a larger number of participants with negative initial colonoscopy (1256 persons, 56.7% of who were men). Again, baseline hyperplastic polyps did not predict incident advanced adenomas. At repeat colonoscopy, no participants had cancer and 16% had at least one adenoma. Only 1.3% of participants had advanced adenomas, more than 50% of which were located in the distal colon. Men were more likely than women to have any adenoma, especially advanced adenoma (RR 1.88 and 3.31, respectively) (Imperiale et al., 2008).

In 2006, two population-based studies confirmed that CRC risk following a negative colonoscopy remained low, for as long as 10-20 years. In a case-control study in the Rhine-Neckar region of Germany, Brenner et al analyzed the records of 380 colonoscopy cases and 485 controls without previous colonoscopy. They found a 74% risk reduction (OR 0.26 [95% CI, 0.16-0.40]) in subjects with negative colonoscopy compared to those without previous colonoscopy. This lower risk persisted even when the colonoscopy had been done up to 20 years previously. Interestingly, risk was lower among subjects with multiple colonoscopies, who more often had a family history of CRC. On the other hand, with less than 20% of multiple-colonoscopy persons reporting previous polypectomy, the possibility of missed polyps on repeat colonoscopy would be very low indeed, thus contributing partly to this particular finding (Brenner et al., 2006). In addition, this study still demonstrated less CRC protection for the right colon compared to the left (OR 0.39 vs. 0.17, respectively), even when colonoscopies without documented completeness were excluded from analysis.

Using Manitoba Health's physician claims database, Singh et al retrospectively analyzed 32,203 individuals with negative colonoscopy. They found that a negative colonoscopy was associated with 31% reduction in the CRC incidence up to 10 years (SIR of 0.66 at 1 year, 0.55 at 5 years, and 0.28 at 10 years). The proportion of right-sided CRC (defined as cecum to hepatic flexure in this study) was significantly higher in the colonoscopy cohort compared to that in the provincial population (47% vs. 28%; $P<0.001$). Colorectal cancer cases were more likely to be right-sided if diagnosed within the initial 2 years, compared to those diagnosed more than 5 years, following the index colonoscopy. There was a non-significant trend toward general practitioners performing the index colonoscopy cases with subsequent CRC detection (Singh et al., 2006).

In yet another population-based retrospective analysis in Saarland, Germany, which examined a larger number of participants (533 with negative colonoscopy and 2701 without previous colonoscopy), Brenner et al arrived at similar conclusions. No cancer was detected in participants within an average of 11.9 years from negative baseline colonoscopy. The prevalence of advanced neoplasms was more than 60% reduced at 15 years, and approximately 50% reduced beyond 16 years, compared to those without colonoscopy (Brenner et al., 2010b).

Certainly, a negative colonoscopy in and of itself is not a tool that can reduce CRC incidence as a colonoscopy with polypectomy can. Its inherent value exists in its ability to reliably predict the sustained low risk of CRC in the near and distant future. Consequently, a negative colonoscopy supports the lengthening of colonoscopic screening intervals up to 10 years or longer, which in turn increases the cost-effectiveness of the CRC screening process in clinical practice.

8. Gender and location in CRC protection by colonoscopy

The weight of evidence suggests that overall, colonoscopy protects against the development of CRC. However, the degree of benefit apparently varies by colonic location and by gender. Studies by Brenner (Brenner et al., 2010a) and Singh (Singh et al., 2010a) demonstrated reduced incidence and mortality of distal, but not proximal CRC. Even in studies, which suggest protection against proximal CRC, that effect appears muted (Brenner et al., 2011).

In addition, there are differences in the CRC incidence and protection by colonoscopy in men and women. In a large meta-analysis consisting of 17 studies involving 924,932 men and women, Nguyen et al provided strong evidence that men are at greater risk for advanced colorectal neoplasia across all age groups. The pooled relative risk for advanced neoplasia for men compared with women was 1.83 (95% CI, 1.69 -1.97) (Nguyen et al., 2009). Although men in general appear to be more likely to develop incident adenomas of all types (Imperiale et al., 2008), Schoenfeld and colleagues urged the use of the full colonoscopy in women for CRC screening in particular due to the increased prevalence of proximal advanced lesions in women (Schoenfeld et al., 2005).

Why colonoscopy might not protect as well against proximal CRC is not well understood. The questions are: (1) Are more missed or early cancers located in the proximal colon? (2) Do cancers arise de novo or from missed or incompletely resected lesions following colonoscopy? (3) What patient or provider factors might contribute to this clinical observation?

Pohl and Robertson found that a significant number of interval cancers came from missed lesions, which could be either cancer or adenomas. They estimated the adenoma prevalence in the screening cohort, adenoma miss rates, cancer prevalence among patients with adenomas based on size, and rates of adenoma-to-cancer transitions from the literature. They then used a model to apply these risk estimates to a hypothetical average-risk population that received screening colonoscopies. They found that the expected rate of persons with CRC from missed cancer and adenomas was 1.8 per 1000 persons within 5 years (range: 0.5-3.5 per 1000 screened persons) (Pohl & Robertson, 2010). This rate would more than double (5.1 per 1000 screened persons) if colonoscopy is applied to an entirely adenoma-bearing population. When this model was extrapolated to average-risk patient populations (Kahi et al., 2009; Lieberman et al., 2007), they found that approximately 65% of the interval cancers might have been related to missed adenomas. When compared against the observed risks in the adenoma-bearing populations (Alberts et al., 2000; Winawer et al., 1993, Pabby et al. 2005), between 70% and 80% of interval cancers might be attributed to a missed lesion.

Bressler et al determined that the rates of missed cancer in the proximal colon were more than twice as high as those in the distal colon. Using the data from Ontario registries, they calculated the rates of interval colorectal cancers in different locations. The interval cancers were defined as cancers found within 6 and 36 months following a colonoscopy. The rates of the right-sided and transverse colon cancers were 5.9% and 5.5%, respectively, while those of the left-sided colon (distal to the splenic flexure) were halved (2.1%-2.3%) (Bressler et al., 2007). The independent risk factors for these interval cancers were older age, diverticular disease, proximal CRC, colonoscopy in an office setting, and colonoscopy by an internist or family physician.

Although women tend to have fewer adenomas than men, their adenomas tend to occur in the proximal colon. Therefore, it is not surprising to find that proximal CRC protection is lower in women than in men.

Additional studies confirm that the issues of gender and CRC location are intertwined. Singh et al in a population-based study using the Manitoba Cancer Registry examined a cohort of 4883 patients with CRC. They classified 388 (7.9%) of these as early or missed cancers, i.e. those that were detected in the time frame of 6-36 months after a colonoscopy, with a range of 4.5% of distal cancers in men to 14.4% of proximal cancers (cecum to splenic flexure) in women (Singh et al., 2010b). In another case-control study in the California Medicaid population with 4458 CRC cases and 43,815 controls, Singh et al again found that despite the overall CRC risk reduction of 45% (RR 0.55 [95% CI, 0.46-0.65]), CRC protection for the left colon after negative colonoscopy (0.16) was disproportionately higher than that for the right side (0.67). The CRC risk reduction for both sexes was equivalent in the left colon (84%), but that for women in the right colon was only 18%, compared to 62% for men (Singh et al., 2007).

Even in patients with negative colonoscopy, differential CRC protection by colonic location was also observed. In a large population-based retrospective analysis, Lakoff et al studied 111,401 patients with negative previous colonoscopy. As in other studies on negative colonoscopy, they found a significant CRC risk reduction up to 14 years of follow-up, compared to the Ontario population (RR 0.21 [95%CI, 0.05-0.36]). However, the sustained reduction in incidence of proximal CRC only started in year 8 (Lakoff et al., 2008).

9. Factors that influence the impact of video colonoscopy

There are several possible explanations for missed or early CRC, particularly in the proximal colon. We can divide these into two categories, operator-independent and operator-dependent. The operator-independent category includes tumor biology, patient-related factors and endoscopic technology. The operator-dependent category includes a set of key skills required for a successful colonoscopy performance, i.e., high adenoma detection rate and cecal intubation rate, adequate instrument withdrawal time and adequate training in both endoscopic techniques and conceptual knowledge of colon cancer.

9.1 Operator-independent factors

The traditional adenoma-to-carcinoma sequence characterized by chromosomal instability or mismatch repair defects explains most, but apparently not all, CRC. Recently, there is a growing body of evidence pointing to other lesions as the precursors in CRC carcinogenesis (Jass, 2001). In 1990, Longacre and Fenoglio-Preiser first coined the term "serrated adenoma" as a distinct form of colonic neoplasia, 11% of which contained foci of intramucosal carcinoma (Longacre & Fenoglio-Preiser, 1990). Mäkinen et al showed that 5.8% of all CRC in their study developed through the sessile serrated adenoma (SSA) pathway. These lesions have a predilection for the proximal colon (51% in the cecum) and excessive mucus production (Mäkinen et al., 2001). Sessile serrated adenomas in the proximal colon tend to be slightly larger, mucus-covered, flatter, and harder to detect than distal lesions (Spring et al., 2006; Torlakovic et al., 2003). Instead of the progressive accumulation of APC, K-ras, DCC and p53 gene mutations in the traditional adenoma-to-cancer sequence (Vogelstein et al., 1988), sessile serrated adenomas are characterized by the CpG island methylator phenotype (CIMP) and three-fold increase in DNA microsatellite instability (MSI) as a result of hypermethylation-related gene silencing and BRAF oncogene mutations (Mäkinen et al., 2001). This carcinogenic pathway may also be associated with more rapid transformation to cancer (Sawhney et al., 2006; Arain et al., 2008). Other studies also showed significantly higher MLH1 and MGMT promoter methylation in the normal proximal colon in older women (Worthley et al., 2010; Menigatti et al., 2009) and K-ras mutations in 80% of hyperplastic polyps in women, compared to 36% in men (Otori et al., 1997), suggesting the intriguing possibility that the epigenetic signatures of cancers may have sex- and segment-specific, early-stage and normal-tissue counterparts.

The failure to detect proximal lesions may also be caused by incomplete colonoscopy, which in turn is associated with patient-related factors such as prior history of pelvic or abdominal surgery (i.e., hysterectomy, gastrectomy), old age and inadequate bowel prep (Lee et al., 2006). For the first two factors, adequate conscious sedation or water immersion technique has been used to improve the colonoscopy performance (Leung et al., 2010). For the third factor, poor colon preparation reduces polyp detection, both large and small, especially in the right colon (Froelich et al., 2005; Harewood et al., 2003). Split-prep protocol has been used to address this problem (Marmo et al., 2010).

Another way of rendering the colonoscopy safe and painless is the use of computer-assisted self-propelled colonoscopes and swallowed video capsules for atraumatic locomotion through the colon. Several different systems have been tested for their feasibility. The Invendoscope™ (Invendo Medical, Kissing, Germany) is a single-use colonoscope based on motor driven inverted sleeve technology with a working channel (Rösch et al., 2008). This system has been shown to nearly painlessly achieve high cecal intubation rate comparable to that of the video colonoscope (Groth et al., 2011). However, no data are currently available on its diagnostic accuracy. The Endotics System (ES) is another robotic device composed of a workstation and a disposable probe, the advancing of which through the colon follows a cyclic sequence of steps (Cosentino et al., 2009). Although taking longer time to complete and having lower cecal intubation rate, the ES has been shown to have comparable sensitivity and specificity for the detection of lesions and require no sedation (Tumino et al., 2010). The Aeroscope (GI View Ltd, Ramat Gan, Israel), a self-propelled, disposable endoscope using low-pressure carbon dioxide to propel a balloon device through the colon, on the other hand, did not reduce abdominal discomfort in healthy volunteers although it did achieve cecal intubation (Vucelic et al., 2006). The Video Capsule Endoscopy (Given Imaging Ltd., Yoqneam, Israel), a pill-size capsule activated upon swallowing, demonstrated lower sensitivity compared to that of standard colonoscopy (Van Gossum et al., 2009).

Regular white light technology may contribute to the under-recognition of the neoplastic lesions in the proximal colon. For paler, smaller, flatter adenomas, the use of high-definition white light and chromoendoscopy with methylene blue or indigo carmine has been shown to improve adenoma detection rate (Rex, 2010). Electronic highlighting such as narrow band imaging (NBI), Fuji Intelligent Chromo Endoscopy (FICE), autofluorescence and I-scan have not consistently proved effective to augment adenoma detection rate.

Another method of increasing the rate of polyp detection is to improve the view through the colonoscopic lens. Wide-angle-view (> 170 degrees) colonoscopy, hooded colonoscopy and the Third-Eye Retroscope are several new technologies being developed to expose hidden mucosa during colonoscopy. They have shown some initial promise in improving adenoma detection and are under active investigation (Rex, 2010).

9.2 Operator-dependent factors

Colonoscopy performance is clearly operator-dependent requiring quality training and experience. Tandem endoscopic studies showed miss rates of 0-6% for adenomas 1 cm or larger, and 12-13% for adenomas 6-9 mm in size, and 15-27% for adenomas 5 mm or smaller (Rex et al., 1997; Hixson et al., 1990). When computed tomography colonography (CTC) was used in segmental unblinding to assess polyp detection during colonoscopy, the miss rates increased to 12% for adenomas 1 cm or larger (Pickhardt et al., 2004).

These miss rates varied among endoscopists, suggesting that skillful colonoscopy performance plays a major role in neoplasia detection and prevention. In a large tandem endoscopic study, Chen et al demonstrated a wide range of adenoma miss rates from 17% to 48% among 26 colonoscopists (Chen et al., 2007). Rex et al in another large study also showed cancer miss rates of 3% for gastroenterologists and 13% for non-gastroenterologists (Rex et al., 1997). Other studies also found that endoscopist quality measures were closely associated with post-colonoscopy or interval colorectal cancer. Colonoscopy by an internist or family physician in the office setting was associated with higher CRC incidence following colonoscopy (Baxter et al., 2011; Bressler et al., 2007). In patients with negative colonoscopy, those who had their procedures performed by a gastroenterologist were less likely to develop CRC (Rabeneck et al., 2010). Interestingly, there was no correlation between high colonoscopy volume and lower CRC incidence, suggesting that ongoing training and tracking of quality indicators for colonoscopy are crucial.

The optimal measures for "high quality" colonoscopy are under debate. Three frequently discussed indicators are adenoma detection rate, cecal intubation rate or endoscopy completion rate, and instrument withdrawal rate. Using the database of the National Colorectal Cancer Screening Program in Poland from 2000 to 2004, Kaminski et al studied a large population of 45,026 subjects who underwent colon cancer screening by 186 endoscopists. They suggested that the higher an adenoma detection rate (ADR) (in this case, 20% or higher), the better CRC protection could be obtained from the screening colonoscopy (Kaminski et al., 2010). The investigators used an ADR of 20% or higher as the gold standard and this ADR is close to those recommended in the US guidelines (15% among women and 25% among men) (Rex et al., 2002). They found that the relative risks of interval cancer following colonoscopy were 10-12 folds higher if the ADR was less than 20%. They also found that the rate of cecal intubation was not significantly associated with the risk of interval cancer.

The need for high cecal intubation or colonoscopy completion rates (95% or higher for screening in healthy adults) is based on repeated observations that CRC protection by colonoscopy is suboptimal in the proximal colon as discussed above. Documentation of cecal intubation has been encouraged as part of ongoing quality improvement program (Rex et al., 2006). However, evidence for a strong association between cecal intubation and reduction in proximal CRC incidence or mortality has yet to be demonstrated.

Likewise, instrument withdrawal rate emerged as an important quality indicator when withdrawal time quicker than 6 minutes was shown to be associated with a lower rate of adenoma detection (Barclay et al., 2006). However, later, in another study, institution-wide policies to keep the colonoscopic withdrawal time within the recommended limits had no effect on polyp detection rate (Sawhney et al., 2008).

10. Conclusion

In summary, the emergence of colonoscopy as the preferred screening test for colorectal cancer by both the public and the medical profession coincides with the substantial decline in the incidence and mortality related to this disease. The impact of colonoscopy on CRC incidence can be seen in various patient populations, including the adenoma cohorts and average-risk cohorts, and this positive protection effect can be long-lasting in individuals with negative colonoscopy as well. However, colonoscopy is imperfect when it comes to CRC protection in the proximal colon, especially in women, although men are more likely to develop incident adenomas. This gender and location disparity can be caused by multiple factors including tumor biology, technological shortcomings, patient-related issues and endoscopist skill level. When colonoscopy fails, often it is due to inadequate lesion detection by the endoscopist. Therefore, the endoscopist can bring about the most significant positive impact on CRC prevention through continuous quality improvement programs.

11. Acknowledgement

We wish to express our sincere thanks to Ms. Eileen Keenan and Ms. Kathleen Lugas for their critical help in preparing the manuscript.

12. References

Alberts, D.; Martinez, M. & Roe, D. et al. (2000). Lack of effect of a high-fiber cereal supplement on the recurrence of colorectal adenomas. *N Engl J Med*, Vol. 342, No. 16, (April 2000), pp. 1156-1162, ISSN 0028-4793

Arain, M.; Sheikh, S. & Thaygarajan, B. et al. (2008). Molecular markers of rapidly growing tumors: another piece to the puzzle. *Am J Gastro*, Vol. 103, (October 2008), pp. S200, ISSN 0002-9270

Atkin,W.; Edwards, R. & Kralj-Hans, I. et al. (2010). Once-only flexible sigmoidoscopy screening in prevention of colorectal cancer: a multicentre randomised controlled trial. *Lancet*, Vol. 375, No. 9726, (May 2010), pp. 1624-1633, ISSN 0140-6736

Barclay, R.; Vicari, J. & Doughty, A. et al. (2006). Colonoscopic withdrawal times and adenoma detection during screening colonoscopy. *N Engl J Med.*, Vol. 355, No. 24, (December 2006), pp. 2533-2541, ISSN 0028-4793

Baxter, N.; Goldwasser, M. & Paszat, L. et al. (2009). Association of colonoscopy and death from colorectal cancer. *Ann Int Med*, Vol. 150, No. 1, (January 2009), pp. 1-8, ISSN 0003-4819

Baxter, N. & Rabeneck, L. (2010). Is the effectiveness of colonoscopy "good enough" for population-based screening? *J Natl Cancer Inst.*, Vol. 102, No. 2, (January 2010), pp. 70-71, ISSN 0027-8874

Baxter, N.; Sutradhar, R. & Forbes, S. et al. (2011). Analysis of administrative data finds endoscopist quality measures associated with post-colonoscopy colorectal cancer. *Gastroenterology*, Vol. 140, No. 1, (January 2011), pp. 65-72, ISSN 0016-5085

Brenner, H.; Arndt, V. & Stürmer, T. et al. (2001). Long-lasting reduction of risk of colorectal cancer following screening endoscopy. *Brit J Cancer*, Vol. 85, No. 7, (September 2001), pp. 972–976, ISSN 0007-0920

Brenner, H.; Chang-Claude, J. & Seiler, C. et al. (2006). Does a negative screening colonoscopy ever need to be repeated? *Gut*, Vol. 55, No. 8, (August 2006), pp. 1145-1150, ISSN 0017-5749

Brenner, H.; Hoffmeister, M. & Stegmaier, C. et al. (2007). Risk of progression of advanced adenomas to colorectal cancer by age and sex: Estimates based on 840,149 screening colonoscopies. *Gut*, Vol. 56, No. 11, (November 2007), pp. 1585-1589, ISSN 0017-5749

Brenner, H.; Hoffmeister, M. & Arndt, V. et al. (2010a). Protection from right- and left-sided colorectal neoplasms after colonoscopy: Population-based study. *J Natl Cancer Inst.*, Vol. 102, No. 2, (January 2010), pp. 89-95, ISSN 0027-8874

Brenner, H.; Haug, U. & Arndt, V. et al. (2010b). Low risk of colorectal cancer and advanced adenomas more than 10 years after negative colonoscopy. *Gastroenterology*, Vol. 138, No. 3, (March 2010), pp. 870-876, ISSN 0016-5085

Brenner, H.; Chang-Claude, J. & Seiler, C. et al. (2011). Protection from colorectal cancer after colonoscopy: A population-based, case-control study. *Ann Int Med.*, Vol. 154, No. 1, (January 2011), pp. 22-30, ISSN 0003-4819

Bressler, B.; Paszat, L. & Chen, Z. et al. (2007). Rates of new or missed colorectal cancers after colonoscopy and their risk factors: A population-based analysis. *Gastroenterology*, Vol. 132, No. 1, (January 2007), pp. 96-102, ISSN 0016-5085

Chen, S. & Rex, D. (2007). Endoscopist can be more powerful than age and male gender in predicting adenoma detection at colonoscopy. *Am J Gastro*, Vol. 102, No. 4, (April 2007), pp. 856-861, ISSN 0002-9270

Citarda, F.; Tomaselli, G. & Capocaccia, R. et al. (2001). Efficacy in standard clinical practice of colonoscopic polypectomy in reducing colorectal cancer incidence. *Gut*, Vol. 48, No. 6, (June 2001), pp. 812-815, ISSN 0017-5749

Classen, M. & Lambert, R. Colorectal Cancer Screening in Europe. (2008). A Survey of the International Digestive Cancer Alliance between November 2004 and March 2007. *Z Gastroenterol.*, Vol. 46, (April 2008), pp. 23-24, ISSN 0044-2771

Cosentino, F.; Tumino, E. & Rubis Passoni, G. et al. (2009). Functional evaluation of the Endotics System, a new disposable self-propelled robotic colonoscope: in vitro tests and clinical trial. *Int J Artif Organs*, Vol. 32, No. 8, (August 8), pp. 517-527, ISSN 0391-3988

Dove-Edwin, I.; Sasieni, P. & Adams, J. et al. (2005). Prevention of colorectal cancer by colonoscopic surveillance in individuals with a family history of colorectal cancer: 16 year, prospective, follow-up study. *BMJ*, Vol. 331, No. 7524, (November 2005), pp. 1047-1049, ISSN: 0959 8138

Edwards, B.; Ward, E. & Kohler, B. et al. (2010). Annual report to the nation on the status of cancer, 1975-2006, featuring colorectal cancer trends and impact of interventions (risk factors, screening, and treatment) to reduce future rates. *Cancer,* Vol. 116, No. 3, (February 2010), pp. 544-573, ISSN 1097-0142

Froelich, F.; Wietlisbach, V. & Gonvers, J. et al. (2005). Impact of colonic cleansing on quality and diagnostic yield of colonoscopy: The European Panel of Appropriateness of Gastrointestinal Endoscopy European Multicenter Study. *Gastrointest Endosc.*, Vol. 61, No. 3, (March 2005), pp. 378-384, ISSN 0016-5107

Groth, S; Rex, D. & Rösch, T. et al. (2011). High cecal intubation rates with a new computer-assisted colonoscope: a feasibility study. *Am J Gastroenterol.*, doi:10.1038/ajg.2011.52, ISSN 0002-9270

Harewood, G.; Sharma, V. & de Garmo, P. (2003). Impact of colonoscopy preparation quality on detection of suspected colonic neoplasia. *Gastrointest Endosc.*, Vol. 58, No. 1, (July 2003), pp. 76-79, ISSN 0016-5107

Hixson, U.; Fennerty, M. & Sampliner, R. et al. (1990). Prospective study of the frequency and size distribution of polyps missed by colonoscopy. *J Natl Cancer Inst.*, Vol. 82, No. 22, (November 1990), pp. 1769-1772, ISSN 0027-8874

Hoff, G. & Dominitz, J. (2010). Contrasting US and European approaches to colorectal cancer screening: which is best? *Gut,* Vol. 59, No. 3, (March 2010), pp. 407-414, ISSN 0017-5749

Hoff, G.; Grotmol, T. & Skovlund, E. et al. (2009). Risk of colorectal cancer seven years after flexible sigmoidoscopy screening: randomised controlled trial. *BMJ*, Vol. 338, (May 2009), pp. b1846, ISSN 1468-5833

Imperiale, T.; Glowinski, E. & Lin-Cooper, C. et al. (2008). Five-year risk of colorectal neoplasia after negative screening colonoscopy. *N Engl J Med,* Vol. 359, No. 12, (September 2008), pp. 1218-1224, ISSN 0028-4793

Jass, J. (2001). Serrated route to colorectal cancer: back street or super highway? *J Pathol,* Vol. 193, No. 3, (March 2001), pp. 283-285, ISSN 1096-9896

Jorgensen, O.; Kronborg, O. & Fenger, C. (1993). The Funen Adenoma Follow-up Study. Incidence and death from colorectal carcinoma in an adenoma surveillance program. *Scand J Gastroenterol.,* Vol. 28, No. 10, (October 1993), pp. 869-874, ISSN 0036-5521

Kahi, C.; Imperiale, T. & Juliar, B. et al. (2009). Effect of screening colonoscopy on colorectal cancer incidence and mortality. *Clin Gastroenterol Hepatol., Vol. 7, No. 7, (July 2009), pp. 770-775,* ISSN *1542-3565*

Kaminski, M.; Regula, J. & Kraszewska, E. et al. (2010). Quality indicators for colonoscopy and the risk of interval cancer. *N Engl J Med,* Vol. 362, No. 19, (May 2010), pp. 1795-1803, ISSN 0028-4793

Lakoff, J.; Paszat, L. & Saskin, R. et al.(2008). Risk of developing proximal versus distal colorectal cancer after a negative colonoscopy: a population-based study. *Clin Gastroenterol Hepatol.*, Vol. 6, No. 10, (October 2008), pp. 1117-1121, ISSN 1542-3565

Lee, S.; Kim, T. & Shin, S. et al. (2006). Impact of prior abdominal or pelvic surgery on colonoscopy outcomes. *J Clin Gastroenterol.,* Vol. 40, No. 8, (September 2006), pp. 711-716, ISSN 0192-0790

Leung, C.; Kaltenbach, T. & Soetikno, R. et al. (2010). Water immersion versus standard colonoscopy insertion technique: randomized trial shows promise for minimal sedation. *Endoscopy*, Vol. 42, No. 7, (July 2010), pp. 557-563, ISSN 0013-726X

Lieberman, D.; Weiss, D. & Bond, G. et al. (2000). Use of colonoscopy to screen asymptomatic adults for colorectal cancer. *N Engl J Med*, Vol. 343, No. 3, (July 2000), pp. 162-168, ISSN 0028-4793

Lieberman, D.; Weiss, D. & Harford, W. et al. (2007). Five-year colon surveillance after screening colonoscopy. *Gastroenterology*, Vol. 133, No. 4, (October 2007), pp. 1077-1085, ISSN: 0016-5085

Longacre, T. & Fenoglio-Preiser, C. (1990). Mixed hyperplastic adenomatous polyps/serrated adenomas: a distinct form of colorectal neoplasia. *Am J Surg Pathol.*, Vol. 14, No. 6, (June 1990), pp. 524-537, ISSN: 0147-5185

Mäkinen, J.; George, S. & Jernvall, P. et al. (2001). Colorectal carcinoma associated with serrated adenoma: prevalence, histologic features, and prognosis. *J Pathol.*, Vol. 193, No. 3, (March 2001), pp. 286-294, ISSN 1096-9896

Marmo, R.; Rotondano, G. & Riccio, G. et al. (2010). Effective bowel cleansing before colonoscopy: a randomized study of split-dosage versus non-split dosage regimens of high-volume versus low-volume polyethylene glycol solutions. *Gastrointest Endosc.*, Vol. 72, No. 2, (August 2010), pp. 313-320, ISSN 0016-5107

Meagher, A. & Stuart, M. (1994). Does colonoscopic polypectomy reduce the incidence of colorectal carcinoma? *Aust N Z J Surg.*, Vol. 64, No. 6, (June 1994), pp. 400-404, ISSN 0004-8682

Menigatti, M.; Truninger, K. & Gebbers, J-O. et al. (2009). Normal colorectal mucosa exhibits sex- and segment-specific susceptibility to DNA methylation at the hMLH1 and MGMT promoters. *Oncogenes*, Vol. 28, No. 6, (February 2009), pp. 899-909, ISSN 0950-9232

Muto, T.; Bussey, H. & Morson, B. (1975). The evolution of cancer of the colon and rectum. *Cancer*, Vol. 36, No. 6, (December 1975), pp. 2251-2270, ISSN 1097-0142

Nguyen, S.; Bent, S. & Chen, Y. et al. (2009). Gender as a risk factor for advanced neoplasia and colorectal cancer: a systematic review and meta-analysis. *Clin Gastroenterol Hepatol.*, Vol. 7, No. 6, (June 2009), pp. 676-681, ISSN 1542-3565

Otori, K.; Oda, Y. & Sugiyama, K. et al. (1997). High frequency of K-ras mutations in human colorectal hyperplastic polyps. *Gut*, Vol. 40, No. 5, (May 1997), pp 660-663, ISSN 0017-5749

Pabby, A.; Schoen, R. & Weissfeld, J. et al. (2005). Analysis of colorectal cancer occurrence during surveillance colonoscopy in the dietary Polyp Prevention Trial. *Gastrointest Endosc.*,Vol. 61, No. 3, (March 2005), pp. 385-391, ISSN 0016-5107

Pickhardt, P.; Nugent, P. & Mysliwiec, P. et al. (2004). Location of adenomas missed by optical colonoscopy. *Ann Int Med.*, Vol. 141, No. 5, (September 2004), pp. 352-359, ISSN 0003-4819

Pohl, H. & Robertson, D. (2010). Colorectal cancers detected after colonoscopy frequently result from missed lesions. *Clin Gastro Hepatol.*, Vol. 8, No. 10, (October 2010), pp. 858-864, ISSN 1542-3565

Prostate, Lung, Colorectal and Ovarian (PLCO) Cancer Screening Trial Web Page (http://dcp.cancer.gov/programs-resources/groups/ed/programs/plco)

Rabeneck, L.; Paszat, L. & Saskin, R. (2010). Endoscopist specialty is associated with incident colorectal cancer after a negative colonoscopy. *Clin Gastroenterol Hepatol.*, Vol. 8, No. 3, (March 2010), pp. 275-279, ISSN 1542-3565

Rex, D.; Cummings, O. & Helper, D. et al. (1996). Five-year incidence of adenomas after negative colonoscopy in asymptomatic average-risk persons. *Gastroenterology*, Vol. 111, No. 5, (November 1996), pp.1178-1181, ISSN 0016-5085

Rex, D.; Cutler, C. & Lemmel, G. et al. (1997). Colonoscopic miss rates of adenomas determined by back-to-back colonoscopies. *Gastroenterology*, Vol. 112, No. 1, (January 1997), pp. 24-28, ISSN 0016-5085

Rex, D.; Bond, J. & Winawer, S. et al. (2002). Quality in the technical performance of colonoscopy and the continuous quality improvement process for colonoscopy: recommendations of the U.S. Multi-Society Task Force on Colorectal Cancer. *Am J Gastroenterol.*, Vol. 97, No. 6, (June 2002), pp.1296-1308, ISSN 0002-9270

Rex, D.; Petrini, J. & Baron, T. et al. (2006). Quality indicators for colonoscopy. *Am J Gastroenterol.*, Vol. 101, No. 4, (April 2006), pp. 873-885, ISSN 0002-9270

Rex, D.& Eid, E. (2008). Considerations regarding the present and future roles of colonoscopy in colorectal cancer prevention. *Clin Gastroenterol Hepatol.*, Vol. 6. No. 5, (May 2008), pp. 506-514, ISSN 1542-3565

Rex, D. (2010). Update on colonoscopic imaging and projections for the future. *Clin Gastroenterol Hepatol.*, Vol. 8, No. 4, (April 2010), pp. 318-321, ISSN 1542-3565

Richardson, L.; Rim, S. & Plescia, M. (2010). Centers for Disease Control and Prevention. Vital Signs: Colorectal Cancer Screening Among Adults Aged 50–75 Years—United States, 2008. *MMWR*, Vol. 59, No. 26, (July 2010), pp. 808-812, ISSN 0149-2195

Robertson, D.; Greenberg, E. & Beach, M. et al. (2005). Colorectal cancer in patients under close colonoscopic surveillance. *Gastroenterology*, Vol. 129, No. 1, (July 2005), pp. 34-41, ISSN 0016-5085

Robertson, D.; Lieberman, D. & Winawer, S. et al. (2007). Interval cancer after total colonoscopy: results from a pooled analysis of eight studies. *Gastroenterology*, Vol. 134, (May 2007), pp. AB111-112, ISSN 0016-5085

Rösch, T.; Adler, A. & Pohl, H. et al. (2008). A motor-driven single-use colonoscope controlled with a hand-held device: a feasibility study in volunteers. *Gastrointest Endosc.*, Vol. 67, No. 7, (June 2008), pp. 1139-1146, ISSN 0016-5107

Sawhney, M.; Farrar, W. & Gudiseva, S. et al. (2006). Microsatellite instability in interval colon cancers. *Gastroenterology*, Vol. 131, No. 6, (December 2006), pp. 1700-1705, ISSN 0016-5085

Sawhney, M.; Cury, M. & Neeman, N. et al. (2008). Effect of institution-wide policy of colonoscopy withdrawal time > or = 7 minutes on polyp detection. *Gastroenterology*, Vol. 135, No. 6, (December 2008), pp. 1892-1898, ISSN 0016-5085

Schatzkin, A.; Lanza, E. & Corle, D. et al. (2000). The Polyp Prevention Trial Study Group. Lack of effect of a low-fat, high-fiber diet on the recurrence of colorectal adenomas. *N Engl J Med*, Vol. 342, No. 16, (April 2000), pp.1149-1155, ISSN 0028-4793

Schoenfeld, P.; Cash, B. & Flood, A. et al. (2005). Colonoscopic screening of average-risk women for colorectal cancer. *N Engl J Med*, Vol. 352, No. 20, (May 2005), pp. 2061-2068, ISSN 0028-4793

Segnan, N.; Senore, C. & Andreoni, B. et al. (2002). Baseline findings of the Italian multicenter randomized controlled trial of "once-only sigmoidoscopy"—SCORE. *J Natl Cancer Inst.*, Vol. 94, No. 23, (December 2002), pp. 1763–72, ISSN 0027-8874

Singh, H.; Turner, D. & Xue, L. et al. (2006). Risk of developing colorectal cancer following a negative colonoscopy examination: Evidence for a 10-year interval between colonoscopies. *JAMA*, Vol. 295, No. 20, (May 2006), pp. 2366-2375, ISSN 0098-7484

Singh, H.; Turner, D. & Xue, L. et al. (2007). Colorectal cancers after a negative colonoscopy. *Gastroenterology*, Vol. 132, (May 2007), pp. A149, ISSN 0016-5085

Singh, H.; Nugent, Z. & Demers, A. et al. (2010a). The reduction in colorectal cancer mortality after colonoscopy varies by site of the cancer. *Gastroenterology*, Vol. 139, No. 4, (October 2010), pp. 1128-1137, ISSN 0016-5085

Singh, H.; Nugent, Z. & Mahmud, S. et al. (2010b). Predictors of colorectal cancer after negative colonoscopy: A population-based study. *Am J Gastroenterol.*, Vol. 105, No. 3, (March 2010), pp. 663–673, ISSN 0002-9270

Spring, K.; Zhao, Z. & Karamatic, R. et al. (2006). High prevalence of sessile serrated adenomas with BRAF mutations: a prospective study of patients undergoing colonoscopy. *Gastroenterology*, Vol. 131, No. 5, (November 2006), pp. 1400-1407, ISSN 0016-5085

Thiis-Evensen, E.; Hoff, G. & Sauar, J. et al. (1999). Population-based surveillance by colonoscopy: effect on the incidence of colorectal cancer. Telemark Polyp Study I. *Scand J Gastroenterol.*, Vol. 34, No. 4, (April 1999), pp. 414-420, ISSN 0036-5521

Torlakovic, E.; Skovland, E. & Snover, D. et al. (2003). Morphologic reappraisal of serrated colorectal polyps. *Am J Surg Pathol.*, Vol. 27, No. 1, (January 2003), pp. 65-81, ISSN 0147-5185

Tumino, E.; Sacco, R. & Bertini, M. et al. (2010). Endotics system vs colonoscopy for the detection of polyps. *World J Gastroenterol.*, Vol. 16, No. 43, (November 2010), pp. 5452-5456, ISSN: 1007-9327

Van Gossum, A.; Munoz-Navas, M. & Fernandez-Urien, I. et al. (2009). Capsule endoscopy versus colonoscopy for the detection of polyps and cancer. *N Engl J Med.*, Vol. 361, No. 3, (July 2009), pp. 264-270, ISSN 0028-4793

Vogelaar, I.; van Ballegooijen, M. & Schrag, D. et al. (2006). How much can current interventions reduce colorectal cancer mortality in the U.S.? *Cancer*, Vol. 107, No. 7, (October 2006), pp. 1624-1633, ISSN 1097-0142

Vogelstein, B.; Fearon, E. & Hamilton, S. et al. (1988). Genetic alterations during colorectal-tumor development. *N Engl J Med*, Vol. 319, No. 9, (September 1988), pp. 525-532, ISSN 0028-4793

Vucelic, B.; Rex, D. & Pulanic, R.; et al. (2006). The aer-o-scope: proof of concept of a pneumatic, skill-independent, self-propelling, self-navigating colonoscope. *Gastroenterology*, Vol. 130, No. 3, (March 2006), pp. 672-677, ISSN 0016-5085

Winawer, S.; Zauber, A. & Ho, M. et al. (1993). Prevention of colorectal cancer by colonoscopic polypectomy. *N Engl J Med*, Vol. 329, No. 7, (December 1993), pp. 1977-1981, ISSN 0028-4793

Worthley, D.; Whitehall, V. & Buttenshaw, R. et al. (2010). DNA methylation within the normal colorectal mucosa is associated with pathway-specific predisposition to cancer. *Oncogene*, Vol. 29, No. 11, (March 2010), pp. 1653-1662, ISSN 0950-9232

Zauber, A.; Winawer, S. & Lansdorp-Vogelaar, I. et al. (2007). Effect of initial polypectomy versus surveillance polypectomy on colorectal cancer mortality reduction: micro-simulation modeling of the National Polyp Study. *Am J Gastroenterol.*, Vol. 102, (October 2007), pp. S558, ISSN 0002-9270.

6

Post-Polypectomy Colonoscopy Surveillance

Sung Noh Hong
Department of Internal Medicine, Konkuk University School of Medicine, Seoul Korea

1. Introduction

Surveillance is becoming common in the practice of colonoscopy because a large number of patients with colorectal polyps are now being discovered as a result of the increased use of colorectal cancer screening, and particularly because of the dramatic increase in screening colonoscopy. Although the term 'colorectal polyp' is not synonymous with colorectal adenoma, two-thirds of colorectal polyps are adenomas and most colorectal cancers arise from them. Therefore, removal of colorectal polyps using colonoscopic polypectomy has been shown to reduce the risk of future colorectal cancer (Winawer et al., 1993; Atkin et al., 2010).

A patient with one colorectal adenoma has a 30 to 50% likelihood of harboring a second synchronous adenoma elsewhere in the colon and rectum at that time, and they have a 30-50% likelihood of developing metachronous adenoma sometime in the future (Winawer et al., 2006; Arditi et al., 2009). Therefore, to minimize the risk for colorectal cancer in the future, patients with adenomas are usually placed into a post-polypectomy surveillance program.

Post-polypectomy surveillance refers to periodically examining the colon to detect and remove missed synchronous and new metachronous adenomas and cancers, by screening or other means, after the detection and removal of a precancerous lesion. Generally, it does not refer to the use of colonoscopy or other procedures to monitor for polyp or cancer recurrence following a diagnosis of colorectal cancer.

This chapter reviews the rationale, the recent literature and the current recommendations for post-polypectomy surveillance, with emphasizing the need to tailor surveillance strategies to the carefully considered individualized assessment of the risk factors as related to the characteristics of the baseline adenoma and those of the individual patient.

2. Risk of colorectal adenoma or cancer following polypectomy

The objective of post-polypectomy surveillance is to reduce the risk of the development of and death from a colorectal cancer by detecting and removing subsequent adenomas and cancers. The largest study on the risk of colorectal cancer after removal of adenoma in the colon or rectum was reported in 2010 from St. Mark's Hospital, London by Atkin et al. and the study involved using flexible sigmoidoscopy screening (Atkin et al., 2010). After 113,195 people were assigned to the control group and 57,237 people were assigned to the intervention group, they were followed for a median of 11.2 years. The incidence of colorectal cancer in the patients who underwent sigmoidoscopy was reduced by 23%

(hazard ratio: 0.77, 95% CI: 0.70-0.84) and mortality was reduced by 31% (hazard ratio: 0.69, CI: 0.59-0.82). On the per-protocol analyses, after adjusting for a self-selection bias for the patients who underwent sigmoidoscopy, the incidence of colorectal cancer in the people attending the screening was reduced by 33% (hazard ratio: 0.67, CI: 0.60-0.76) and the mortality was reduced by 43% (hazard ratio: 0.57, CI: 0.45-0.72). The relative colorectal cancer risk after polypectomy in all the previously published studies has ranged from 0.2 (range: 0.1–0.6) in the National Polyp Study to 1.3 (range: 0.6–2.3) in the Funen Adenoma follow-up Study (Winawer et al., 1993; Meagher and Stuart 1994; Citarda et al., 2001; Lund et al., 2001; Bertario et al., 2003; Loeve et al., 2005; Atkin et al., 2010). The difference can partially be explained by the inclusion or exclusion of patients with large sessile polyps and other factors too such as the patient characteristics at baseline, the duration of follow-up, the patient compliance and the quality of the initial colonoscopy and polypectomy. The risk of colorectal cancer for patients after polypectomy is lower than that in the general population.

2.1 Concept of the advanced adenoma as a surrogate marker of colorectal cancer

Based on the studies on the prevalence of adenoma from autopsy, the studies on follow-up colonoscopy after polypectomy and the lifetime cumulative incidence of colorectal cancer, it appears that only about 5% of colorectal adenomas undergo malignant transformation (Muto et al., 1975; Stryker et al., 1987; Vogelstein et al., 1988; Center et al., 2009; Hong et al., 2010). These follow-up experiences as well as the increasing information about the molecular genetics for the adenoma-carcinoma sequence are increasingly shifting the emphasis away from simply finding and harvesting large numbers of clinically insignificant adenomas toward strategies that focus on ways to reliably detect and resect the less common, but clinically much more dangerous advanced adenoma.

Colorectal carcinogenesis is a multistep process that occurs over many years and it results from the progressive accumulation of genetic and epigenetic alterations. An adenoma is a monoclonal derivative of a single epithelial stem cell that either inherits or acquires the first of these many genetic alterations. Each additional genetic "hit," which is probably caused by environmental carcinogenic factors, leads to a new clone of daughter cells with a growth advantage that allows the clone to take over the developing polyp. The reason most small simple tubular adenomas stay small and clinically benign is because they never develop the additional genetic alterations needed to make them advance (Vogelstein et al., 1988).

Observational studies also reported the different behavior of small tubular adenomas and advanced adenomas. Most previous studies of the natural history of small colorectal adenomas showed no increase in size, no changes that would have necessitated treatment within a couple of years and that malignant transformation is rare. Hoff et al. reported that 215 polyps less than 5 mm in diameter were left *in situ* in 112 persons for a 2 year follow-up period to ascertain their growth rate. At the end of the 2 years, 49% of the adenomas had increased in size and 14% had regressed. Although the total adenoma mass had increased by 36%, none had grown to a size greater than 5mm and none had developed high-grade dysplasia or cancer (Hoff et al., 1986). On the other hand, Eide reported that the risk of developing cancer in a 1cm sized adenoma was 3% per year in a Norwegian population (Eide 1986). Stryker et al. showed the considerable malignant potential of large adenomas. Before the availability of colonoscopy, 226 patients who had large (>l cm) polyps detected with a barium enema, but who refused their removal by surgery were followed for up to 20 years. Follow-up of these untreated patients showed that 37% of the polyps enlarged, 21 invasive cancers developed at a polyp site and 11 cancers developed at another site. The cumulative risk of cancer at 5, 10 and 20 years was 2.5, 8 and 24%, respectively (Stryker et al., 1987).

Based on a large volume of high-quality scientific evidence published during the past decade, the concept of the advanced adenoma as a surrogate biological indicator of the cancer risk has been established (Winawer and Zauber 2002). Although colorectal cancer would be a more ideal outcome measure, the advanced adenoma was adopted as an early outcome measure of efficacy because a much longer period of time would be required for conclusions to be drawn if cancer was used as the outcome measure.

The recent guidelines for surveillance after polypectomy have adopted the concept of advanced adenoma and the guidelines have introduced the concept of risk stratification of patients at the time of polypectomy into those who are more likely or less likely to develop subsequent serious neoplasia (Bond 2000; Davila et al., 2006; Winawer et al., 2006; Sung et al., 2008; Arditi et al., 2009; Schmiegel et al., 2009; Cairns et al., 2010). However, a uniform definition of an advanced adenoma has not yet been clearly established, but most definitions include that advanced adenoma is an adenoma with high-grade dysplasia or an adenoma that is >10 mm in size or it has a villous component (≥25%), and advanced neoplasia is advanced adenoma and invasive cancer. A synchronous adenoma is an adenoma that is diagnosed at the same time as that of an index colorectal neoplasm. Thirty to fifty percent of colons with one adenoma will contain at least one other synchronous adenoma. A metachronous adenoma is an adenoma that is diagnosed at least 3 to 6 months after the diagnosis of a previous adenoma.

2.2 Colonoscopy is the procedure of choice for post-polypectomy surveillance

Colonoscopy is the preferred modality for post-polypectomy surveillance. It offers the advantages of complete visualization of the entire colon, detection and removal of polyps, and diagnostic sampling of cancers. An early controlled, single-blinded study that compared the accuracy between colonoscopy and a double contrast barium enema performed in the same patients demonstrated a sensitivity of double-contrast barium enema and colonoscopy for detecting polyps of 67% and 94%, respectively (Durdey et al., 1987; Winawer et al., 2000).

Computed tomography (CT) colonography is now being studied for the surveillance of patients with colorectal cancer or polyps. CT colonography has already been shown to be more accurate than a double-contrast barium enema for detecting polyps as well as having similar or more accuracy than colonoscopy for detecting large (≥ 1cm) polypoid adenomas, although the accuracy rapidly drops for medium-sized and small polyps (Kim et al. 2007; Benson et al., 2010). However, a major limitation of CT colonography compared with conventional colonoscopy is that, as with a barium enema, this modality has only diagnostically usefulness. Whenever a suspicious lesion or clinically significant neoplasia is found, the patient must undergo a subsequent colonoscopy to confirm and resect the lesion. Considering a patient with one colorectal adenoma has a 30-50% likelihood of developing new metachronous adenoma, the need to do two expensive tests would make such surveillance costly and inconvenient.

3. Quality of baseline colonoscopy

The quality of the baseline colonoscopy is important to clearly visualize synchronous and to predict the risk for subsequent neoplasia. To assess the quality of colonoscopy, several direct and indirect quality measures have been proposed, including the bowel preparation status and other parameters for the performance of colonoscopy, and the parameters include the cecal intubation rate, the withdrawal time and the adenoma detection rate. Until now, there is a lack of objective data related to any of these measures to assess the most important outcome of screening colonoscopy, which is the subsequent incidence of advanced adenoma or colorectal cancer. However, the US Multi-Society Task Force defined a high-quality colonoscopy as a colonoscopy that reaches the cecum, it has little fecal residue and it has a minimum time of withdrawal from the cecum of 6–10 minutes (Rex et al., 2002). With the current recommendations suggesting that the postpolypectomy surveillance colonoscopy intervals should lengthen to improve the efficacy of the utilization of resources, the need for high-quality colonoscopy is of paramount importance.

3.1 Bowel preparation

Even small amounts of fecal material can obscure colorectal adenomas, advanced adenoma and cancers. In a retrospective evaluation of more than 5,000 colonoscopies performed over a 3.5-year period, Leaper et al. identified 17 patients with a missed colorectal cancer. Poor bowel preparation was noted in 6 of these patients, which suggested that the cleansing quality may have an impact on the diagnostic yield during a colonoscopy.(Leaper et al., 2004) In a larger retrospective study, Harewood et al. analyzed the impact of the adequacy of bowel-preparation on the detection of polypoid lesions for approximately 93,000 colonoscopies recorded in the Clinical Outcome Research Initiative database. Suspected neoplasms were identified in 26,490 colonoscopies (29%) overall, with higher detection rates for those cases with adequate preparation (rated excellent or good by the endoscopist) versus those cases with inadequate preparation (fair or poor) (29% vs. 26%, respectively, $P<.0001$). Although significant lesions (a polyp >9 mm or a mass lesion) were detected in approximately 7% of the colonoscopies, regardless of preparation quality ($P = .82$), lesions ≤ 9 mm were more likely to be detected when the bowel preparation was adequate versus inadequate (22% vs. 19%, respectively $P<.0001$) (Harewood et al., 2003). Although the risk of advanced neoplasia increases with polyp size, high-grade dysplasia and carcinoma can occur in adenomas of any size. High-grade dysplasia was reported in 0.9 to 3.4% of the adenomas ≤5 mm and in 3.6 to 12.5% of the adenomas 5 or 6 mm to 10 mm in size.
In addition, a prospective study by Froehlich et al. reported that the detection of neoplasia, including polyps of any size as well as large lesions (>10 mm), was associated with the quality of bowel preparation; polyps were detected in 29% of the patients with high-quality cleansing versus 24% of the patients with low-quality cleansing ($P<.007$). Identifying polyps of any size significantly depended on the cleansing quality (intermediate-quality vs. low-quality preparation: OR: 1.73, 95% CI: 1.28-2.36; high-quality vs. low-quality preparation: OR: 1.46, 95% CI: 1.11-1.93). For polyps ≥ 10 mm in size, the OR was 1.83 (95% CI: 1.11-3.05) for intermediate-quality cleansing and 1.72 (95% CI: 1.11-2.67) for high-quality cleansing, respectively (Froehlich et al., 2005). Furthermore, flat and depressed lesions are rarer than protruding lesions, but they more frequently contain advanced neoplasia, including invasive carcinoma. Parra-Blanco et al. reported that the number of flat lesions detected in patients with inadequate bowel preparation was significantly lower than that in patients with adequate bowel preparation (9 vs. 28, respectively, $P = .002$) (Parra-Blanco et al., 2006).

3.2 Adenoma detection rate

In one of the most important studies of the past year, Kaminski et al. demonstrated that the adenoma detection rate for individual endoscopists, which is the most commonly proposed proxy for quality in colorectal cancer screening, is indeed an independent predictor of the risk for subsequent colorectal cancer after screening colonoscopy. Among 45,026 patients who were enrolled in a national screening colonoscopy program, 42 interval colorectal cancers were identified by a search of national and regional cancer registries in Poland. Most patients with cancer had no family history of colorectal cancer (83.3%) and no polyps identified on the screening examination (92.9%). Only one cancer (2.4%) was attributed to incomplete polyp resection at the time of the screening procedure. The 186 contributing endoscopists had a median adenoma detection rate of 12.2%. The 42 interval cancers occurred after procedures by 32 endoscopists, with three endoscopists contributing three cases each and four contributing two cases each. A strong association between the adenoma detection rates and the subsequent identification of interval cancers was noted (P=0.008), with significant hazard ratios for those endoscopists with adenoma detection rates of less than 11%, 11-14.9%, and 15-19.9%, as compared with those endoscopists with adenoma detection rates over 20% (P = 0.02 for all comparisons). The adenoma detection rate is an independent predictor of the risk of interval colorectal cancer after screening colonoscopy (Kaminski et al., 2010).

3.3 Withdrawal time

Numerous published series have assessed correlations between the proportion of patients with identified polyps or adenomas and the colonoscopic withdrawal time. Barclay et al compared the rates of detecting neoplastic lesions among 12 gastroenterologists who had mean colonoscopic withdrawal times of less than 6 minutes with the rates of those gastroenterologists who had mean withdrawal times of 6 minutes or more. There were large differences among the gastroenterologists in the adenoma detection rates (9.4% to 32.7%) and in their withdrawal times of the colonoscope from the cecum to the anus (range: 3.1 to 16.8 minutes). As compared with the colonoscopists with mean withdrawal times of less than 6 minutes, those colonoscopists with mean withdrawal times of 6 minutes or more had higher rates of detecting any neoplasia (28.3% vs. 11.8%, respectively P<0.001) and advanced neoplasia (6.4% vs. 2.6%, respectively, P=0.005) (Barclay et al., 2006). Furthermore, most series have also shown significant associations between the speed of withdrawal and the polyp or adenoma detection rates, and some series have shown associations between the speed of withdrawal and the detection of high-risk lesions, based on size or histology.

3.4 Cecal intubation

Cecal intubation is defined as insertion of the colonoscope tip into the cecal caput so that the medial wall of the cecum proximal to the ileocecal valve can be fully inspected. The targets for successful cecal intubation rates are 90% for all colonoscopies and 95% for screening colonoscopies. However, because almost all the previous studies excluded the colonoscopy with incomplete cecal intubation from analysis, there is very scare information about the effect of incomplete colonoscopy on the detection of advanced neoplasia with surveillance colonoscopy. In the Funen adenoma follow-up study by Jorgensen and colleagues, the 53 patients with incomplete initial colonoscopy had at least 1 complete colonoscopy during surveillance; advanced neoplasia was detected in 6 of these patients. The area of new advanced neoplasia had been covered by the initially incomplete colonoscopy in three of the six patients, and later the area was covered in four of the six, before advanced neoplasia was detected. Newly detected advanced neoplasia was associated with incomplete colonoscopy at the initial examination (OR: 2.5; 95% CI: 1.0-6.3) (Jorgensen et al., 1995).

3.5 Completeness of polypectomy

In the absence of magnifying endoscopy combined with dye spraying, it is often not possible to determine the histological type of a polyp by endoscopic inspection. Diminutive polyps (<5 mm) may be indistinguishable from hyperplastic polyp and adenomas. In addition, the unusual large hyperplastic polyp may mimic an adenoma. For this reason, all polyps should be considered for removal. Magnifying endoscopy is likely to become increasingly available and an endoscopic diagnosis may reduce the requirement to remove minute polyps in patients with multiple lesions. Diminutive polyps may be too numerous to be completely cleared. In subjects with multiple small polyps, a sample of at least three should be biopsied for histological study. The cancer risk is related to the number of adenomas, so the documentation of the polyp type has prognostic value and surveillance implications. Hot biopsy and electrocoagulation have been used to eradicate diminutive polyps, but destruction of the specimen makes it difficult to histologically review it, and hot biopsy and electrocoagulation may leave residual polyp behind. Cold snare polypectomy is an effective alternative and it does not compromise the histology(Deenadayalu and Rex 2005).

Lesions less than 2 cm in diameter can readily be transected with one application of the snare with submucosal injection. Inclusion of a small portion of normal mucosal adjacent to the confines of the polyp does not pose a problem, providing that this portion of normal mucosa is also resting on the submucosal fluid-filled bleb. However, sessile polyps greater than 2cm in diameter may require piecemeal removal, but this will make histological evaluation difficult or it may be impossible to completely remove them in a piecemeal fashion. Residual neoplastic tissue has been reported in up to one-third of cases after piecemeal resection of sessile polyps greater than 2cm in diameter. The area may be tattooed with sterile India ink to facilitate follow-up evaluation. Tattooing will also identify the site for subsequent surgical resection. A repeat clearing colonoscopy to insure complete polypectomy is essential after piecemeal resection of large sessile polyps. Such polyps often contain appreciable amounts of villous tissue with a high malignant potential and they tend to recur locally after colonosoopic resection even in cases where the initial polypcctomy appeared to be complete. A repeat clearing colonoscopy should be performed in 3-6 months to confirm that the resection was complete (Winawer et al., 2006; Cairns et al., 2010). In order to decrease the incidence of recurrent polyp at the polypectomy site, the base and edges of the polyp can be treated with a thermal modality. Although many endoscopists treat small residual fragments of adenoma following removal of large polyps with a thermal modality, this has not been studied for any device except the argon plasma coagulator (Zlatanic et al., 1999). If polyp tissue persists after two or three examinations, then patients with low surgical morbidity should usually be referred for surgical resection. When patients are found to have these large sessile polyps, they need to be educated at the time of the initial diagnosis about the importance of complying with the entire course of management and follow-up. Most experienced colonoscopists have witnessed tragic cases in which a patient was partially treated by piecemeal snare polypectomy and was then lost to follow-up, and the patient returned later with an advanced cancer at the polyp site.

4. Predictors of subsequent advanced adenomas

The increased risk of recurrent adenomas after polypectomy is the result of lesions missed during the initial colonoscopy as well as a true increased risk of developing de-novo neoplastic lesions due to environmental and genetic risk factors that are particular to the patient. In other words, the characteristics of initial adenoma and the patient serve as a marker for an increased risk of colorectal neoplasia. Although multiple studies have tried to identify the risk factors for metachronous neoplasia at the time of surveillance, the studies differed with respect to the classification levels of the risk factors and on the definition of advanced neoplasia. In addition, the studies also covered different periods of follow-up evaluation and they used different measures of effect such as ORs, relative risks, hazard ratios and standardized incidence ratios. To clarify these issues, Martinez and colleagues published the pooled analysis using individual data from 8 prospective studies (The Antioxidant Polyp Prevention Study, National Polyp Study, Calcium Polyp Prevention Study, Wheat Bran Fiber study, Veterans Affairs Cooperative Study, Aspirin Folate Trial and Ursodeoxycholic Acid study) that included 9167 men and women aged 22 to 80 with previously resected colorectal adenomas to quantify their risk of developing subsequent advanced adenoma or cancer, as well as to identify factors associated with the development of advanced colorectal neoplasia during surveillance (Martinez et al., 2009).

4.1 Characteristics of baseline adenomas

4.1.1 Multiplicity

Multiplicity at baseline has been shown to predict subsequent detection of advanced adenomas. The pooled analysis of prospective studies showed that the number of adenomas at baseline was related to an increased risk (OR: 1.32, 95% CI: 1.25–1.40) for advanced adenomas at the time of surveillance. Of the randomized controlled trials, with excluding the studies included in the pooled analysis, Funen's adenoma follow-up study and the European fiber and calcium study showed that multiplicity conferred an increased risk for advanced neoplasia at the time of surveillance. The Erlangen Registry of Colorectal Polyps by Nusko and colleagues showed that individuals with 2 or more adenomas at baseline were more likely than those with 1 adenomas at baseline to have an adenoma detected at the time of surveillance (OR: 1.54, 95% CI: 1.12–2.12).

The observational prospective cohort studies also showed that multiplicity was a risk factor for subsequent advanced adenomas and cancer. Noshirwani and colleagues reported that the number of adenomas at baseline was related to an increased risk (OR: 1.25, 95% CI: 1.13–1.38) for advanced adenomas at surveillance in a cohort from the Cleveland Clinic. However, the Study of Colonoscopy Utilization described by Pinsky and Bertario et al. failed to show a significant association between baseline multiplicity and the detection of advanced adenoma at the time of follow-up evaluation.

Study	Number of index adenoma	Total patients (N)	Patients with Metachronous Advanced Neoplasia (N)	Adjusted OR/RR/HR (95% CI)
Jorgensen (The Funen Adenoma Follow-up Study) 1995	1	not mentioned		1
	2	not mentioned		1.3 (0.6-3.0)
	≥3	not mentioned		3.0 (1.2-7.1)
Noshirwani (Cleveland Clinic Foundation Adenoma Registry) 2000	per 1 increase	697	63	1.25 (1.13-1.38)

Nusko (Erlangen Registry of Colorectal Polyps) 2002	1	not mentioned		1
	≥ 2	not mentioned		1.54 (1.12–2.12)
Bertario 2003	1	736	7	1
	≥ 2	350	7	2.0(0.7–5.8)
Bonithon-Kopp (European Fiber-Calcium Intervention trial) 2004	1	360	18	1
	2	109	8	1.4 (0.59–3.51)
	≥ 3	83	15	3.6 (1.64–7.89)
Martinez (Pooled anaylsis) 2009	1	5465	497	1
	2	2054	271	1.39 (1.17–1.66)
	3	890	146	1.85 (1.46–2.34)
	4	326	68	2.41 (1.71–3.40)
	≥5	377	94	3.87 (2.76–5.42)
Pinsky (Study of Colonoscopy Utilization) 2009	1–2 small tubular adenoma	not mentioned		1
	≥ 3 small tubular adenoma	not mentioned		1.5 (0.8–2.6)
The below studies were included in the pooled analysis (Martinez et al. 2009)				
Winawer (National Polyp Study) 1993	1	541	6	1
	2	200	4	1.5 (0.4-5.6)
	≥ 3	197	18	6.9 (2.6-18.3)
van Stolk (Antixoidant Polyp Prevention Trial) 1998	1 or 2	393	13	1
	≥ 3	84	5	1.13 (0.40–3.18)
Martinez (Wheat bran fiber trial) 2001	1	742	86	1
	2	284	28	0.76 (0.43–1.36)
	≥3	261	32	1.01 (0.54–2.10)

Table 1. Multiplicity of adenoma as a risk factor for advanced neoplasia at surveillance

4.1.2 Size

An adenoma size larger than 1 cm also was shown to predict metachronous advanced adenomas in a pooled analysis of prospective studies by Martinez (OR, 1.68; 95% CI, 1.39-2.02). However, other randomized controlled trials, including Funen's adenoma follow-up study and the European fiber and calcium study, did not find adenoma size at baseline to be an independent predictor of advanced neoplasia at the time of surveillance. Adenoma size was important in the prospective observational cohort studies that assessed advanced neoplasia. Noshirwani's study, the Erlangen Registry of Colorectal Polyps and the Study of Colonoscopy Utilization showed that a baseline adenoma of 1 cm or larger, as compared with a baseline adenoma 1cm or smaller, conferred an OR of 3.68 (95% CI: 2.01-6.76), 1.81 (95% CI: 1.42-2.31) and 1.5 (95% CI: 1.03–2.3), respectively, for subsequent advanced neoplasia. Bertario found that patients with adenomas larger than 2 cm, as compared with adenomas 2 cm or smaller, at baseline had a hazard ratio of 4.0 (95% CI: 1.1–14.4) for the development of follow-up advanced adenomas.

Study	Size of index adenoma (mm)	Total patients (N)	Patients with Metachronous Advanced Neoplasia (N)	Adjusted OR/RR/HR (95% CI)
Jorgensen (The Funen Adenoma Follow-up Study) 1995	≤5	not mentioned		1
	6-10	not mentioned		1.2 (0.5-2.9)
	>10	not mentioned		1.2 (0.5-2.9)
Noshirwani (Cleveland Clinic Foundation Adenoma Registry) 2000	< 10	not mentioned		1
	≥ 10	not mentioned		3.68 (2.01-6.76)
Nusko (Erlangen Registry of Colorectal Polyps) 2002	≤10	not mentioned		1
	> 10	not mentioned		1.81 (1.42-2.31)
Bertario 2003	≤10	700	6	1
	10-20	256	4	1.9 (0.5-6.6)
	> 20	107	4	4.0 (1.1-14.4)
Bonithon-Kopp (European Fiber-Calcium Intervention trial) 2004	<10	243	19	1
	≥ 10	309	22	1.06 (0.54-2.06)
Martinez (Pooled anaylsis) 2009	<5	2540	209	1
	5-10	3115	287	1.17 (0.95-1.42)
	10-20	2487	415	2.27 (1.84-2.78)
	≥ 20	672	138	2.99 (2.24-4.00)
	pooled	not mentioned		1.56 (1.39-1.74)
Pinsky (Study of Colonoscopy Utilization) 2009	<10	not mentioned		1
	≥10 TA	not mentioned		1.5 (1.03-2.3)
The below studies were included in the pooled analysis (Martinez et al. 2009)				
Winawer (National Polyp Study) 1993	≤ 5	228	3	1
	6-10	354	8	1.3 (0.3-5.2)
	> 10	356	17	2.2 (0.6-7.8)
van Stolk (Antixoidant Polyp Prevention Trial) 1998	< 10	258	11	1
	≥ 10	219	7	0.49 (0.16-1.51)
Martinez (Wheat bran fiber trial) 2001	< 5	395	36	1
	6-10	543	52	0.88 (0.52-2.14)
	10	349	58	2.27 (1.25-4.14)

Table 2. Size of adenoma as a risk factor for advanced neoplasia at the time of surveillance

4.1.3 Histology

The histologic type of adenoma at baseline also was shown to predict metachronous advanced adenomas in a pooled analysis of prospective studies by Martinez (OR: 1.40, 95% CI: 1.17-1.68). However, in the randomized trials, the histologic type of adenoma at baseline was not a significant predictor of advanced neoplasia. In the observational cohorts, villous or tubulovillous adenoma was a significant predictor of advanced neoplasia in the Study of Colonoscopy Utilization, but not in the study by Norshirwani.

Study	Histology of adenoma at the index polyp	Total patients (N)	Patients with Metachronous Advanced Neoplasia (N)	Adjusted OR/RR/HR (95% CI)
Jorgensen (The Funen Adenoma Follow-up Study) 1995	Tubular	not mentioned		1
	Tubulovillous	not mentioned		1.2 (0.6-2.7)
Noshirwani (Cleveland Clinic Foundation Adenoma Registry) 2000	Tubular	not mentioned		1
	Others	not mentioned		1.37 (0.72-2.62)
Bertario 2003	Tubular	772	10	1
	Tubulovillous	205	3	1.5 (0.4–5.6)
	Villous	80	1	1.2 (0.2–10.2)
Bonithon-Kopp (European Fiber-Calcium Intervention trial) 2004	Tubular	455	31	1
	Tubulovillous/villous	97	10	1.67 (0.76–3.67)
Martinez (Pooled anaylsis) 2009	Tubular	7268	749	1
	Tubulovillous/villous	1899	336	1.28 (1.07–1.52)
Pinsky (Study of Colonoscopy Utilization) 2009	Tubular	not mentioned		1
	Tubulovillous/villous	not mentioned		2.2 (1.5–3.1)
The below studies were included in the pooled analysis (Martinez et al. 2009)				
Martinez (Wheat bran fiber trial) 2001	Tubular	842	92	1
	Tubulovillous	317	41	1.10 (0.64–1.87)
	Villous	59	9	0.41 (0.15–1.13)
	Unspecified/incipient	69	4	0.47 (0.09–2.62)
Lieberman (VA Cooperative Study Group 380) 2007	No neoplasia	298	7	1
	Villous adenoma	81	13	6.05 (2.48-14.71)

Table 3. Tubulovillous/villous adenoma as a risk factor for advanced neoplasia at the time of surveillance

4.1.4 Degree of dysplasia

By definition, all adenomas have some level of dysplasia. In the past, dysplasia has been classified as mild, moderate, severe or carcinoma in situ. Currently, severe dysplasia or carcinoma in situ is considered the equivalent of high-grade dysplasia and mild or moderate dysplasia is considered the equivalent of low-grade dysplasia. High-grade dysplasia at baseline was not a significant predictor of advanced neoplasia in the pooled analysis of prospective studies (OR: 1.08, 95% CI: 0.82-1.41) and randomized controlled studies. However, high-grade dysplasia is related to a larger adenoma size and villous component at baseline. Although the VA Cooperative Study by Lieberman and colleagues was included in the pooled analysis, the VA Cooperative Study determined that 10.9% of the patients with high-grade dysplasia in adenomas of any size at baseline had advanced neoplasia over the 5-year surveillance period, as compared with 0.6% in those with tubular adenomas less than 1.0 cm in size and that lacked high-grade dysplasia.

Study	Degree of atypia of the index polyp	Total patients (N)	Patients with Metachronous Advanced Neoplasia (N)	Adjusted OR/RR/HR (95% CI)
Jorgensen (The Funen Adenoma Follow-up Study) 1995	Mild	not mentioned		1
	Moderate	not mentioned		1.0 (0.4-2.2)
	Severe	not mentioned		2.1 (0.6-7.1)
Bertario 2003	Low/moderate	1050	11	1
	Severe	36	1	3.3 (0.7-15.5)
Bonithon-Kopp (European Fiber-Calcium Intervention trial) 2004	Mild	308	17	1
	Moderate/Severe	244	24	1.86 (0.96-3.64)
Martinez (Pooled anaylsis) 2009	Low grade dysplasia	6485	719	1
	High grade dysplasia	683	118	1.05 (0.81-1.35)
The below studies were included in the pooled analysis (Martinez et al. 2009)				
Lieberman (VA Cooperative Study Group 380) 2007	no neoplasia	298	7	1
	High grade Dysplasia	46	8	6.87 (2.61-18.07)
	CRC	23	8	13.56 (5.54-33.18)

Table 4. High-grade dysplasia of adenoma as a risk factor for advanced neoplasia at the time of surveillance

4.1.5 Location

The pooled analysis by Martinez reported that a proximal adenoma at baseline was associated with an increased risk for subsequent advanced adenomas. The OR was 1.68 (95% CI: 1.39–2.02) for any proximal adenomas at baseline vs distal adenomas only at baseline. Similarly, Bonithon-Kopp reported an OR of 2.63 (95% CI: 1.31–5.3) for subsequent advanced neoplasia for patients with a proximal location of baseline adenomas compared with no proximal location of baseline adenomas. In the observational cohort study of

Pinsky, the risk of metachronous neoplasia at surveillance was significant higher for patients with adenomas on the proximal colon only at baseline than for patients with adenomas on the distal colon only.

Study	Location of index adenoma	Total patients (N)	Patients with Metachronous Advanced Neoplasia (N)	Adjusted OR/RR/HR (95% CI)
Bertario 2003	Right colon	317	2	0.7 (0.1–7.6)
	Left colon	641	11	2.0 (0.3–16.1)
	Rectum	128	1	1
Bonithon-Kopp (European Fiber-Calcium Intervention trial) 2004	No distal location	50	2	1
	Distal location	502	39	3.37 (0.74–15.3)
	No proximal location	438	23	1
	Proximal location	114	18	2.63 (1.31–5.3)
Martinez (Pooled anaylsis) 2009	Distal	4434	395	1
	Proximal only	2620	330	Any proximal: 1.68 (1.43–1.98)
	Both	1754	325	
Pinsky (Study of Colonoscopy Utilization) 2009	Distal colon only	not mentioned		1
	Proximal colon only	not mentioned		1.8 (1.1–2.7)
The below studies were included in the pooled analysis (Martinez et al. 2009)				
Martinez (Wheat bran fiber trial) 2001	Distal colon	701	68	1
	Proximal colon	349	44	1.65 (1.02–2.67)
	Both	234	33	2.69 (1.34–5.42)

Table 5. Location of adenoma as a risk factor for advanced neoplasia at the time of surveillance

4.1.6 Shape of adenoma

The flat adenoma may be a more aggressive pathway in colorectal carcinogenesis. However, O'Brien reclassified the histopathologically sessile adenomas from the National Polyp Study cohort as flat (defined as an adenoma thickness ≤1.3 mm and <2× the normal mucosa thickness) or polypoid and O'Brien compared between the initial and surveillance pathology. Flat adenomas identified in the National Polyp Study cohort at baseline were not associated with a higher risk for advanced adenomas at the time of surveillance.

4.1.7 Serrated polyps

Recent studies have shown that, aside from classic adenomas, serrated polyps (sessile serrated adenomas, mixed mucosal polyps and traditional serrated adenomas) are of special significance. These lesions are also associated with an elevated risk of malignant degeneration via the so called serrated cancer development pathway (Hiraoka et al., 2010; Leggett et al., 2010; Lu et al., 2011). However, in contrast, after the removal of singular hyperplastic polyps, no special follow-up examination is required (Imperiale et al., 2008).

4.2 Patient's characteristics
4.2.1 Age

Pooled analysis and several prospective observational studies by Bertario and Yamaji reported an increasing risk for subsequent neoplasia with increasing age. However, age was frequently used as a control variable in the analyses without an explicit risk factor presented for the age effect.

Study	Age at the time of polypectomy (years)	Total patients (N)	Patients with Metachronous Advanced Neoplasia (N)	Adjusted OR/RR/HR (95% CI)
Jorgensen (The Funen Adenoma Follow-up Study) 1995	≤60	not mentioned		1
	>60	not mentioned		1.5 (0.8-3.0)
Noshirwani (Cleveland Clinic Foundation Adenoma Registry) 2000	per 10-year increase	not mentioned		1.10 (0.82-1.45)
Bertario 2003	<60	503	5	1
	60–69	339	5	2.1 (0.6–7.5)
	≥70	244	4	4.1 (1.0–16.0)
Yammaji 2004	< 40	154	6	1
	40-49	804	52	2.3 (0.7–7.6)
	50-59	2397	213	3.6 (1.1–12)
	≥ 60	62	12	5.5 (1.6–19)
Martinez (Pooled anaylsis) 2009	< 40	154	6	0.41 (0.18–0.94)
	40-49	804	52	0.67 (0.48–0.93)
	50-59	2397	213	1
	60-69	3676	460	1.39 (1.16–1.68)
	70-79	2074	328	1.72 (1.40–2.11)
	≥ 80	62	12	2.70 (1.31–5.57)
	< 40	154	6	0.41 (0.18–0.94)
Laiyemo 2009, USA	≤65	not mentioned		1
	> 65	not mentioned		1.3 (0.7–2.5)

Table 6. Age at the time of polypectomy as a risk factor for advanced neoplasia at the time of surveillance

4.2.2 Gender

Gender was also frequently used as a control variable in the analyses without an explicit risk factor presented for the gender effect. The pooled analysis and the observational study by Bertario reported an increased risk for males for advanced neoplasia at the time of surveillance.

Study	Gender	Total patients (N)	Patients with Metachronous Advanced Neoplasia (N)	Adjusted OR/RR/HR (95% CI)
Jorgensen (The Funen Adenoma Follow-up Study) 1995	Female	not mentioned		1
	Male	not mentioned		1.1 (0.6-2.5)
Noshirwani (Cleveland Clinic Foundation Adenoma Registry) 2000	Female	not mentioned		1
	Male	not mentioned		1.48 (0.74-2.93)
Bertario 2003, Italy	Female	487	2	1
	Male	599	12	6.5 (1.4–29.9)
Yammaji 2004, Japan	Female	not mentioned		1
	Male	not mentioned		0.9 (0.5–1.5)
Martinez (Pooled anaylsis) 2009	Female	2642	267	1
	Male	6525	815	1.40 (1.19–1.65)
Laiyemo (Continued Follow-Up Study of the Polyp Prevention Trial) 2009	Female	not mentioned		1
	Male	not mentioned		2.0 (0.9–4.6)
Pinsky (Study of Colonoscopy Utilization) 2009	Female	not mentioned		1
	Male	not mentioned		1.2 (0.9–1.8)

Table 7. Gender as a risk factor for advanced neoplasia at the time of surveillance

4.2.3 Family history of colorectal cancer in first degree relatives

A family history of colorectal cancer in first degree relatives is an established risk factor for the development of colorectal cancer. However, few studies have specifically addressed the relationship between a family history and metachronous advanced adenomas in postpolypectomy patients. The Erlangen Registry of Colorectal Polyps reported that a parental history of colorectal cancer is associated with subsequent advanced neoplasia, but the pooled analysis, Bertario's study and the Continued Follow-Up Study of the Polyp Prevention Trial by Laiyemo did not find a significant association between the subsequent advanced neoplasia and a family history of colorectal cancer in first degree relatives.

4.2.4 History of previous polyps

Both the pooled analysis and Bonithon-Kopp study noted that a history of polyps before the baseline adenoma was associated with an increased risk for advanced neoplasia at the time of surveillance. Although it is not always possible to determine whether prior polyps are adenomatous polyps, the presence of prior polyps can be considered as an additional risk factor.

Study	Family history of colorectal cancer	Total patients (N)	Patients with Metachronous Advanced Neoplasia (N)	Adjusted OR/RR/HR (95% CI)
Nusko (Erlangen Registry of Colorectal Polyps) 2002	No	not mentioned		1
	Yes	not mentioned		2.32 (1.77-3.04)
Bertario 2003, Italy	No	787	10	1
	Yes	299	4	1.3 (0.4-4.1)
Martinez (Pooled anaylsis) 2009	No	6547	759	1
	Yes	2089	255	1.17 (0.99-1.38)
Laiyemo (Continued Follow-Up Study of the Polyp Prevention Trial) 2009	No	not mentioned		1
	Yes	not mentioned		1.0 (0.5-2.0)

Table 8. A family history of colorectal cancer in first degree relatives as a risk factor for advanced neoplasia at the time of surveillance

Study	History of previous polyp	Total patients (N)	Patients with Metachronous Advanced Neoplasia (N)	Adjusted OR/RR/HR (95% CI)
Bonithon-Kopp (European Fiber-Calcium Intervention trial) 2004	No	468	29	not mentioned
	Yes	84	12	
Martinez (Pooled anaylsis) 2009	No	6941	722	1
	Yes	2057	329	1.76 (1.48-2.09)

Table 9. A history of previous polyp as a risk factor for advanced neoplasia at the time of surveillance

4.2.5 Race

The pooled analysis of prospective studies by Martinez reported that the race of patients with polyp removal was associated with a different risk for subsequent advanced neoplasia. Compared to the white race, the black race showed an increased risk for subsequent advanced neoplasia (OR: 1.08, 95% CI: 0.79–1.47), whereas other races showed a tendency for a decreased risk for subsequent advanced neoplasia (OR: 0.83, 95% CI: 0.60–1.16).

5. Risk stratification for the metachronous advanced adenoma risk

The totality of evidence suggests that multiplicity (3 or more adenomas), size (1 cm or more), villous features, high-grade dysplasia, a proximal location and a history of previous polyp are the predictors of future advanced neoplasia. Race, age, gender and a family

history of colorectal cancer also may predict metachronous advanced neoplasia, but this has not been well studied. Analysis of the relative importance of each of these predictors is complicated by their interrelationships.
The current guidelines from the major organizations, including the US Multi-Society Task Force on Colorectal Cancer (USMTF), the American College of Gastroenterology (ACG), the American Society of Gastrointestinal Endoscopy (ASGE), and the British Society of Gastroenterology (BSG), have accepted the risk stratification listed in Table 10 (Bond 2000; Davila et al., 2006; Winawer et al., 2006; Cairns et al., 2010).
There is a consensus among many of the studies that the group at a lower risk for subsequent advanced neoplasia has only 1 or 2 tubular adenomas that are less than 1 cm in size and low-grade dysplasia and they are located only in the distal colon. In the colonoscopy based studies, the patients have been followed-up for only 5-6 years after colonoscopic polypectomy to assess their subsequent risk for neoplasia.

Term	Definition
Low risk group	All of the following: 1 or 2 adenomas Size < 1 cm Tubular histology No high-grade dysplasia
High risk group	Any of the following: Multiple adenomas (≥ 3) Size ≥ 1 cm Villous or tubulovillous histology High-grade dysplasia
Higher risk group	Any of the following: >10 small adenomas Piecemeal resection of large sessile adenoma

Table 10. Risk stratification for subsequent advanced neoplasia

6. Post-polypectomy surveillance interval

Based on risk stratification, the major organisations have suggested the post-polypectomy colonoscopy surveillance interval (Table11). All the guidelines rely on periodic colonoscopy as the primary method of surveillance. The surveillance interval is based on the risk of metachronous advanced neoplasia as predicted by the findings on initial colonoscopy. Most of the guidelines recommend repeat colonoscopy in 5-10 years for low-risk patients (only one or two small adenomas, <1 cm in size); for such patients, the BSG advises either repeat colonoscopy in 5 years or no surveillance at all (the patients can continue average-risk screening). For the patients at high risk (advanced neoplasm or 3-10 small adenomas), colonoscopy should be repeated in 3 years, with subsequent colonoscopies every 5 years if the preceding colonoscopy was negative. In most of the guidelines, an advanced neoplasm is defined as a villous or tubulovillous adenoma, an adenoma with intermediate-grade or high-grade dysplasia, or a tubular adenoma 1 cm in size or larger. The USMTF guidelines specify that the colonoscopy intervals can be extended to 10 years if the preceding colonoscopy did not show adenomas. In patients with numerous (>10) adenomas but there was no overt adenomatous polyposis syndrome, colonoscopy should be repeated in less than 3 years, with the exact interval to be determined by the endoscopist. For patients with large sessile adenomas that are difficult to completely remove in one session, a repeat colonoscopy after a short interval (2–6 months) is recommended. Subsequent intervals are customized according to the level of suspicion for residual adenomatous tissue at the polypectomy site. If a sessile polyp is very extensive or it has high-grade dysplastic features, then surgical resection should be considered. After it is certain that all adenomatous tissue has been removed, surveillance with 3–5 year intervals can be resumed.

	Organization	First surveillance interval	Second surveillance interval if surveillance colonoscopy shows no adenomas
Low risk group			
1–2 tubular adenomas, <1cm and lowe-grade dysplasia	USMTF	5–10 years	-
	ACG	5 years*	5 years
	ASGE	No earlier than 5 years	No earlier than 5 years
	BSG	5 years or no surveillance	No surveillance
High risk group			
3-10 adenomas, ≥ 1 cm, tubulovillous /villous adenoma or High-grade dysplasia	USMTF	3 years	5 years
	ACG	3 years†	5 years
	ASGE	3 years	No earlier than 5 years
	BSG	3 years‡	3 years§
Higher risk group			
>10 small adenomas	USMTF	<3 years	
	ACG	-	-
	ASGE	<3 years	5 years
	BSG	1 year¶	3 years‡
Large sessile adenoma	USMTF	2–6 months	Customised
	ACG	3–6 months	-
	ASGE	2–6 months	Customised
	BSG	3 month	1 year‖

Abbreviation: US Multi-Society Task Force on Colorectal Cancer, USMTF; American College of Gastroenterology, ACG; American Society of Gastrointestinal Endoscopy, ASGE; British Society of Gastroenterology, BSG.

*The ACG guidelines note that selected low-risk patients might not need surveillance at all, but they do not further elaborate. †The ACG guidelines consider patients with 1–2 small adenomas and a positive family history in a first-degree relative to be at intermediate risk. ‡The BSG guidelines define intermediate-risk patients as those with 3–4 small adenomas or at least one adenoma ≥1 cm in size. §The BSG guidelines recommend ceasing surveillance if two consecutive follow-up colonoscopies are negative. ¶The BSG guidelines define high risk patients as those with ≥5 adenomas or ≥3 adenomas with at least one of which is ≥1 cm in size. ‖The BSG guidelines recommend repeating colonoscopy in 1 year after confirmation of complete removal, and then every 3 years.

Table 11. Summary of the post-polypectomy guidelines

Over the past few decades, the recommended intervals between surveillance colonoscopies have been extended, on the basis of accumulating data that showed longer surveillance intervals are safe. For example, the National Polyp Study showed no difference in the adenoma risk between patients who had repeat colonoscopy at 1 year versus those who had colonoscopy at 3 years, while the Funen Adenoma Study showed no statistically significant difference in the adenoma recurrence rates at 4 years colonoscopy compared with 2 years colonoscopy. Depending on the patient's and physician's preference, surveillance may be discontinued if the life expectancy is under 10 years (USMTF) or if the patient is over 75 years old (BSG). For most guidelines, the surveillance recommendations are relaxed after one or two negative follow-up colonoscopies. However, the ACG considers those patients with a history of adenomas to be at a lifelong risk for metachronous lesions and the ACG recommends colonoscopies at least every 5 years indefinitely. It is important to note that these surveillance interval recommendations are based on the assumption that the baseline colonoscopy is of high quality with good bowel preparation, thorough removal of polyps has been done, there is an adequate examination time and complete visualization of all colonic mucosa up to and including the caecum.

Surveys have shown that the patients' compliance with physicians' recommendations for surveillance is high (up to 85%), and particularly in the presence of multiple or larger polyps (Klabunde et al., 2003; Mysliwiec et al., 2004; Kang et al., 2006). Also, patients are often interested in chemopreventive measures such as antioxidants, fiber, and calcium or other dietary supplements, although the efficacy of all these agents has not been unequivocally shown. The effect of surveillance colonoscopy on the quality of life has not been directly studied, although patients probably derive benefit if we extrapolate the results from quality-of-life studies on screening colonoscopy. Unfortunately, many clinicians do not adhere to the surveillance guidelines and they often do colonoscopies more frequently than is recommended. This over-surveillance is probably due to concerns about missed lesions or interval cancers, which can occur even in patients who are under close surveillance. Improved adherence to guidelines could be achieved by the use of reminder devices and algorithms for continuous improvement. Other screening measures, such as the use of interval testing of faecal occult blood, might also allow practitioners to feel more comfortable with longer surveillance intervals (Bampton et al., 2005).

7. Conclusion

Identifying the high risk subjects is important, as is ensuring that the subjects accept and comply with the recommended surveillance program. Two important factors, in addition to the individual patient factors, have a profound effect on the cancer risk: these are the quality of performing the examination, and ensuring complete removal of large sessile lesions. In addition to the potentially therapeutic value of polyp removal, colonoscopy is an opportunity to identify a small, high risk group of patients who require careful surveillance to prevent the development of cancer. It is also an opportunity to identify a much larger group of patients who can be informed with some confidence that their cancer risk is low. The overall effectiveness of an adenoma surveillance program for preventing colorectal cancer depends on each colonoscopy being undertaken slowly, carefully and thoroughly with a fail-safe system in place for recalling the higher risk patients

Further research will help define the best surveillance intervals, as well as the role of technical innovations such as CT colonography, chromoendoscopy and narrow-band imaging.

8. Acknowledgment

I would like to express sincere thanks to Ewe Chung Chung, who has given me the most support and encouragement.

9. References

Arditi, C., Peytremann-Bridevaux, I., Burnand, B., Eckardt, V.F., Bytzer, P., Agreus, L., Dubois, R.W., Vader, J.P., Froehlich, F., Pittet, V., Schussele Filliettaz, S., Juillerat, P. and Gonvers, J.J. (2009) Appropriateness of colonoscopy in Europe (EPAGE II). Screening for colorectal cancer. *Endoscopy*, Vol.41, No.3, (March 2009), pp. 200-208, ISSN 1438-8812

Atkin, W.S., Edwards, R., Kralj-Hans, I., Wooldrage, K., Hart, A.R., Northover, J.M., Parkin, D.M., Wardle, J., Duffy, S.W. and Cuzick, J. (2010) Once-only flexible sigmoidoscopy screening in prevention of colorectal cancer: a multicentre randomised controlled trial. *Lancet*, Vol.375, No.9726, (May 2010), pp. 1624-1633, ISSN 1474-547X

Bampton, P.A., Sandford, J.J., Cole, S.R., Smith, A., Morcom, J., Cadd, B. and Young, G.P. (2005) Interval faecal occult blood testing in a colonoscopy based screening programme detects additional pathology. *Gut*, Vol.54, No.6, (June 2005), pp. 803-806, ISSN 0017-5749

Barclay, R.L., Vicari, J.J., Doughty, A.S., Johanson, J.F. and Greenlaw, R.L. (2006) Colonoscopic withdrawal times and adenoma detection during screening colonoscopy. *New England Journal of Medicine*, Vol.355, No.24, (December 2006), pp. 2533-2541, ISSN 1533-4406

Bensen, S., Mott, L.A., Dain, B., Rothstein, R. and Baron, J. (1999) The colonoscopic miss rate and true one-year recurrence of colorectal neoplastic polyps. Polyp Prevention Study Group. *American Journal of Gastroenterology*, Vol.94, No.1, (January 1999), pp. 194-199, ISSN 0002-9270

Benson, M., Dureja, P., Gopal, D., Reichelderfer, M. and Pfau, P.R. (2010) A comparison of optical colonoscopy and CT colonography screening strategies in the detection and recovery of subcentimeter adenomas. *American Journal of Gastroenterology*, Vol.105, No.12, (December 2010), pp. 2578-2585, ISSN 1572-0241

Bertario, L., Russo, A., Sala, P., Pizzetti, P., Ballardini, G., Andreola, S. and Spinelli, P. (2003) Predictors of metachronous colorectal neoplasms in sporadic adenoma patients. *International Journal of Cancer*, Vol.105, No.1, (May 2003), pp. 82-87, ISSN 0020-7136

Bond, J.H. (2000) Polyp guideline: diagnosis, treatment, and surveillance for patients with colorectal polyps. Practice Parameters Committee of the American College of Gastroenterology. *American Journal of Gastroenterology*, Vol.95, No.11, (November 2007), pp. 3053-3063, ISSN 0002-9270

Bonithon-Kopp, C., Piard, F., Fenger, C., Cabeza, E., O'Morain, C., Kronborg, O. and Faivre, J. (2004) Colorectal adenoma characteristics as predictors of recurrence. *Diseases of the Colon and Rctum*, Vol.47, No.3, (March 2004), pp. 323-333, ISSN 0012-3706

Cairns, S.R., Scholefield, J.H., Steele, R.J., Dunlop, M.G., Thomas, H.J., Evans, G.D., Eaden, J.A., Rutter, M.D., Atkin, W.P., Saunders, B.P., Lucassen, A., Jenkins, P., Fairclough, P.D. and Woodhouse, C.R. (2010) Guidelines for colorectal cancer screening and surveillance in moderate and high risk groups (update from 2002). *Gut,* Vol.59, No.5, (May 2010), pp. 666-689, ISSN 1468-3288

Center, M.M., Jemal, A. and Ward, E. (2009) International trends in colorectal cancer incidence rates. *Cancer epidemiology, biomarkers & prevention,* Vol.18, No.6 (June 2009), pp. 1688-1694, ISSN 1538-7755

Citarda, F., Tomaselli, G., Capocaccia, R., Barcherini, S., Crespi, M. (2001). Efficacy in standard clinical practice of colonoscopic polypectomy in reducing colorectal cancer incidence. *Gut,* Vol.48, No.6 (June2001), pp. 812-815, ISSN 0017-5749

Davila, R.E., Rajan, E., Baron, T.H., Adler, D.G., Egan, J.V., Faigel, D.O., Gan, S.I., Hirota, W.K., Leighton, J.A., Lichtenstein, D., Qureshi, W.A., Shen, B., Zuckerman, M.J., VanGuilder, T. and Fanelli, R.D. (2006) ASGE guideline: colorectal cancer screening and surveillance. *Gastrointestinal Endoscopy,* Vol.63, No.4 (April 2006), pp. 546-557, ISSN 0016-5107

Deenadayalu, V. P. and Rex, D. K. (2005). Colon polyp retrieval after cold snaring. *Gastrointestinal Endoscopy,* Vol.62, No.2 (August 2005), pp. 253-256, ISSN 0016-5107

Durdey, P., Weston, P.M. and Williams, N.S. (1987) Colonoscopy or barium enema as initial investigation of colonic disease. *Lancet,* Vol.2, No.8558, pp. 549-551, ISSN 0140-6736

Eide, T.J. (1986) Risk of colorectal cancer in adenoma-bearing individuals within a defined population. *International Journal of Cancer,* Vol.38, No.2 (August 1986), pp. 173-176, ISSN 0020-7136.

Farrar, W.D., Sawhney, M.S., Nelson, D.B., Lederle, F.A. and Bond, J.H. (2006) Colorectal cancers found after a complete colonoscopy. *Clinical Gastroenterolenterology and Hepatology,* Vol. 4, No.10 (October 2006), pp. 1259-1264, ISSN 1542-3565

Froehlich, F., Wietlisbach, V., Gonvers, J.J., Burnand, B. and Vader, J.P. (2005) Impact of colonic cleansing on quality and diagnostic yield of colonoscopy: the European Panel of Appropriateness of Gastrointestinal Endoscopy European multicenter study. *Gastrointestinal Endoscopy,* Vol.61, No.3 (March 2005), pp. 378-384, ISSN 0016-5107

Harewood, G. C., Sharma, V. K. and de Garmo, P. (2003) Impact of colonoscopy preparation quality on detection of suspected colonic neoplasia. *Gastrointestinal Endoscopy,* Vol.58, No.1 (July 2003), pp 76-79, ISSN 0016-5107

Heresbach, D., Barrioz, T., Lapalus, M.G., Coumaros, D., Bauret, P., Potier, P., Sautereau, D., Boustiere, C., Grimaud, J.C., Barthelemy, C., See, J., Serraj, I., D'Halluin, P.N., Branger, B. and Ponchon, T. (2008) Miss rate for colorectal neoplastic polyps: a prospective multicenter study of back-to-back video colonoscopies. *Endoscopy,* Vol.40, No. 4 (April 2008), pp. 284-290, ISSN 1438-8812

Hiraoka, S., Kato, J., Fujiki, S., Kaji, E., Morikawa, T., Murakami, T., Nawa, T., Kuriyama, M., Uraoka, T., Ohara, N. and Yamamoto, K. (2010) The presence of large serrated polyps increases risk for colorectal cancer. *Gastroenterology,* Vol.139, No.5 (November, 2010), pp. 1503-1510, ISSN 1528-0012

Hixson, L.J., Fennerty, M.B., Sampliner, R.E. and Garewal, H.S. (1991) Prospective blinded trial of the colonoscopic miss-rate of large colorectal polyps. *Gastrointestinal Endoscopy,* Vol.37, No.2 (March-April 1991), pp. 125-127 ISSN 0016-5107

Hoff, G., Foerster, A., Vatn, M.H., Sauar, J. and Larsen, S. (1986) Epidemiology of polyps in the rectum and colon. Recovery and evaluation of unresected polyps 2 years after detection. *Scandinavian Journal of Gastroenterololgy*, Vol.21, No. 7 (September 1986), pp. 853-862, ISSN 0036-5521

Hofstad, B., Vatn, M.H., Andersen, S.N., Huitfeldt, H.S., Rognum, T., Larsen, S. and Osnes, M. (1996) Growth of colorectal polyps: redetection and evaluation of unresected polyps for a period of three years. *Gut*, Vol.39, No.3 (September 1996), pp. 449-456, ISSN 0017-5749

Hong, S.N., Kim, J.H., Choe, W.H., Han, H.S., Sung, I.K., Park, H.S. and Shim, C.S. (2010) Prevalence and risk of colorectal neoplasms in asymptomatic, average-risk screenees 40 to 49 years of age. *Gastrointestinal Endoscopy*, Vol.72, No.3 (September 2010), pp. 480-489, ISSN 0016-5107

Imperiale, T.F., Glowinski, E.A., Lin-Cooper, C., Larkin, G.N., Rogge, J.D. and Ransohoff, D.F. (2008) Five-year risk of colorectal neoplasia after negative screening colonoscopy. *New England Journal of Medicine*, Vol.359, No.12 (September 2008), pp. 1218-1224. ISSN 1533-4406

Ji, J.S., Choi, K.Y., Lee, W.C., Lee, B.I., Park, S.H., Choi, H., Kim, B.W., Chae, H.S., Park, Y.M. and Park, Y.J. (2009) Endoscopic and histopathologic predictors of recurrence of colorectal adenoma on lowering the miss rate. *Korean Journal of Internal Medicine*, Vol.24, No.3 (September 2009), pp. 196-202, ISSN 1226-3303

Jorgensen, O.D., Kronborg, O. and Fenger, C. (1995) A randomized surveillance study of patients with pedunculated and small sessile tubular and tubulovillous adenomas. The Funen Adenoma Follow-up Study. *Scandinavian Journal of Gastroenterololgy*, Vol. 30, No. 7 (July 1995), pp. 686-692, ISSN 0036-5521

Kaminski, M.F., Regula, J., Kraszewska, E., Polkowski, M., Wojciechowska, U., Didkowska, J., Zwierko, M., Rupinski, M., Nowacki, M.P. and Butruk, E. (2010) Quality indicators for colonoscopy and the risk of interval cancer. *New England Journal of Medicine*, Vol.362, No.19 (May 2010), pp. 1795-1803. ISSN 1533-4406

Kang, M.S., Park, D.I., Park, J.H., Kim, H.J., Cho, Y.K., Sohn, C.I., Jeon, W.K. and Kim, B.I. (2006) A Survey on the Interval of Post-polypectomy Surveillance Colonoscopy. *Korean Journal of Gastrointestinal Endoscopy*, Vol.33, No.3 (n.d.), pp.339-345.

Kim, D.H., Pickhardt, P.J., Taylor, A.J., Leung, W.K., Winter, T.C., Hinshaw, J.L., Gopal, D.V., Reichelderfer, M., Hsu, R.H. and Pfau, P.R. (2007) CT colonography versus colonoscopy for the detection of advanced neoplasia. *New England Journal of Medicine*, Vol.357, No.14 (October 2007), pp. 1403-1412. ISSN 1533-4406

Kim, H.S. (2009) Postpolypectomy Colonoscopy Surveillance. *Korean Journal of Gastrointestinal Endoscopy* Vo.39, No.3(n.d.), pp. 257-64

Kim, J.B., Han, D.S., Lee, H.L., Kim, J.P., Jeon, Y.C., Sohn, J.H. and Hahm, J.S. (2004) The recurrence rate of colon polyp after polypectomy and the interval of surveillance colonoscopy: predictors of early development of advanced polyp. *Korean Journal of Gastroenterology*, Vol.44, No.3 (n.d.), pp. 77-83

Klabunde, C. N., Frame, P. S., Meadow, A., Jones, E., Nadel, M. and Vernon, S. W. (2003) A national survey of primary care physicians' colorectal cancer screening recommendations and practices. *Preventive medicine*, Vol.36, No.3 (March 2003), pp. 352-62, ISSN 0091-7435.

Laiyemo, A.O., Pinsky, P.F., Marcus, P.M., Lanza, E., Cross, A.J., Schatzkin, A. and Schoen, R.E. (2009) Utilization and yield of surveillance colonoscopy in the continued follow-up study of the polyp prevention trial. *Clinical Gastroenterolenterology and Hepatology*, Vol. 7, No.5 (May 2009), pp. 562-567, ISSN 1542-3565

Leaper, M., Johnston, M. J., Barclay, M., Dobbs, B. R. and Frizelle, F. A. (2004) Reasons for failure to diagnose colorectal carcinoma at colonoscopy. *Endoscopy* Vol.36, No.6 (June 2004), pp. 499-503, ISSN 0013-726X

Lee, B.H. and Jeong, S.Y. (2002) Korean National Recommendation Guidelines on Screening and Surveillance for Early Detection of Colorectal Cancers. *Journal of Korean Medical Association*, Vol. 45, No.3 (n.d.), pp. 981-991

Leggett, B. and Whitehall, V. (2010) Role of the serrated pathway in colorectal cancer pathogenesis. *Gastroenterology*, Vol.138, No.6 (June 2010), pp. 2088-2100, ISSN 1528-0012

Levin, B., Lieberman, D.A., McFarland, B., Andrews, K.S., Brooks, D., Bond, J., Dash, C., Giardiello, F.M., Glick, S., Johnson, D., Johnson, C.D., Levin, T.R., Pickhardt, P.J., Rex, D.K., Smith, R.A., Thorson, A. and Winawer, S.J. (2008) Screening and surveillance for the early detection of colorectal cancer and adenomatous polyps, 2008: a joint guideline from the American Cancer Society, the US Multi-Society Task Force on Colorectal Cancer, and the American College of Radiology. *Gastroenterology*, Vol.134, No.5 (May 2008), pp. 1570-1595, ISSN 1528-0012

Lieberman, D.A., Weiss, D.G., Harford, W.V., Ahnen, D.J., Provenzale, D., Sontag, S.J., Schnell, T.G., Chejfec, G., Campbell, D.R., Kidao, J., Bond, J.H., Nelson, D.B., Triadafilopoulos, G., Ramirez, F.C., Collins, J.F., Johnston, T.K., McQuaid, K.R., Garewal, H., Sampliner, R.E., Esquivel, R. and Robertson, D. (2007) Five-year colon surveillance after screening colonoscopy. *Gastroenterology*, Vol.133, No. 4 (October 2007), pp. 1077-1085, ISSN 1528-0012

Loeve, F., M. van Ballegooijen, Snel, P., Habbema, J. D. (2005). Colorectal cancer risk after colonoscopic polypectomy: a population-based study and literature search. *European Journal of Cancer*, Vol. 41, No.3 (February 2005), pp. 416-422. ISSN 0959-8049.

Lu, F.I., van Niekerk de, W., Owen, D., Tha, S.P., Turbin, D.A. and Webber, D.L. (2010) Longitudinal outcome study of sessile serrated adenomas of the colorectum: an increased risk for subsequent right-sided colorectal carcinoma. *The American Journal of Surgical Pathology*, Vol.37, No.7 (July 2010), pp. 927-937, ISSN 0147-5185

Lund, J.N., Scholefield, J.H., Grainge, M.J., Smith, S.J., Mangham, C., Armitage, N.C., Robinson, M.H. and Logan, R.F. (2001) Risks, costs, and compliance limit colorectal adenoma surveillance: lessons from a randomised trial. *Gut*, Vol.49, No.1 (July 2001), pp. 91-96, ISSN 0017-5749

Martinez, M.E., Baron, J.A., Lieberman, D.A., Schatzkin, A., Lanza, E., Winawer, S.J., Zauber, A.G., Jiang, R., Ahnen, D.J., Bond, J.H., Church, T.R., Robertson, D.J., Smith-Warner, S.A., Jacobs, E.T., Alberts, D.S. and Greenberg, E.R. (2009) A pooled analysis of advanced colorectal neoplasia diagnoses after colonoscopic polypectomy. *Gastroenterology*, Vol.136, No.3 (March 2009), pp. 832-841, ISSN 1528-0012

Martinez, M.E., Sampliner, R., Marshall, J.R., Bhattacharyya, A.K., Reid, M.E. and Alberts, D.S. (2001) Adenoma characteristics as risk factors for recurrence of advanced adenomas. *Gastroenterology*, Vol.120, No.5 (April 2001), pp. 1077-1083, ISSN 1528-0012

Meagher, A. P. and M. Stuart (1994) Does colonoscopic polypectomy reduce the incidence of colorectal carcinoma? *The Australian and New Zealand journal of surgery,* Vol. 64, No.6 (June 1994), pp. 400-404, ISSN 0004-8682

Muto, T., Bussey, H.J. and Morson, B.C. (1975) The evolution of cancer of the colon and rectum. *Cancer,* Vol.36, No.6 (December 1975), pp. 2251-2270. ISSN 0008-543X

Mysliwiec, P. A., Brown, M. L., Klabunde, C. N. and Ransohoff, D. F. (2004) Are physicians doing too much colonoscopy? A national survey of colorectal surveillance after polypectomy. *Annals of Internal Medicine,* Vol. 141, No.4 (August, 2004), pp. 264-271, ISSN 1539-3704.

Noshirwani, K.C., van Stolk, R.U., Rybicki, L.A. and Beck, G.J. (2000) Adenoma size and number are predictive of adenoma recurrence: implications for surveillance colonoscopy. *Gastrointestinal Endoscopy,* Vol.51, No.4 (April 2000), pp. 433-437, ISSN 0016-5107

Nusko, G., Mansmann, U., Kirchner, T. and Hahn, E.G. (2002) Risk related surveillance following colorectal polypectomy. *Gut,* Vol.51, No.3 (September 2002), pp. 424-428, ISSN 0017-5749

Parra-Blanco, A., Nicolas-Perez, D., Gimeno-Garcia, A., Grosso, B., Jimenez, A., Ortega, J. and Quintero, E. (2006) The timing of bowel preparation before colonoscopy determines the quality of cleansing, and is a significant factor contributing to the detection of flat lesions: a randomized study. *World Journal of Gastroenterology,* Vol.12, No.38 (October 2006), pp. 6161-1666, ISSN 1007-9327

Pinsky, P.F., Schoen, R.E., Weissfeld, J.L., Church, T., Yokochi, L.A., Doria-Rose, V.P. and Prorok, P. (2009) The yield of surveillance colonoscopy by adenoma history and time to examination. *Clinical Gastroenterolenterology and Hepatology,* Vol. 7, No.1 (January 2009), pp. 86-92, ISSN 1542-3565

Rapuri, S., Spencer, J. and Eckels, D. (2008) Importance of postpolypectomy surveillance and postpolypectomy compliance to follow-up screening--review of literature. *International Journal of Colorectal Disease,* Vol.23, No.5 (May 2008), pp. 453-459, ISSN 1432-1262

Rex, D.K., Bond, J.H., Winawer, S., Levin, T.R., Burt, R.W., Johnson, D.A., Kirk, L.M., Litlin, S., Lieberman, D.A., Waye, J.D., Church, J., Marshall, J.B. and Riddell, R.H. (2002) Quality in the technical performance of colonoscopy and the continuous quality improvement process for colonoscopy: recommendations of the U.S. Multi-Society Task Force on Colorectal Cancer. *The American Journal of Surgical Pathology,* Vol.97, No.6 (July 2002), pp. 1296-1308, ISSN 0147-5185

Schmiegel, W., Pox, C., Arnold, D., Porschen, R., Rodel, C. and Reinacher-Schick, A. (2009) Colorectal carcinoma: the management of polyps, (neo)adjuvant therapy, and the treatment of metastases. *Deutsches Arzteblatt international,* Vol.106, No. 51-52 (December 2009), pp. 843-648, ISSN 1866-0452

Stryker, S.J., Wolff, B.G., Culp, C.E., Libbe, S.D., Ilstrup, D.M. and MacCarty, R.L. (1987) Natural history of untreated colonic polyps. *Gastroenterology,* Vol.93, No.5 (November 1987), pp. 1009-1013, ISSN 1528-0012

Sung, J.J., Lau, J.Y., Young, G.P., Sano, Y., Chiu, H.M., Byeon, J.S., Yeoh, K.G., Goh, K.L., Sollano, J., Rerknimitr, R., Matsuda, T., Wu, K.C., Ng, S., Leung, S.Y., Makharia, G., Chong, V.H., Ho, K.Y., Brooks, D., Lieberman, D.A. and Chan, F.K. (2008) Asia

Pacific consensus recommendations for colorectal cancer screening. *Gut*, Vol.57, No.8 (August 2008), pp. 1166-1176, ISSN 0017-5749

Vogelstein, B., Fearon, E.R., Hamilton, S.R., Kern, S.E., Preisinger, A.C., Leppert, M., Nakamura, Y., White, R., Smits, A.M. and Bos, J.L. (1988) Genetic alterations during colorectal-tumor development. *New England Journal of Medicine*, Vol.319, No.9 (September 1988), pp. 525-532. ISSN 1533-4406

Winawer, S.J., Stewart, E.T., Zauber, A.G., Bond, J.H., Ansel, H., Waye, J.D., Hall, D., Hamlin, J.A., Schapiro, M., O'Brien, M.J., Sternberg, S.S. and Gottlieb L.S. (2000) A comparison of colonoscopy and double-contrast barium enema for surveillance after polypectomy. National Polyp Study Work Group. *New England Journal of Medicine*, Vol.342, No.24 (June 2000), pp. 1766-1772, ISSN 1533-4406

Winawer, S.J., Zauber, A.G., Ho, M.N., O'Brien, M.J., Gottlieb, L.S., Sternberg, S.S., Waye, J.D., Schapiro, M., Bond, J.H., Panish, J.F. (1993) Prevention of colorectal cancer by colonoscopic polypectomy. The National Polyp Study Workgroup. *New England Journal of Medicine*, Vol.329, No.27 (December 1993), pp. 1977-1981. ISSN 1533-4406

Winawer, S.J., Zauber, A.G., O'Brien, M.J., Ho, M.N., Gottlieb, L., Sternberg, S.S., Waye, J.D., Bond, J., Schapiro, M., Stewart, E.T. (1993) Randomized comparison of surveillance intervals after colonoscopic removal of newly diagnosed adenomatous polyps. The National Polyp Study Workgroup. *New England Journal of Medicine*, Vol.328, No.13 (April 1993), pp. 901-906. ISSN 1533-4406

Winawer, S.J. and Zauber, A.G. (2002) The advanced adenoma as the primary target of screening. *Gastrointestinal endoscopy clinics of North America*, Vol.12, No.1, pp.1-9, ISSN 1052-5157

Winawer, S.J., Zauber, A.G., Fletcher, R.H., Stillman, J.S., O'Brien, M.J., Levin, B., Smith, R.A., Lieberman, D.A., Burt, R.W., Levin, T.R., Bond, J.H., Brooks, D., Byers, T., Hyman, N., Kirk, L., Thorson, A., Simmang, C., Johnson, D. and Rex, D.K. (2006) Guidelines for colonoscopy surveillance after polypectomy: a consensus update by the US Multi-Society Task Force on Colorectal Cancer and the American Cancer Society. *Gastroenterology*, Vol.130, No.6 (May 2006), pp. 1872-1885, ISSN 1528-0012

Zlatanic, J., Waye, J. D., Kim, P. S., Baiocco, P. J. and Gleim, G. W. (1999). Large sessile colonic adenomas: use of argon plasma coagulator to supplement piecemeal snare polypectomy. *Gastrointestinal Endoscopy*, Vol.49, No.6 (June 1999), pp. 731-735, ISSN 0016-5107

7

Endoscopic Manifestations and Mucosal Patterns Associated to Collagenous Colitis

Daniel Gustavo Cimmino and José Manuel Mella
Endoscopy Unit and Gastroenterology Unit, Hospital Alemán, Buenos Aires, Argentina

1. Introduction

Microscopic colitis (MC) are clinical pathologic entities characterized by secretory-like aqueous chronic diarrhea, in its large majority without hematochezia. From the first descriptions of MC[1], normal endoscopic and radiological findings have been a pathognomonic feature. It is thought that up to 20% of adults with chronic diarrhea who have an endoscopically normal colonoscopy may have MC.

Most common MC are collagenous colitis and lymphocytic colitis. They are two morphologically distinct entities of MC. They are similar in presentation but differ histologically. Endoscopic biopsy is required for the diagnosis of MC[2]. As there are usually no mucosal abnormalities, the biopsies taken must be random. However, several authors have described different mucosal abnormalities related to the MC, most of them related to collagenous colitis.

Our aims were to review the medical literature and to describe the mucosal patterns and mucosal abnormalities that have been associated with the microscopic colitis, especially those related to the collagenous colitis.

1.1 Search

A MEDLINE search (1966-December 2010), was done using the terms "Colitis, Microscopic"[Mesh] or "Colitis, Collagenous"[Mesh] or "Colitis, Lymphocytic"[Mesh] and "Endoscopy, Digestive System"[Mesh] or "Endoscopy, Gastrointestinal"[Mesh] or "Colonoscopy"[Mesh] to find relevant articles. The search was carried out without restrictions or limits. The selection process of the articles was done independently by both authors. Agreement was measured using kappa coefficient (k). First, relevant studies were selected by the title (k 0.80, CI95% 0.63-0.97) and differences were resolved by consensus. Then, the fulltexts of selected articles were read.

2. Role of endoscopy in microscopic colitis

Endoscopy is essential for the diagnosis of microscopic colitis[2]. The diagnosis of microscopic colitis is based on mucosal biopsies taken during colonoscopy at the appropriate sites. It is essential to take colonic biopsies when endoscopic examinations are carried out in the clinical context of chronic diarrhea, even if the functional nature of the diarrhea is suspected.

By definition, the colonic mucosa has an endoscopically normal appearance in microscopic colitis. However, some authors have reported endoscopic abnormalities and mucosal patterns in patients with MC (see below).

2.1 Colorectal biopsy samples: where and how much?

Histological abnormalities in MC are generally pancolonic as they can be distributed throughout the colon as well as limited to the right colon[3]. In collagenous colitis, thickening of the subepitelial collagen band is in some cases more marked in the proximal colon than in the distal colon. The two endoscopically normal sites in which biopsies should be taken for optimal diagnosis of MC are the ascending colon and the sigmoid colon. Three to four biopsies should be taken per site.

3. Mucosal patterns and mucosal lesions associated to microscopic colitis

In the colonoscopy, the colonic mucosa has usually a normal aspect or it can present minimum and unspecific abnormalities such as erythema patches, edema or alterations in the vascular pattern.

In our search, we found several case reports and case series of endoscopic findings that would suggest the presence of this type of colitis, most of the findings related to collagenous colitis. In Table 1 there is a summary of the different endoscopic manifestations of the collagenous colitis and the authors of these findings.

Author	**Colorectal findings in collagenous colitis**
Richieri *et al* [4] (1993)	mucosal tears
Katsinelos *et al* [16](1997)	multiple red spots
Sato *et al* [17] (1998)	spindle network pattern
Cruz–Correa *et al* [5] (2002)	mucosal tears
Buchman *et al* [18] (2004)	pseudomembranous collagenous colitis
Koulaouzidis *et al* [6] (2006)	mucosal tears and scars
Tysk *et al* [7] (2006)	mucosal tears, longitudinal mucosal lacerations
Smith *et al* [13] (2007)	mucosal tears on insufflattion, colonic perforation
Allende *et al* [14] (2008)	bleeding linear ulcers, colonic perforations
Hashimoto *et al* [8] (2008)	linear ulcers, scar–like areas; crowded vascularity of the colonic mucosa and dilated, circling or winding blood capillaries
Dunzendorfer *et al* [21] (2008)	mucosal tears
Umeno *et al* [10] (2008)	linear mucosal defects
Couto *et al* [9] (2009)	scars; mucosal tears, superficial lacerations or "cat scratches" enhanced with air insufflation during colonoscopy
Hashimoto *et al* [19] (2009)	mucosa similar to ischemic colitis
Cimmino *et al* [20] (2010)	colorectal mosaic pattern
Nomura *et al* [11] (2010)	linear mucosal defects

Table 1. Summary of the mucosal abnormalities associated with collagenous colitis.

3.1 Mucosal tears

Mucosal tears were the most frequent endoscopic findings in our search. The terms "linear mucosal defects" have been used by several authors to describe mucosal tears and sharp longitudinal ulcers (characteristic colonoscopic findings in patients with collagenous colitis). One of the first descriptions of mucosal tears that we found data were from 1993 (Richieri *et al.*[4]) and 2002 (Cruz-Correa *et al.*[5]).

In 2006, Koulaouzidis *et al.*[6] described discrete linear mucosal breaks in the caecum after gentle insufflation, suggesting that this mucosal tears in the colon could occur spontaneously in patients with collagenous colitis.

In the same year, Curl Tysk *et al.*[7] reviewed the medical literature and reported longitudinal mucosal lacerations in the colon of patients with collagenous colitis (Figure 1 and 2), emphasizing that these lesions may be a sign of underlying collagenous colitis, and that mucosal biopsies should be obtained to confirm the diagnosis. Based on the previous reports that they had found, they advised that these lesions might be associated with an increased risk of colonic perforation, and that the colonoscopist should be aware that the risk of perforation is likely to be increased.

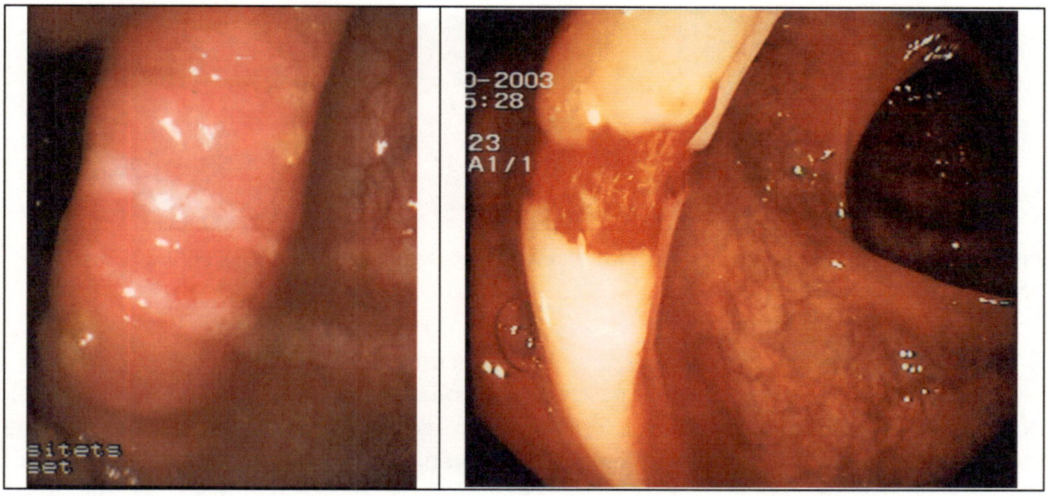

Fig. 1. Mucosal tears in patients with collagenous colitis (Courtesy of Dr Curt Tysk [7])

In 2008, Hashimoto *et al* [8] described a surprising finding in a patient with chronic diarrhea: a 20 cm long linear ulcer or scar like area of mucosal damage without bleeding in the descending colon. The biopsies taken revealed that it was a collagenous colitis.

In 2009, Couto *et al* [9] suggested that the scars found in the colonic mucosa were signs of scaring of previous spontaneous mucosal tears, superficial lacerations or "cat scratches" enhanced with air insufflation during colonoscopy in patients with collagenous colitis.

3.1.1 Drugs associated with mucosal tears

Umeno *et al* [10] and Nomura *et al* [11] have associated the presence of these linear mucosal defects to the drug lansoprazole, a proton bomb inhibitor. They found that linear mucosal defects and friable mucosa may be characteristic colonoscopic findings in cases of lanzoprale-associated collagenous colitis (Figure 2).

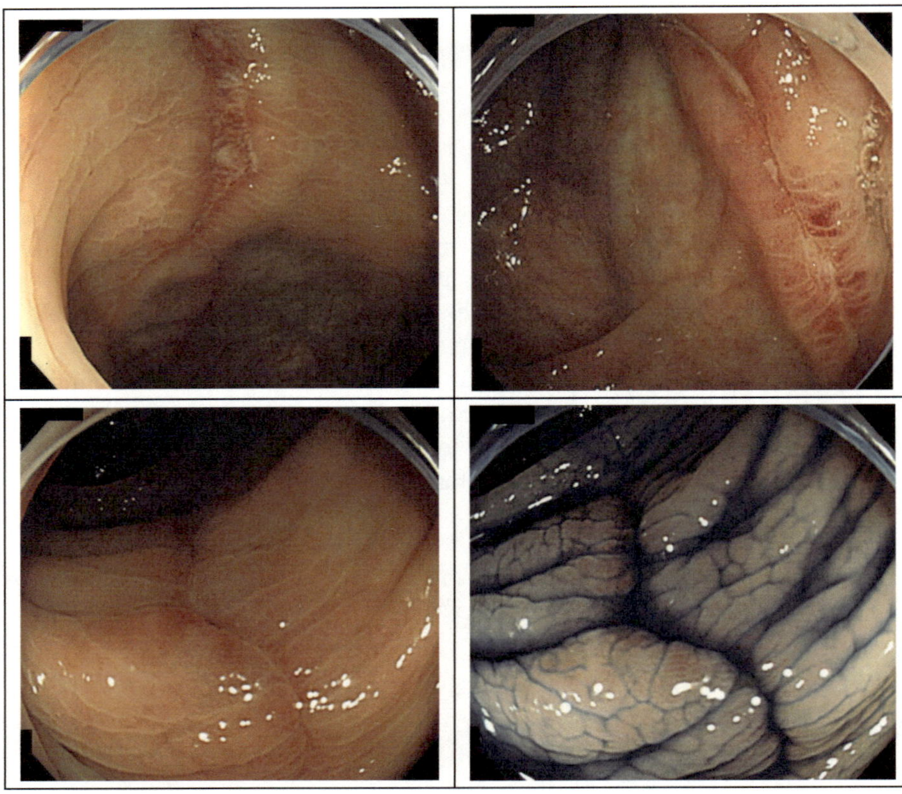

Fig. 2. Mucosal tears in patients with lansoprazole associated-collagenous colitis (Courtesy of Dr Eiki Nomura[11])

3.1.2 Risk of colonic perforation in patients with collagenous colitis

Several authors have suggested that patients with collagenous colitis have an increased risk of colonic perforation during the colonoscopy procedure. Most of them agree that the mucosal tears might be the initial lesion of the perforations.

Sherman *et al* [12] and Smith *et al* [13] found mucosal tears (linear "fractures" of the colon) following diagnostic colonoscopies in patients with severe collagenous colitis. They theorized that the stiffness of the colon in areas of collagenous colitis with submucosal fibrosis could made it susceptible to linear "fractures" during colonoscopic air insufflation with subsequent transmural air dissection. They urged extreme caution if these lesions were recognized at colonoscopy and recommended aborting the examination and obtaining plain radiographs to detect free intraperitoneal air.

Allende *et al* [14] published the largest series up to date about 12 patients with collagenous colitis complicated with colonic perforations. In their series the most outstanding colonoscopic findings were bleeding linear ulcers. They observed that the colon in collagenous colitis perforates not only with colonoscopy, but also with barium enema. Colonoscopic perforations were more common than barium enema, probably due to its higher intraluminal pressures. They thought that marked collagenous colitis severity was implicated as a risk factor for perforation. They found that the right colon was the most

common perforation site, corresponding to its preferential involvement by collagenous colitis and predisposing physical properties of the right colonic wall.
In 2010, Hussain *et al* [15] published a systematic review about the colonic perforations in patients with collagenous colitis. They did an exhaustive and systematic search and found 21 case reports of colonic perforation, mainly following colonoscopy. The site of colonic perforations and mucosal tears were predominantly in the right colon.

3.2 Other mucosal abnormalities

In 1997, Katsinelos *et al* [16] reported the presence of multiple red spots in the lower part of the ascending colon in a patient with chronic diarrhea. The histological examinations of the biopsies taken from this pathological area showed it was a collagenous colitis.
In 1998, Sato *et al* [17] reported a spindle network pattern after indigo carmine dye-spraying, in association with collagenous colitis.
In 2004, Alan Lewis Buchman *et al* [18] described an interesting endoscopic manifestation of collagenous colitis in two patients with chronic diarrhea: pseudomembrane formations (Figure 3) in the absence of Clostridium *difficile* infection. They used the term of "pseudomembranous collagenous colitis".

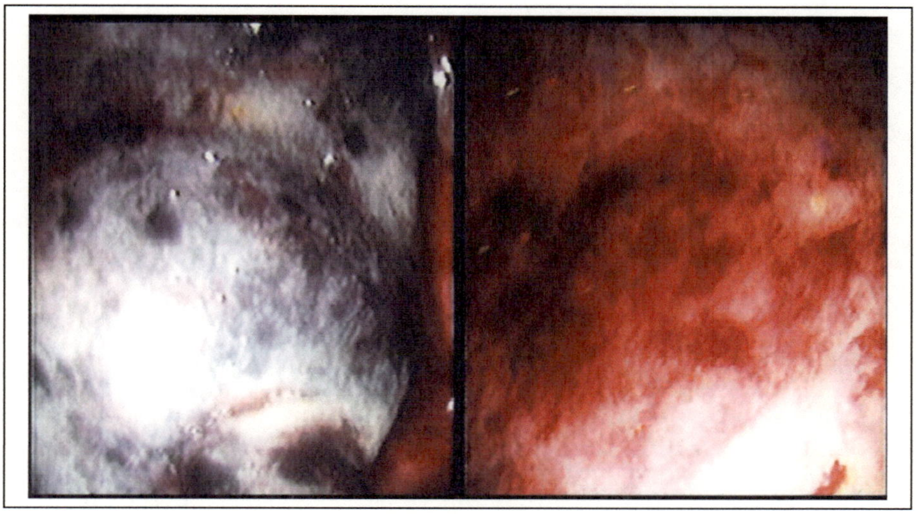

Fig. 3. Pseudomembranes in a patient with collagenous colitis (Courtesy of Dr Alan Buchman [18])

In 2008, Hashimoto *et al* [8] reported numerous crowded, small, dilated, circling or winding blood vessels on the mucosal surface of the entire colon, especially the transverse colon (appearing like a spider web) in association with this type of colitis.
In 2009, Hashimoto *et al* [19] found an actively hemorrhagic linear ulcer and a linear ulcer scar in a woman with abrupt onset of lower abdominal pain and heavy blood in her stool. Histopathological examination of biopsy samples taken showed subepithelial collagen bands and the diagnosis of collagenous colitis was made. They thought it was a case of lansoprazole-associated collagenous colitis with a unique presentation similar to an ischemic colitis.

In 2010, Cimmino *et al* [20] described a mosaic pattern as an endoscopic finding in the collagenous colitis (Figure 4). They compared the presence of this mosaic pattern in patients with chronic diarrhea, and they found that the presence of this colorectal mosaic pattern would have a high specificity (99%) and a high positive likelihood ratio (LR+ 17) for the diagnosis of collagenous colitis in patients with chronic diarrhea who undergo a colonoscopy.

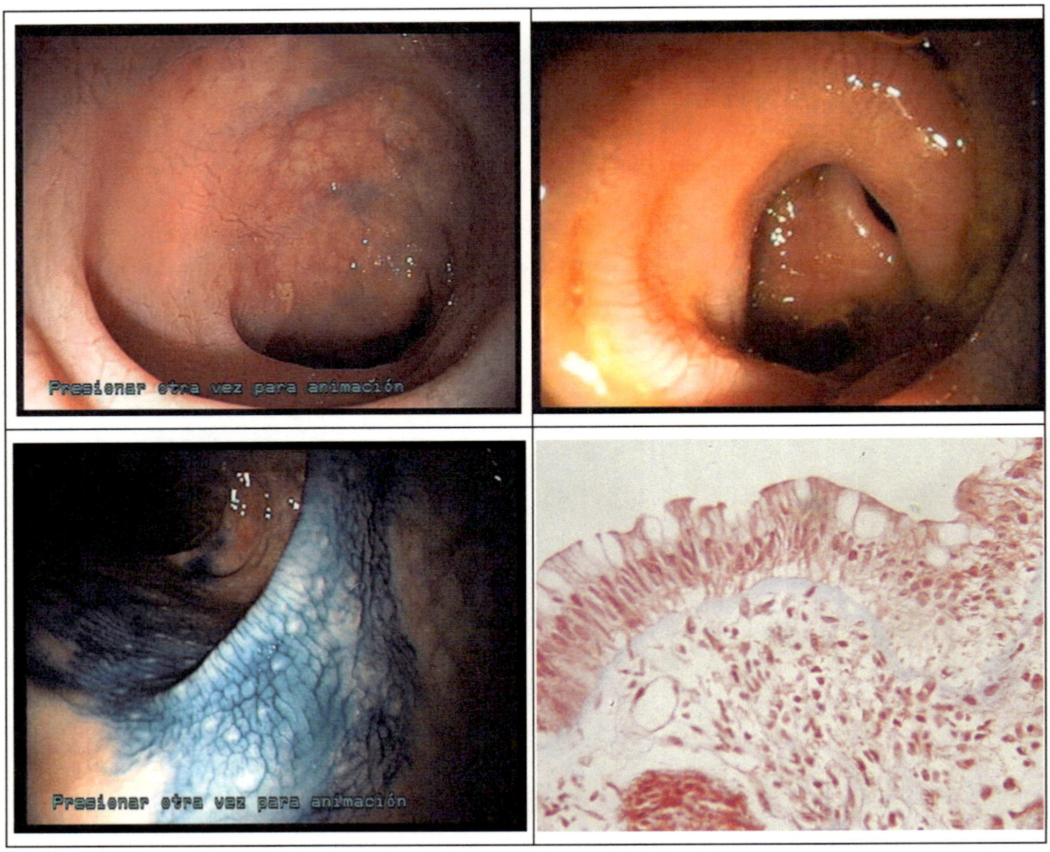

Fig. 4. Colorectal mosaic pattern in patients with collagenous colitis (Courtesy of Dr Cimmino [20])

4. The future of endoscopy in microscopic colitis

Endomicroscopy is a newly developed endoscopic modality, which allows in vivo microscopy of the mucosal layer in about 1000-times magnification with subcellular resolution during ongoing gastrointestinal endoscopy. This technique enables subsurface imaging of living tissue during ongoing endoscopy and allows confocal microscopy in addition to standard video endoscopy.

Kiesslich *et al* [22] showed that endomicroscopy allows localization and measurement of the amount of collagenous bands in the mucosal layer, offering the possibility of targeted biopsies, which would be a new approach in collagenous colitis.

5. Summary

The term microscopic colitis includes the collagenous colitis and the lymphocitic colitis, both entities are characterized by chronic diarrhea and normal colonoscopy, and the diagnosis is confirmed by biopsies taken at random. In recent years, abnormalities in the mucosa, mainly related with collagenous colitis, have been described. In Table 1 we summaries the mucosal patterns and the endoscopic manifestations which have been associated with collagenous colitis. Most of the reports mentioned the mucosal tears as the most frequent abnormality. Scars following mucosal lacerations were also a frequent finding. The risk of colonic perforations seems to be slightly higher in patients with collagenous colitis during colonoscopy. The main reason appears to be the lacerations done during air insufflations in the procedure. Other endoscopics findings were blood vessels alterations, pseudomembranes and mosaic pattern.

6. Conclusion

Several mucosal patterns and mucosal abnormalities have been reported in association with collagenous colitis. Knowledge of these endoscopic manifestations of the collagenous colitis could help to a better understanding of this disease and to target the colonic biopsies.

7. Acknowledgment

We want to thank Dr. Curl Tysk, Dr. Eiki Nomura and Dr. Alan Lewis Buchman for providing us the pictures and photos of their endoscopic findings. They have been very kind.

8. References

[1] Lindstrom CG. "Collagenous colitis" with watery diarrhoea – a new entity? Pathol Eur 1976;11:87.

[2] Beaugerie L, Napoleon B, Ponchon T, Boyer J, Canard JM, Dalbies P, Escourrou J, Greff M, Lapuelle J, Letard JC, Marchetti B, Palazzo L, Rey JF, Sautereau D; Société Française d'Endoscopie Digestive. Guidelines of the French Society for Digestive Endoscopy (SFED). Role of endoscopy in microscopic colitis. Endoscopy. 2005 Jan;37(1):97-8.

[3] Thijs WJ, van Baarlen J, Kleibeuker JH, Kolkman JJ. Microscopic colitis: prevalence and distribution throughout the colon in patients with chronic diarrhoea. Neth J Med. 2005 Apr;63(4):137-40.

[4] Richieri JP, Bonneau HP, Cano N, Di Costanzo J, Martin J. Collagenous colitis: an unusual endoscopic appearance. Gastrointest Endosc 1993; 39:192-4.

[5] Cruz-Correa M, Milligan F, Giardiello FM. Collagenous colitis with mucosal tear on endoscopic insufflation: a unique presentation. Gut 2002;51:600-600

[6] Koulaouzidis A, Henry JA, Saeed AA. Mucosal tears can occur spontaneously in collagenous colitis. Endoscopy 2006; 38:549.

[7] Wickbom A, Lindqvist M, Bohr J, Ung KA, Bergman J, Eriksson S, Tysk C. Colonic mucosal tears in collagenous colitis. Scand J Gastroenterol 2006; Jun;41(6): 726-9.

[8] Hashimoto Y, Endo Y, Kuroki Y, Yoshikumi H, Yoshiba M. Collagenous colitis with unique colonoscopic findings. Endoscopy. 2008 Sep;40 Suppl 2:E162.

[9] Couto G, Bispo M, Barreiro P, Monteiro L, Matos L. Unique endoscopy findings in collagenous colitis. Gastrointest Endosc. 2009 May;69(6):1186-8.

[10] Umeno J, Matsumoto T, Nakamura S, Jo Y, Yada S, Hirakawa K, Yoshimura R, Yamagata H, Kudo T, Hirano A, Gushima M, Yao T, Nakashima Y, Iida M. Linear mucosal defect may be characteristic of lansoprazole-associated collagenous colitis. Gastrointest Endosc. 2008 Jun;67(7):1185-91.

[11] Nomura E, Kagaya H, Uchimi K, Noguchi T, Suzuki S, Suzuki M, Onodera H, Tateno H. Linear mucosal defects: a characteristic endoscopic finding of lansoprazole-associated collagenous colitis. Endoscopy. 2010;42 Suppl 2:E9-10.

[12] Sherman A, Ackert JJ, Rajapaksa R, et al. Fractured colon: an endoscopically distinctive lesion associated with colonic perforation following colonoscopy in patients with collagenous colitis. J Clin Gastroenterol 2004; 38:341–345.

[13] Smith RR, Ragput A. Mucosal tears on endoscopic insufflation resulting in perforation: an interesting presentation of collagenous colitis. J Am Coll Surg. 2007 Nov;205(5):725.

[14] Allende DS, Taylor SL, Bronner MP. Colonic perforation as a complication of collagenous colitis in a series of 12 patients. Am J Gastroenterol. 2008 Oct;103(10):2598-604.

[15] Hussain Z, Kelly S, Clarke A, Adams S, Miller G. Colonic perforation in collagenous colitis: a systematic review of a rare complication and guidance on management. Surg Endosc. 2010 Dec;24(12):2930-4.

[16] Katsinelos P, Katsos I, Patsiaoura K, Xiarchos P, Goulis I, Eugenidis N. A new endoscopic appearance of collagenous colitis. Endoscopy 1997;Feb;29(2):135.

[17] Sato S, Benoni C, Tóth E, Veress B, Fork FT. Chromoendoscopic appearance of collagenous colitis--a case report using indigo carmine. Endoscopy 1998;Sep;30(7):S80–1.

[18] Buchman AL, Rao S. Pseudomembranous collagenous colitis. Dig Dis Sci. 2004 Nov-Dec;49(11-12):1763-7.

[19] Yusuke H, Jun T, Naotaka M, Yuichi T, Yutaka E, Kazuaki I. Lansoprazole-associated collagenous colitis: unique presentation, similar to ischemic colitis. Endoscopy. 2009;41 Suppl 2:E281-2.

[20] Daniel G. Cimmino, José M. Mella, Lisandro Pereyra, Pablo A.E. Luna, Gabriel Casas, Ignacio Caldo, Federico Popoff, Silvia Pedreira, Luis A. Boerr. "A colorectal mosaic pattern might be an endoscopic feature of collagenous colitis". Journal of Crohn's and Colitis 2010, 4:139-143

[21] Dunzendorfer T, Wilkins S, Johnson R. Mucosal tear in collagenous colitis. Clin Gastroenterol Hepatol. 2009 Sep; 7(9):e57.

[22] Kiesslich R, Hoffman A, Goetz M, Biesterfeld S, Vieth M, Galle PR, Neurath MF. In vivo diagnosis of collagenous colitis by confocal endomicroscopy. Gut. 2006 Apr;55(4): 591-2.

8

Endoscopic Approach in Ulcerative Colitis

Rogério Saad-Hossne[1] and Fábio V. Teixeira[2]
[1]*Medical School - UNESP Botucatu, São Paulo,*
[2]*Medical School - UNESP Botucatu and GI Surgeon and consultant of UNIGASTRO e Clínica GASTROSAUDE, Marília, São Paulo, Brazil*

1. Introduction

The term inflammatory bowel disease (IBD) is frequently used in the medical literature to define a set of diseases involving the digestive tract, particularly the small and the large intestine. The major IBDs are Crohn's Disease (CD) and ulcerative colitis (UC).

Ulcerative colitis is a chronic inflammatory disease characterized by diffuse mucosal inflammation limited to the colon. UC affects 500,000 individuals in the United States with an incidence of 12 per 100,000 per year. The lifetime risk of a severe exacerbation of UC requiring hospitalization is 15%. Patients with extensive disease (macroscopic disease proximal to the splenic flexure) are more likely to develop acute severe colitis. Approximately 4% to 9% of UC patients will require colectomy within the first year of diagnosis; the risk of colectomy following that is 1% per year. The vast majority of UC patients will require medical therapy throughout their lifetime.

Ulcerative colitis, usually, involves the rectum at presentation and may extend proximally in a symmetrical, circumferential, and continuous pattern to involve parts or all of the large intestine. The disease course of UC is characterized by exacerbations and remissions, which may occur spontaneously or in response to treatment changes, superimposed infection. The diagnosis of inflammatory bowel disease is based on clinical history in combination with the results of various tests, once a single pathognomonic test allowing for a diagnostic definition is not available. Hence, the following can be cited: radiology, laboratory and hematological tests, and endoscopy combined with histology in particular.[1-3]

With this respect, endoscopy has revolutionized the management of patients with IBD by increasingly enabling the identification and study of lesions. Some more recent advances in endoscopic techniques can be cited, such as double-balloon enteroscopy and the capsule endoscopy, which allow for evaluating areas of the small intestine that have not been thoroughly studied to this date, in addition to digital chromoendoscopy.

Improvement in IBD diagnostic capacity has direct implications in the diagnosis and follow-up of patients that have or are suspected to have IBD as well as in better understanding their pathogenesis, which consequently influences treatment.

Great changes have occurred in IBD treatment and management in the last few decades due to the introduction of biological agents in its therapeutic arsenal. Biological therapy, represented by its major drugs - anti-TNF antibodies - has rapidly become the top of a mountain whose base is represented by other drugs that have been used in the treatment of inflammatory bowel disease for several decades.

These new drugs directly interfere with the individual's immune response by decreasing the activation of T cells and inducing apoptosis of defense cells, thus controlling this complex mechanism which is still not fully known and triggers diseases such as ulcerative colitis and Crohn's Disease.
Some time ago, it was believed that the most important objective in treatment would be the patient's clinical remission, normally based on symptom and sign scores, in CD (CDAI - Crohn's disease activity index < 150 points), and in UC (Mayo Score < 5 points). However, after the advent of biological therapy, which induces healing of the inflamed intestinal mucosa, such objectives have changed, that is, in addition to seeking sustained clinical remission, mucosal healing should also be sought.
Due to these characteristics and to the fact that such healing can be maintained for long periods, it is believed that the development and prognosis of IBD will also change.
As previously pointed out, mucosal healing is one of the objectives of clinical trials and of daily clinical practice. For this reason, endoscopy, and colonoscopy in particular, assumes a major role in these patients' follow-up by enabling the direct visualization of the mucosa as well as the removal of fragments for histological analysis.

2. Indications

The diagnosis of UC can be suggested initially by sigmoidoscopy in great number of cases during first attack of UC, fewest biopsies usually are sufficient to confirm the diagnosis and indicate the initial therapy. In patients with diarrhea, mucus, active and flares, this exam can be performed in unprepared bowel so the earliest signs of UC can be detected; other reason to do the sigmoidoscopy without bowel prep is to decrease the hyperemia that is often present after enemas.
In this active fase, colonoscopy is not recommended for fear of perforation and the risk of cause great distention in colon. Only after this acute and active fase the colonoscopy can be performed to establish the extent of the disease and to exclude other disease and Crohn's disease.
The initial aim points in colonoscopy are to evaluate both the extension and intensity of UC. In a second moment, to evaluate the response to the treatment. Thus, the colonoscopy is useful to make the diagnosis, to follow the evolution and response and finally prevent colorectal cancer (displasia).
The most recent studies confirm that the mucosal healing is the end point of treatment, so the indications of colonoscopy do not resume in diagnostic only. In TABLE 1, are the most important indications of colonoscopy in UC.

Acute	Sub acute	chronic
Diagnosis	Extension	Treatment response
Biopsy	Intensity	Displasia surveillance
Differential diagnosis	Biopsy	Cancer surveillance
	Treatment response	

Table 1. Indications of colonoscopy in ulcerative colitis

3. Bowel preparation

Correct diagnostic of colonoscopy depends on the quality of the colonic preparation or cleansing. The ideal preparation should reliably empty the colon of fecal material in a rapid fashion and do not cause histological alteration or gross of the rectal and colonic mucosa.

For patients, the preparation should not cause discomfort and shifts in electrolytes and fluids; those are the ideal bowel preparation, unfortunately none of the preparations available meet them.

Recently, the American Society of Colon and Rectal Surgeons (ASCRS), the American Society for Gastrointestinal Endoscopy (ASGE), and the Society of American Gastrointestinal and Endoscopic Surgeons (SAGES) made a document: "A Consensus Document on Bowel Preparation Before Colonoscopy". [4] Based on this document the recommendations are (grade of recommendation supported by evidence-based medicine):

1. Diet- Dietary modifications, such as a clear liquid diet, alone are inadequate for colonoscopy. However, they have proven to be a beneficial adjunct to other mechanical cleansing methods (Grade IIB).
2. Enemas - Use enemas in patients who present to endoscopy with a poor distal colon preparation and in patients with a defunctionalized distal colon.
3. High-Volume Gut Lavage - Neither high-volume nor unbalanced solutions, such as mannitol, should be used for colonic preparation (Grade IA). In addition, caution should be exercised when using nasogastric tubes for the administration of any bowel preparation infusion (Grade VD).
4. Rectal Pulsed Irrigation - administered immediately before the procedure combined with magnesium citrate given the evening before the procedure is a reasonable alternative to full-volume (4-liters) PEG in those individuals who cannot tolerate per oral administration of PEG (Grade IIB).
5. PEG - Faster, more effective, and better-tolerated method for cleansing the colon than a restricted diet combined with cathartics, high-volume gut lavage, or mannitol/NaP (Grade IA). PEG is safer than osmotic laxatives/NaP for patients with electrolyte or fluid imbalances, such as renal or liver insufficiency, congestive heart failure, or liver failure and is, therefore, preferable in these patient groups (Grade IA). Divided-dose PEG regimens (2–3 liters given the night before the colonoscopy and 1–2 liters on the morning of procedure) are acceptable alternative regimens that enhance patient tolerance (Grade IIB). Cleansing preparations for colonoscopies performed in the afternoon should instruct that at least part of the PEG solution be given the morning before the procedure (Grade IIB). Enemas, bisacodyl, and metaclopramide as adjuncts to the full volume of PEG have not been demonstrated to improve colonic cleansing or patient tolerance and are, therefore, unnecessary (Grade IIB).
6. NaP - Aqueous NaP colonic preparation is an equal alternative to PEG solutions except for pediatric and elderly patients, patients with bowel obstruction, and other structural intestinal disorders, gut dysmotility, renal or failure, congestive heart failure, or liver failure (Grade IA). Dosing of aqueous NaP should be 45 ml in divided doses, 10 to 12 hours apart with one of the doses taken on the morning of the procedure (Grade IIB). Aqueous NaP is the preferable form of NaP at this time (Grade IIB). Apart from anecdotal reports, the addition of adjuncts to the standard NaP regimen has not demonstrated any dramatic effect on colonic cleansing preparation. Carbohydrate-electrolyte solutions such as E-Lyte\ may improve safety and tolerability.

In those patients with possible underlying IBD, NaP preparations may cause mucosal abnormalities that mimic Crohn's disease [5-7]. However, the frequency of this problem is rare and may not mitigate against using NaP. This caveat is most important in the initial colonoscopic evaluation of patients with symptoms suspect for colitis.
We may conclued that bowel preparation is safe for patients with UC and must be avoid in acute phases.

4. Macroscopic characteristics of ulcerative colitis

The macroscopic characteristic of UC is symmetrical and continuous inflammation, which begins in the rectum and extends proximally without interruption during the whole extension of the disease. When present, this aspect is easily made visible by colonoscopy.
The figure 1 shows the initial endoscopic signs of UC:

1. Reduction or loss of normal vascular patterns.
2. Loss or distortion of vascular markings and relief, and, many times, this aspect may be the only endoscopic alteration in patients with UC in its quiescent phase
3. Mucosal erythema and edema

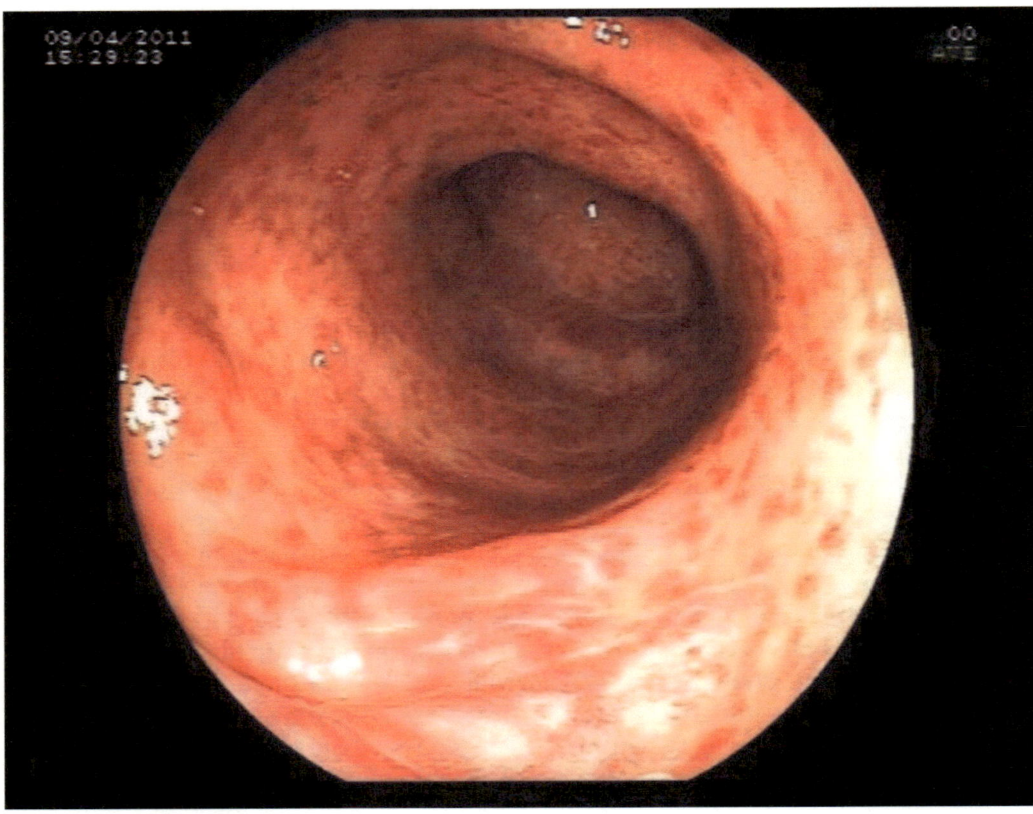

Fig. 1. Mucosal friability, loss of vascular pattern, eythema and edema

As the disease progresses, the mucosal pattern changes, becomes extremely friable, and shows a granular aspect. The disease, then, enters the most severe phase, when the mucosa is covered with yellowish and sometimes mucopurulent exudate, with intense ulceration of the adjacent mucosa. (FIGURE 2) Such exulceration and ulceration pattern is mainly characterized by a serpiginous, linear, dotted or annular aspect, or even an association of such aspects. As to size, they may vary from millimeters to centimeters, and may, at times, be deep, depending on the phase and inflammation intensity.

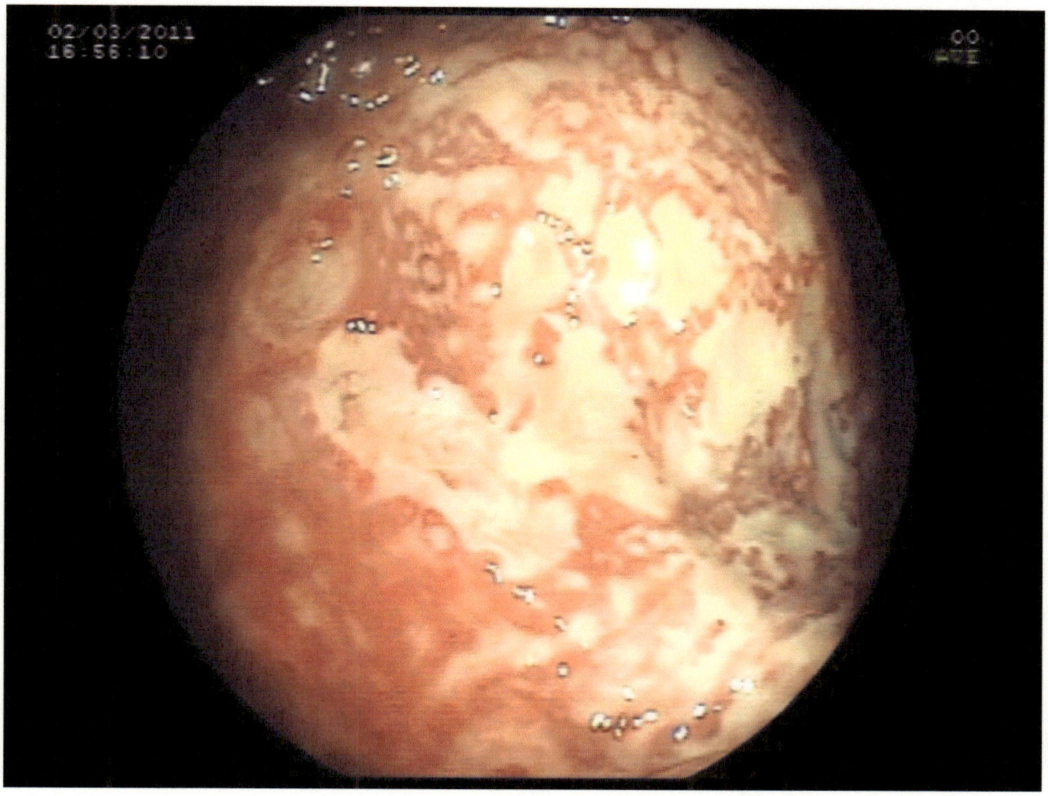

Fig. 2. Colonic mucosa with intense ulceration covered with yellowish and mucopurulent exudates

In the active and acute phase of the disease, a simple touch to these lesions by the instrument may cause bleeding due to mucosal friability. Another important aspect is that when such edema is intense and diffuse, it may lead to lumen narrowing. The differential diagnosis is made by adenomatous polyps, which can only be differentiated under microscopy. Another important differential diagnosis is made by CD. Crohn´s colitis endoscopic features includes: skip lesions(pathchy inflammation adjacent to normal mucosa), rectal sparing, aphtous ulcerations and cobblestone appearance of the mucosa due to the presence of deep linear ulcers.

The inflammation/cicatrization process may lead to the onset of pseudopolyp images, which, in reality, are healthy mucosal areas amidst areas of an intense inflammatory process. (FIGURE 3) They can be characterized by endoscopy with small, bright and soft lesions that may develop to large pedunculated or sessile lesions. Also, they may be detected both in the acute and chronic phases of the disease and are largely suggestive of UC, showing the appearance of cobble-like shapes both by colonoscopy and opaque enema.

Other endoscopic aspects that can be made visible in patients with a chronic form of the disease are:

1. Loss of normal haustration patterns
2. Loss of normal colon architecture, with muscle hypertrophy
3. Colon shortening
4. Luminal diameter reduction
5. Stenosis. In this case, the differential diagnosis is made from cancer.

With this regard, some UC endoscopic activity scales have been developed with the purpose to classify and quantify such inflammatory activity in the colonic mucosa. The scale proposed and used by the Mayo Clinic is noteworthy.

Stool frequency	
0	Normal
1	1-2 stools/day more than normal
2	3-4 stools/day more than normal
3	>4 stools/day more than normal
Rectal bleeding[a]	
0	None
1	Visible blood with stool less than half the time
2	Visible blood with stool half of the time or more
3	Passing blood alone
Mucosal appearance at endoscopy[b]	
0	Normal or inactive disease
1	Mild disease (erythema, decreased vascular pattern, mild friability)
2	Moderate disease (marked erythema, absent vascular pattern, friability, erosions)
3	Severe disease (spontaneous bleeding, ulceration)
Physician rating of disease activity	
0	Normal
1	Mild
2	Moderate
3	Severe

[a]A score of 3 for bleeding required patients to have at least 50% of bowel motions accompanied by visible blood and at least one bowel motion with blood alone.

[b]The mucosal appearance at endoscopy is not included in the Partial Mayo Score.

Table 2. Mayo score for ulcerative colitis *

* from: Cima RR, Pemberton JH. Medical and surgical management of chronic ulcerative colitis. Arch Surg. 2005;140(3):300-10

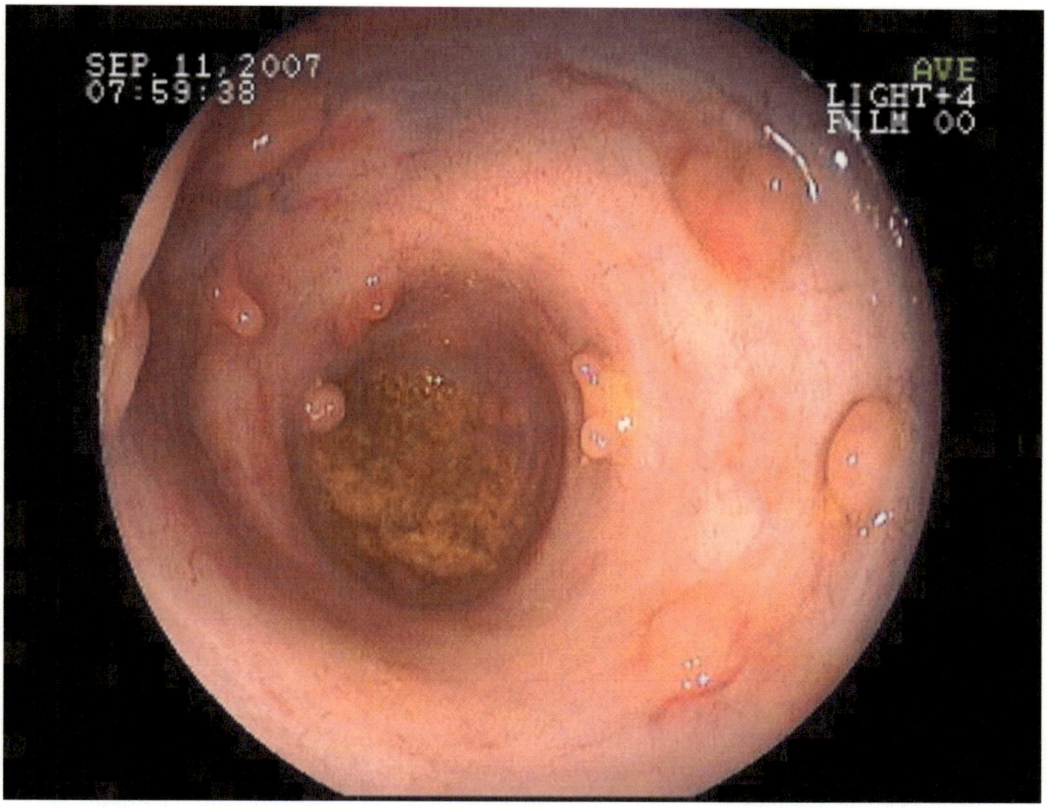

Fig. 3. Pseudopolyps and colonic mucosal healing after infliximab treatment

5. Histology

The histological analysis of biopsy has the following aims: confirm the UC diagnosis, graduate the inflammatory response and third, confirm the presence of displasia or cancer.

An early and accurate diagnosis is necessary. It is important to distinguish between IBD and acute self-limited colitis and a differential diagnosis between UC and CD. The histopathological diagnosis of UC should, therefore, be based on discriminating histological features which are sufficiently reproducible and suitable in routinely processed biopsy specimens.

In cases where the clinical picture is unclear, the histomorphologic analysis often plays a pivotal role in determining the diagnosis and thus the management. By contrast, a biopsy analysis may be indeterminate, and thus the clinical progression of the disease must inform its treatment.

Great changes have occurred in IBD treatment and management in the last few decades due to the introduction of biological agents in its therapeutic arsenal. Thus, mucosal healing is one of the objectives of clinical trials and of daily clinical practice. FIGURE 3 For this reason, colonoscopy assumes a major role in these patients' follow-up by enabling the direct visualization of the mucosa as well as the removal of fragments for histological analysis.[11-19]

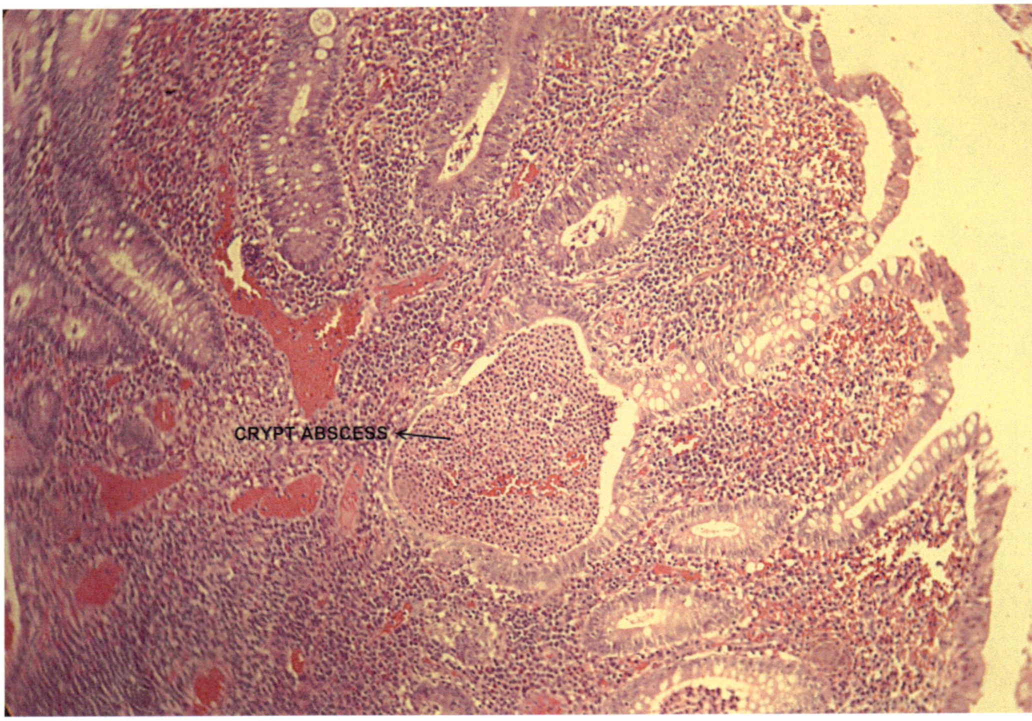

Fig. 4. Photomicrography of a colectomy specimen (pancolitis): we observe distortion of crypt architecture, inflammation of crypts (cryptitis) and crypt abcess (arrow) Courtesy of Prof. Dr. Marcus M. Matsushita, professor of the Pathology Department of the Hospital Universitário - ABHU, Medical School of the University of Marilia, São Paulo, Brazil. www.unimar.br

6. Dysplasia and Colorectal Cancer (CRC) surveillance

Dysplasia is considered the best marker of cancer risk in UC. The clinical management depends on the endoscopic and histological identification of dysplasia in mucosal biopsy specimens of the colon by pathologists with particular expertise in gastrointestinal disorders. The dysplasia can be divided in two groups: low-grade dysplasia (LGD) and high-grade dysplasia (HGD), not all patients with LGD will progress through detectable HGD. Patients with HGD have higher risk of progression to colorectal cancer.[19]

Rubin and colleagues in Seattle showed that among a group of colectomy specimens obtained from UC patients, 33 biopsies per examination was the number of nontargeted biopsies required to exclude dysplasia with 90% confidence. [19] It has being reported that 80% to 90% of UC patients with cancer have dysplasia when analyzed the colectomy specimen. However, colorectal cancer can develop in patients without a prior history of dysplasia. [14-15,19]

In a meta-analysis with 116 published studies, Eaden and colleagues found that the overall prevalence of CRC in any patient with UC is 3.7% which increases to 5.4% for those with pancolitis. [18] The cumulative risk for CRC of any patient with UC is 2% at 10 years, 8% at 20 years, and 18% at 30 years. Increasing duration of disease is as one of the most important risk factors for the development of cancer in UC, which is significant after 9 years of disease and increases in subsequent years.[13-19] The extension of the disease is also a risk factor for cancer. Most cancers arise in patients when the whole colon is affected (pancolitis). Patients with UC beyond the distal sigmoid and rectum are at increase risk of CRC and risk is intermediate in patients with left-sided disease and lower in patients with proctitis.[14-19]

Recently, we have published the Brazilian consensus for management of IBD. Supported by evidence-based medicine, we recommend that the screening should be performed using colonoscopy every 3 years in the 2nd decade, every 2 years in the 3rd decade and yearly in the 4th decade of illness together with 4-quadrant biopsies of non-inflamed mucosal at every 10 cm of colon, in the whole colon in association with biopsies of suspected areas. [14]

7. Chromoendoscopy

Because of the limitations of what could be seen with traditional colonoscopies emitting white light, adjunct techniques have been investigated in colitis and sporadic polyp surveillance practices that have the potential to enable endoscopists to better visualize the colorectal mucosa. It has being demonstrated a higher diagnostic accuracy for dysplasia diagnosis in biopsies targeted by chromoendoscopy when compared to biopsies obtained with standard colonoscopy.[17] Chromo colonoscopy with biopsy of suspected area is a valid alternative to multiple biopsies.[14] There are a stronger correlation between the endoscopic assessment of colonic inflammation and histopathologic findings. In this scenario, chromoendoscopy allow for the differentiation between nonneoplastic and neoplastic lesions with a sensitivity and specificity of 93%.

It became apparent that adding an adjunct technique would enable us to identify more patients with dysplasia. Unfortunately, however, there are no longitudinal data showing that chromoendoscopy actually lessens either the incidence of dysplasia on follow-up colonoscopy or cancer-related morbidity or mortality. On the other hand, once this technique are inexpensive, safe, and relatively easy to perform, it should be have an important role in surveillance of dysplasia and cancer in UC patients.

8. Narrow Band Imaging (NBI)

Narrow band imaging (NBI) and Multi-Band Imaging (MBI)* are real-time, on-demand endoscopic imaging techniques designed to enhance visualization of the vascular network and surface texture of the mucosa in an effort to improve tissue characterization, differentiation, and diagnosis. [17] NBI and MBI were developed to be an alternative to chromoendoscopy. The techniques may allow contrast enhancement of tissue surface structures helping in the endoscopic diagnosis. In contrast, neither NBI nor MBI have being studied extensively as chromoendoscopy.[17]

It has being reported in the literature that, in ulcerative colitis, the role of NBI is not as promising as observed in other scenarios. [8-10] On the other hand, in an uncontrolled study consisting of 46 patients with ulcerative colitis, the relative frequency of dysplasia was higher in areas of tortuous pattern (8%) than in those of honeycomb-like or villous pattern (0.4%), as seen under NBI with magnification. The tortuous pattern determined by NBI may be a clue for the identification of dysplasia during surveillance of UC. [9,16]

9. References

[1] Meyers S, Janowitz HD. The "natural history" of ulcerative colitis: an analysis of the placebo response. J Clin Gastro- enterol 1989;11(1):33–37

[2] Loftus EV Jr, Silverstein MD, Sandborn WJ, Tremaine WJ, Harmsen WS, Zinsmeister AR. Ulcerative colitis in Olmsted County, Minnesota, 1940-1993: incidence, prevalence, and survival. Gut 2000;46(3):336–343

[3] Kappelman MD, Rifas-Shiman SL, Kleinman K, et al. The prevalence and geographic distribution of Crohn's disease and ulcerative colitis in the United States. Clin Gastroenterol Hepatol 2007;5(12):1424–1429

[4] Rejchrt S, Bures J, Siroky M, Kopacova M, Slezak L, Langr F. A prospective, observational study of colon- ic mucosal abnormalities associated with orally administered sodium phosphate for colon cleansing before colonoscopy. Gastrointest Endosc 2004;59: 651 - 654.

[5] Zwas FR, Cirillo NW, el-Serag HB, Eisen RN. Colonic mucosal abnormalities associated with oral sodium phosphate solution. Gastrointest Endosc 1996;43:463 - 6

[6] Wong NA, Penman ID, Campbell S, Lessells AM. Microscopic focal cryptitis associated with sodium phosphate bowel preparation. Histopathology 2000; 36:476 - 8

[7] Matsumoto T, Esaki M, Fujisawa R, Nakamura S, Yao T, Iida M. Chromoendoscopy, narrow-band imaging colono- scopy, and autofluorescence colonoscopy for detection of diminutive colorectal neoplasia in familial adenomatous polyposis. Dis Colon Rectum 2009;52(6):1160–1165

[8] Tung SY, Wu CS, Su MY. Magnifying colonoscopy in differentiating neoplastic from nonneoplastic colorectal lesions. Am J Gastroenterol 2001;96(9):2628–2632

[9] Song LM, Adler DG, Conway JD, et al; ASGE TECH-NOLOGY COMMITTEE. Narrow band imaging and multiband imaging. Gastrointest Endosc 2008;67(4):581– 589

[10] Cima RR, Pemberton JH. Medical and surgical management of chronic ulcerative colitis. Arch Surg. 2005 Mar;140(3):300-10

[11] Lichtenstein GR, Rutgeerts P. Importance of mucosal healing in ulcerative colitis. Inflamm Bowel Dis. 2010;16(2):338-46.

[12] Frøslie KF, Jahnsen J, Moum BA, Vatn MH; IBSEN Group. Mucosal healing in inflammatory bowel disease: results from a Norwegian population-based cohort. Gastroenterology. 2007;133(2):412-22.

[13] Fratila OC, Craciun C. Ultrastructural evidence of mucosal healing after infliximab in patients with ulcerative colitis. J Gastrointestin Liver Dis. 2010;19(2):147-53.

[14] Consensus guidelines for the management of inflammatory bowel disease. Brazilian Study Group of Inflammatory Bowel Diseases. Arq Gastroenterol. 2010;47(3):313-25.

[15] Ekbom A, Helmick C, Zack M, Adami HO. Ulcerative colitis and colorectal cancer. A population-based study. N Engl J Med. 1990;323(18):1228-33.

[16] Lukas M. Inflammatory bowel disease as a risk factor for colorectal cancer. Dig Dis. 2010;28(4-5):619-24.

[17] Matsumoto T, Kudo T, Jo Y, et al. Magnifying colonoscopy with narrow band imaging system for the diagnosis of dysplasia in ulcerative colitis: a pilot study. Gastrointest Endosc 2007;66:957-65.

[18] Eaden JA, Abrams KR, Mayberry JF. The risk of colorectal cancer in ulcerative colitis: a meta-analysis. Gut. 2001;48(4):526-35.

[19] Rubin DT, Rothe JA, Hetzel JT, Cohen RD, Hanauer SB. Are dysplasia and colorectal cancer endoscopically visible in patients with ulcerative colitis? Gastrointest Endosc. 2007 Jun;65(7):998-1004.

9

Pathological Issues of Ulcerative Colitis/Dysplasia

Tomita S.[1], Fujii S.[2] and Fujimori T[1]
[1]*Department of Surgical and Molecular Pathology, DOKKYO Medical University School of Medicine*
[2]*Center for Gastrointestinal Endoscopy, Kyoto-Katsura Hospital*
Japan

1. Introduction

The first ulcerative colitis (UC)-associated carcinoma (colitic cancer) appears to have been 14-year history of UC (Fujii et al., 2002, as cited in Crohn & Rosenberg, 1925). It is widely accepted that inflammation plays important roles in the development of various cancers, and indeed, patients with UC show an increased incidence of colorectal neoplasia, and UC-associate dysplasia/neoplasia represents a major cause of increased mortality in such patients. In order to improve the prognosis of patients with UC-associated dysplasia/neoplasia, diagnosis at an early or precancerous stage is crucial. Predisposition to colorectal dysplasia/neoplasia in UC is generally considered to depend on 2 risk factors, namely the presence of long-standing disease and extensive colitis (Fujii et al., 2008, as cited in Ekbom, et al., 1990, and Eaden et al., 2001). Thus, colitic cancers are believed to arise through a chronic inflammation-dysplasia-carcinoma sequence, and therefore early detection of precancerous dysplasia is very important for optimizing the prognosis of patients with long-standing UC. In a clinical setting, UC patients are monitored for dysplasia endoscopically on a regular basis, but it is difficult to discriminate UC-associated dysplasia/neoplasia from inflamed regenerating epithelium even by pathological examination. Therefore, surveillance colonoscopy with multiple random biopsies has been widely recommended for patients with long-standing and extensive UC. However, because UC-associated dysplasia/neoplasia is often difficult to detect endoscopically and to discriminate from inflammatory regenerative epithelium histologically, it remains a matter of contention whether conventional surveillance colonoscopy is effective for the early detection of UC-associated dysplasia/neoplasia. Here we describe the ulcerative colitis/dysplasia based on pathology and discuss relevant issues in arriving at the correct differential diagnosis based on morphological, immunohistochemical and molecular findings.

2. Risk factor and clinicopathological characteristics of dysplasia/neoplasia development in the patients with ulcerative colitis

The reported prevalence rates of colitic cancer range from 1 to 10% of all patients with UC. This increased risk, above that of the general population, appears approximately 8–10 years after the onset of the disease. The risk increases with the duration of disease and is greater in persons with extensive colitis (Fujii et al., 2002, as cited in Dobbins, 1984). A cumulative incidence of colorectal cancer was 5–10% with UC of 20 years duration and 12–20% with UC of 30 years duration (Fujii et al., 2002, as cited in Levin, 1995). The risk of colorectal cancer in patients with left-sided colitis was considered to increase 20 years after the onset of UC. Moreover incidence of colitic cancer in patients with left-sided disease did not differ from that in patients with pancolitis. In order to detect UC-associated dysplasia/neoplasia and the early stages of cancer, surveillance colonoscopy has been recommended for patients with long-standing and extensive UC. In Japan, possibly because the number of UC patients with dysplasia/neoplasia is smaller than that in Western countries. We reviewed Japanese case reports of UC-associated dysplasia/neoplasia published between 1990 and 2002 (Fujii et al., 2003b). Of 118 patients with UC-associated neoplasia, 41 underwent surveillance colonoscopy (surveillance group), 64 did not (nonsurveillance group), and the remaining 13 cases were unknown as to surveillance status. The 64 UC associated neoplasias including colitic cancer (UC associated carcinoma) in the nonsurveillance group were found by colonoscopy that was undertaken because of developing symptomatic episode, or for the evaluation of inflammation activities. The depth of tumor invasion, incidence of lymph node metastasis, incidence of liver metastasis, and stage in the two groups are shown in Table 1.

	Surveillance (41)	Nonsurveillance (64)
Depth of neoplastic invasion		
Tis	11	11
T1	12	5
T2	5	6
T3	10	30
T4	0	6
Unknown	3	6
Lymph node metastasis		
Positive	4	25
Negative	25	23
Unknown	12	16
Liver metastasis, positive	1	4
Peritoneal dissemination, positive	0	7
Dukes' stage		
A	22	15
B	2	8
C	4	25
Unknown	13	16

Table 1. Clinicopathological features of neoplasias in the surveillance and nonsurveillance groups (adapted from Fujii et al., 2003b)

Regarding depth of tumor invasion, early colorectal cancer, defined as tumor invading the lamina propria and/or muscularis mucosae and/or submucosa, was more frequent in the surveillance group than in the nonsurveillance group (60.5% vs. 27.6%). The incidence of lymph node metastasis was lower in the surveillance group than in the nonsurveillance group (13.8% vs. 52.1%). Four out of the five tumors associated with liver metastasis and, all seven tumors associated with peritoneal dissemination were in the nonsurveillance group. The distribution of Dukes' stages in the two groups was: A/B/C, 78.6%/7.1%/14.3% in the surveillance group, compared with 31.2%/16.7%/52.1% in the nonsurveillance group. Similar to Western countries, surveillance colonoscopy in Japan contributes to the early detection of UC-associated dysplasia/neoplasia. The surveillance colonoscopy appears to contribute to the early detection and excellent prognosis of UC-associated dysplasia/neoplasia. But it still remains questionable whether surveillance colonoscopy with multiple-step biopsy effectively enables the early detection of UC-associated dysplasia/neoplasia.

3. The morphological, immunohistochemical and molecular finding of ulcerative colitis/dysplasia

Morphological futures of macroscopic and endoscopic images, UC-associated dysplasia/neoplasias in the precancerous and early stages show various changes. Such dysplasia/neoplasias are often flat, plaque-like, and superficially elevated or even depressed, and frequently appear as faintly red, mildly discoloured, finely villous, and granular (Fig.1).

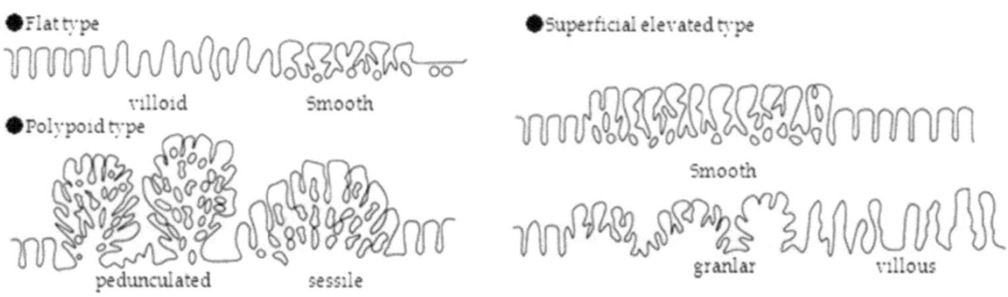

Fig. 1. Morphological classification of dysplastic epithelium in ulcerative colitis. (adapted from Fujii et al., 2002)

Macroscopic and endoscopic changes are not clear, and are sometimes missed in chronically inflamed epithelium. Detecting UC-associated dysplasia/neoplasias in the precancerous and early stages is difficult by macroscopy (Fig.2), endoscopy (Fig.3a), and stereomicroscopic finding (Fig.3b). We retrospectively verified the percentage of UC-associated dysplasia/neoplasias that was detectable endoscopically before surgical resection (Yamagishi et al., 2009). When classified UC-associated dysplastic/neoplastic lesions according to macroscopic appearance, 79.1% lesions were of flat-type. In detail, 92.5% dysplasias, 80.9% Tis carcinomas, 60% T1 carcinomas were of flat (flat and superficial elevated type), whereas 6 of 7 (85.7%) T2-4 carcinomas were protruding (polypoid type). In each T category, the detection rare of lesions tends to be high in the protruding appearance (Table 2). Most of the undetectable lesions were the flat or flat-elevated type macroscopically. Thus, endoscopic detection of UC-associated dysplasia/neoplasias at the precancerous and early stage appears to be difficult. Therefore, improvements to the current methods of colonoscopy are needed in order to detect UC-associated dysplasia/neoplasias more effectively and accurately. On the other hand, several Japanese investigators reported that observation of the configuration of the outlet of the colorectal surface lesion using high-resolution endoscopy, chromoendoscopy (Fujii et al., 2008, as cited in Rembacken, et al., 2000, and Kudo et al., 1994), increasingly useful for diagnosing and treating colorectal neoplasia. Recent reported the usefulness of high-resolution endoscopy, chromoendoscopy, and new endoscopic system (NBI, FICE, i-scan) for detecting UC associated dysplasia • neoplasia (East et al., 2006).

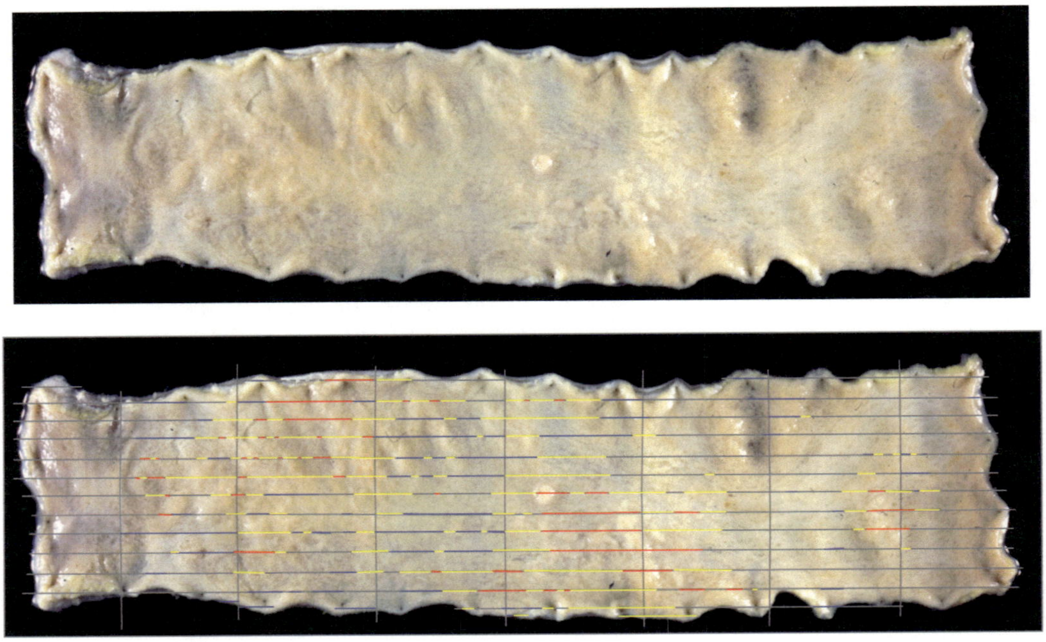

Fig. 2. Macroscopic appearance of ulcerative colitis/dysplasia, post formalin-fixed. Most of the endoscopic undetectable lesions were the flat and superficial elevated type macroscopically. (Red bar: UC-IV, Yellow bar: UC-III, Blue bar: UC-IIb)

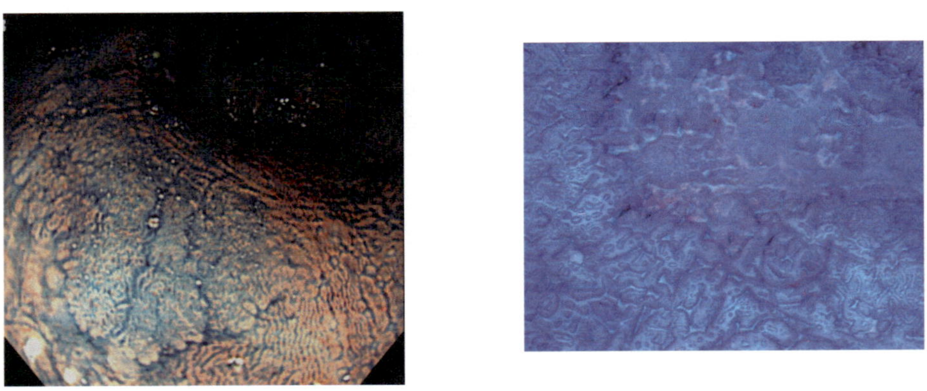

(a) Endoscopic finding (b) Stereomicroscopic finding

Fig. 3. Endoscopic finding of the UC-III lesion. In non-dysplastic epithelium, circle and/or oval pits were scattered in the area (a). Stereomicroscopic finding of the UC-III lesion. The mucosal surface shows packed distribution of oval and/or club-like shape and/or branch-like shaped pit (b).

T grade	P value		Protruding	Flat	*P value
Dysplasia(n=40)					
Detectable	19		3	16	0.058
Undetectable	21		0	21	
Tis(n=15					
Detectable	10	0.205[a]	3	7	0.171
Undetectable	5		0	5	
T1(n=5)					
Detectable	2	0.751[a]	2	0	<0.05
Undetectable	3	0.292[b]	0	3	
Advanced (n=7)					
Detectable	7	<0.05 [a]	6	1	ND
		0.082 [b]			
Undetectable	0	<0.05 [c]	0	0	
[a] Compared with dysplasia, [b] Compared with Tis, [c] Compared with T1.					
* Relationship between detection and macroscopic appearance. NF: not determined					

Table 2. Relationship between detection and macroscopic appearance of UC-associated lesions (adapted from Yamagishi et al., 2009)

3.1 Histological diagnosis of ulcerative colitis/dysplasia

UC associated dysplasia was a precursor of colitic cancer in UC, several studies have shown that UC-associated dysplasia correlates with the presence of colitic cancer. The existence of carcinoma at the time of colectomy in UC patients with high-grade dysplasia, as determined by a preoperative rectal biopsy. A presence of dysplasia could identify patients likely either to have or to develop colitic cancer. Thus, dysplasia is not only a precursor of colitic cancer, but may also be a marker for the existence of colitic cancer in other areas of the colorectum. Gastrointestinal surgical pathologist have been diagnosis inflammatory grade and epithelial injury on UC patient using by Matts grading system (Table 3) , The Inflammatory Bowel Disease Morphology Study Group in Western countries attempted to verify a standardized terminology and classification for the assessment of dysplasia in UC (Table 4). However, in Japan, the interpretation of'dysplasia' in UC varies from one pathologist to another. Therefore, the Research Committee on Inflammatory Bowel Disease of the Ministry of Health and Welfare of Japan proposed a new classification for UC associated dysplasia/neoplasia in 1993 (Table 5).

Grade 1	Normal appearance.
Grade 2	Some infiltration of the mucosa or lamina propria with either round cells or polymorphs.
Grade 3	Much cellular of the mucosa or lamina propria and submucosa.
Grade 4	Presence of crypt abscess, with much infiltration of all layers of the mucosa.
Grade 5	Ulceration, erosion, or necrosis of the mucosa, with cellular infiltration of some or all its layer.

Table 3. The value of rectal biopsy in the diagnosis of ulcerative colitis (adapted from Matts , 1961).

Negative	
	Normal mucosa
	Inactive (quiescent) colitis
	Active colitis
Indefinite	
	Probably negative (probably inflammatory)
	Unknown
	Probably positive (probably dysplasia)
Positive	
	Low-grade dysplasia
	High-grade dysplasia

Table 4. Biopsy classification of dysplasia in inflammatory bowel disease (adapted from Riddle et al., 1983).

Category	Description
UC-I	Inflammatory change
UC-II	Indefinite
UC-IIa	Probably inflammatory
UC-IIb	Probably neoplastic
UC-III	Neoplastic but not carcinoma
UC-IV	Carcinoma
UC: ulcerative colitis.	

Table 5. Histological classification of the neoplasia epithelium arising in ulcerative colitis (adapted from Konishi et al., 1993).

Matts grading system (Table 3) and UC associated dysplasia/neoplastic classification (Table 4 & 5) are used for clinical and research purposes and applies to both colectomy and biopsy specimens. The histological characteristics of each stage of UC-associated dysplasia/ neoplasia with inflammatory lesion (Fig 4). However, it is difficult and sensitive to discriminate between UC-associated dysplasia and regenerative epithelium by the conventional Hematoxylin and Eosin staining section. Histological diagnosis of UC-associated dysplasia/neoplasia is based on a combination of architectural and cytological alterations. The architectural alterations often result in glandular arrangements, e.g., club-shaped villi, crawling glands or bifid formation at the base of the crypts. The cytological alterations comprise cellular and nuclear pleomorphism, nuclear hyperchromatism, loss of nuclear polarity, marked nuclear stratification, dystrophic goble cells and failure of maturation from the crypt base to the surface.

3.2 Immunohistochemical finding of ulcerative colitis/dysplasia

Pathologically, it is not rare those surgical pathologists are unable to distinguish between from UC-associated dysplasia/neoplasia and inflammatory regenerative epithelium using by hematoxylin and eosin staining. Furthermore, there are differences in the diagnostic criteria that different surgical pathologist use for dysplasia/neoplasia. In order to improve the accuracy of pathological diagnosis, it will be necessary to use ordinary method for immunohistochemical technique.

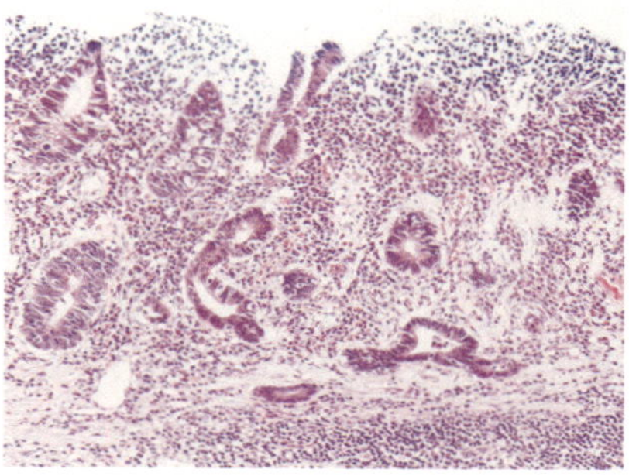

(a) Crawling crypts.

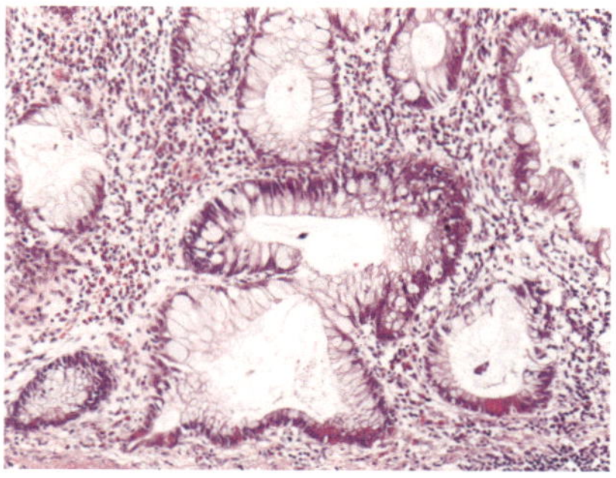

(b) Dystrophic goblet cell

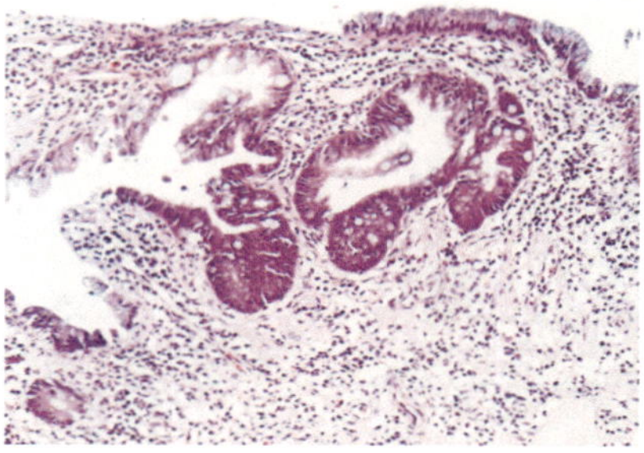

(c) Distorted crypts with cellular atypia

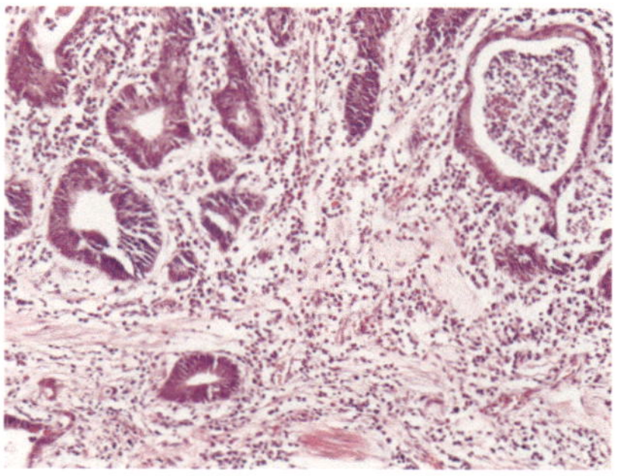

(d) Invasive crypt and crypt abscess

Fig. 4. Histological appearance of UC-associated dysplasia/neoplasia on Hematoxylin and Eosin staining section. There are marked distorted and crawling crypts. This epithelium could be interpreted as UC-IIb with Matts grade 3 (a). There are a lot of goblet cells, so-called dystrophic goblet cell. This epithelium could be interpreted as UC-IIb with Matts grade 3 (b). There are marked distorted crypts with cellular atypia. This epithelium could be interpreted as UC-III with Matts grade 3 (c). Neoplastic crypts with submucosal invasion. This epithelium could be interpreted as UC-IV with Matts grade 4 including crypt abscess. (d).

3.2.1 P53 protein nuclear accumulation

Several reports have shown that the rate of the tumor suppressor *p53* gene alteration is high in UC-associated dysplasia/neoplasia (Lashner et al., 1999). Immunohistochemical analysis of P53 protein is a useful and easy method for detecting *p53* gene alterations. In our study, 59.5% of neoplastic lesions (UC-III and IV) and 40.0% of lesions that were probably neoplastic (UC-IIb) displayed nuclear accumulation of P53 protein (Fujii et al., 2003a). Thus, immunohistochemical analysis of P53 could be a useful marker of UC associated dysplasia/neoplasia in cases where discriminating between neoplasia and regenerative epithelium is difficult (Fig 5) (Table 6).

3.2.2 Increased expression of DNA Methyltransferase -1

Neoplastic progression in UC occurs in a histologically stepwise manner, from chronic epithelial inflammation to dysplasia/neoplasia, and the process of neoplastic progression involves accumulation of genetic and epigenetic alterations. Some of these alterations are

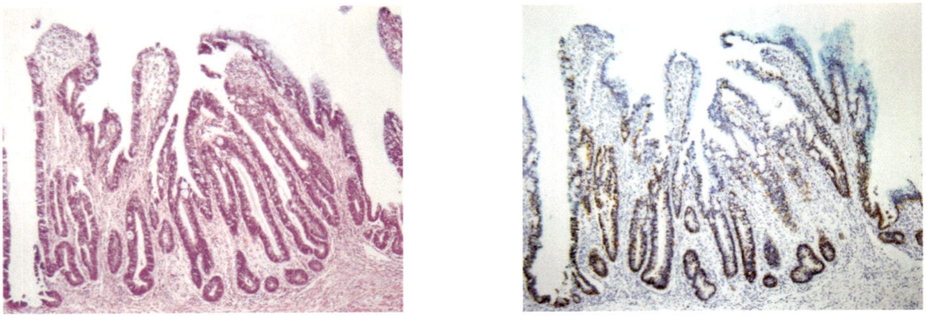

(a) Hematoxylin and Eosin (b) P53 protein

Fig. 5. Mucin droplets are well preserved but have lost their normal polarity, being present apically or basally or lateral to the nucleus (a). This epithelium could be interpreted as UC-IIb. Immunohistochemistry analysis revealed normal accumulated P53 protein in the nucleus (b).

Histological diagnosis	n	Positive staining(%)
Inflammatory change (UC-I)	5	0(0)
Indefinite, probably inflammatory (UC-IIa)	38	0(0)
Indefinite, probably neoplastic (UC-IIb)	35	14(40.0)
Neoplastic but not carcinoma (UC-III)	24	14(58.3)
Carcinoma (UC-IV)	18	11(61.1)

Table 6. Relation between nuclear accumulations of P53 protein and histological diagnosis (adapted from Fujii et al., 2003a)

known to occur in both the neoplastic and nonneoplastic epithelium of UC patients with neoplasia, and are considered to be widespread and to occur early in the process of neoplastic progression. In several types of neoplasia, aberrant methylation of promoter-region CpG islands, as an epigenetic modification of DNA, is associated with transcriptional inactivation of tumor suppressor genes and plays a crucial role in the development and progression of neoplasia (Hsieh et al., 1998). DNA methylation results from a methyl transfer reaction performed by the three active DNA methyltransferases (DNMTs): DNMT1, DNMT3a and DNMT3b (Okano et al., 1999). Of these, DNMT1 is the most abundant DNMT targeted to replication foci and has a preference for hemimethylated DNA substrates. Recent investigations have shown that DNMT1 is overexpressed in tumorigenic cells and several types of human tumors, and that increased expression of DNMT1 is dependent on cell proliferation. We reported that the immunoreactive DNMT1 expression gradually increased from rectal epithelium of UC patients without neoplasia to nonneoplastic rectal epithelium of UC patients with neoplasia ($p < 0.001$), and to colorectal neoplasia ($p < 0.001$) (Fujii et al., 2010). Among 31 neoplasias, there was no difference in the immunoreactive DNMT1 expressions between dysplasia and invasive cancer. Expression of DNMT1 in non-neoplastic epithelium may precede or be a relatively early event in UC-associated carcinogenesis (Fig. 6).

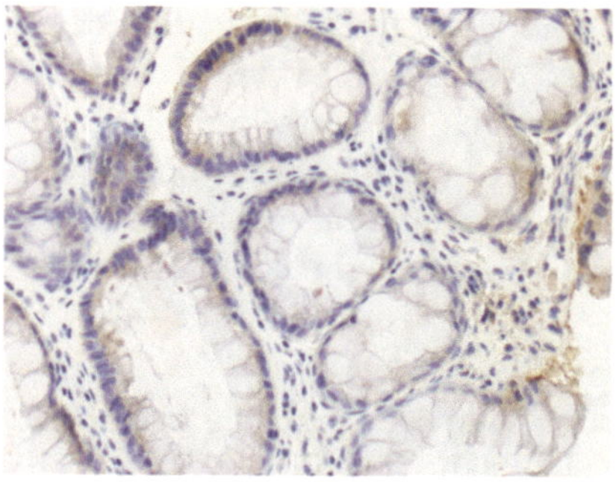

(a) Non-neoplastic epithelium without colitic cancer

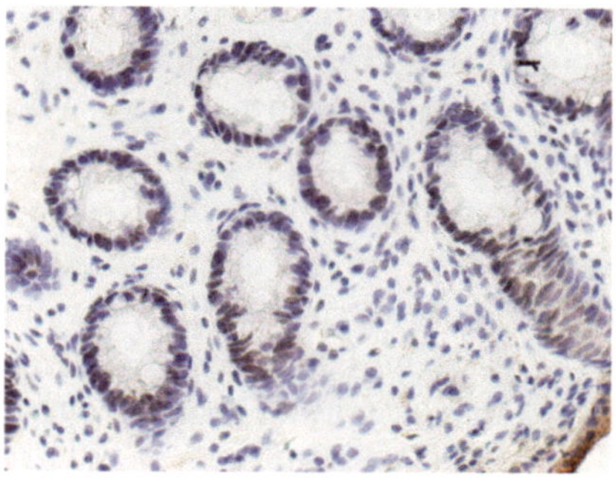

(b) Non-neoplastic epithelium with colitic cancer

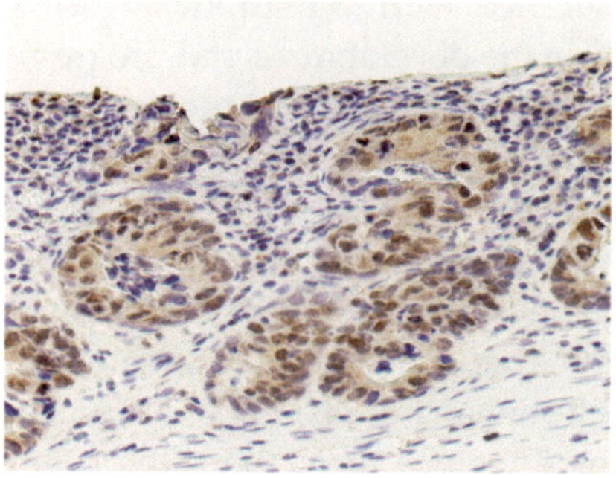

(c) Colitic cancer.

Fig. 6. Immunohistochemical staining for DNMT1 protein in non-neoplastic rectal epithelium from UC patients without neoplasia (a), non-neoplastic rectal epithelium from UC patients with neoplasia (b) and colorectal neoplasia (c).

3.3 Molecular alterations of ulcerative colitis/dysplasia

Numerous reports have revealed molecular alterations (e.g., *K-Ras* gene mutation, *p16* gene hypermethylation, *p14* gene hypermethylation, *p53* gene mutation, DNA aneuploidy, chromosomal instability, microsatellite instability, age-related methylation, telomere length shortening) of nonneoplastic epithelium in UC patients with neoplasia (Brentnail et al., 1994, Holzmann et al., 2001, Fujii et al., 2005). Several of these reports have indicated higher frequencies of molecular alterations to nonneoplastic epithelium in UC patients with dysplasia/neoplasia than in nonneoplastic epithelium in UC patients without neoplasia, suggesting that these molecular alterations may be applicable as new markers for identifying individuals with UC at increased risk of neoplasia.

3.3.1 P53 gene abnormalities

In the *p53* gene, point mutations have been reported in 40–50% and LOH in 80% of sporadic colorectal cancers (Baker et al., 1990). However, these genetic alterations of the *p53* gene have only been found in approximately 10% of sporadic adenomas. These data suggest that genetic alterations in the *p53* gene are involved in the progression from adenoma to cancer. Alterations in *p53* gene were reported in both UC-associated dysplasia and colitic cancer at an incidence of about 50–80%.The point mutations in *p53* gene were detected in 48% of case of UC-associated dysplasia, and that both point mutation and allelic loss were found in more than 80% of cases of colitic cancer (Brentnail et al., 1994. When the *p53* gene has a nonsense mutation or frameshift, the P53 protein does not accumulate in the nucleus despite the alteration. In fact, 92.9% of the neoplastic lesions that displayed negative immunohistochemical staining for P53 protein demonstrated a *p53* gene mutation within exons 5–8 under PCR singlestranded conformation polymorphism (Fujii et al., 2003a). This suggests that screening for *p53* gene mutation using PCR single-stranded conformation polymorphism is more accurate than immunohistochemistry for discriminating between UC-associated neoplasia and regenerative epithelium.

3.3.2 Age-related methylation and methylation analysis of ER Gene

In several neoplasias, aberrant methylation of promoter region Chg. islands, as an epigenetic modification of DNA, is associated with transcriptional inactivation of tumor suppressor genes and plays a crucial role in the development and progression of neoplasia (Hsieh et al., 1998). In normal colorectal epithelium, some genes are methylated with aging, and this alteration is known as age-related methylation. A methylation of the estrogenic receptor (ER) Chg. Island increased with age in no neoplastic colorectal epithelium and that the same methylation occurred in most sporadic colorectal neoplasias (Isa et al. 1994). They concluded that methylation of the *ER* gene in aging colorectal epithelium could represent one of the earliest events predisposing to sporadic colorectal carcinogenesis. Therefore, in our recent study (Fujii et al., 2005 and Tominaga et al., 2005), we analysed *ER* gene methylation in multiple samples taken from 6 regions throughout the colorectum: the rectum, sigmoid colon, descending colon, transverse colon, ascending colon and cecum (Fig. 7). Non-neoplastic colorectal epithelia from patients with longstanding and extensive UC, including 8 UC patients with neoplasia and 10 patients without, were evaluated. The combined bisulfite restriction analysis method (COBRA) was used to determine the methylation status of the *ER* gene. The mean methylation level of the *ER* gene was 25.4% in the nonneoplastic epithelia from UC patients with neoplasia, whereas it was only4.0 % in those without neoplasia (P < 0.001). The methylation level of the ER gene in UC patients with neoplasia was significantly higher than in UC patients without neoplasia throughout the colorectum except for the cecum. In UC patients with neoplasia, the mean ER methylation level in the distal colon was significantly higher than in the proximal colon (P < 0.001) Analysis of *ER* gene methylation may have potential as a useful marker for identifying individuals at increased risk of neoplasia among those with longstanding and extensive UC.

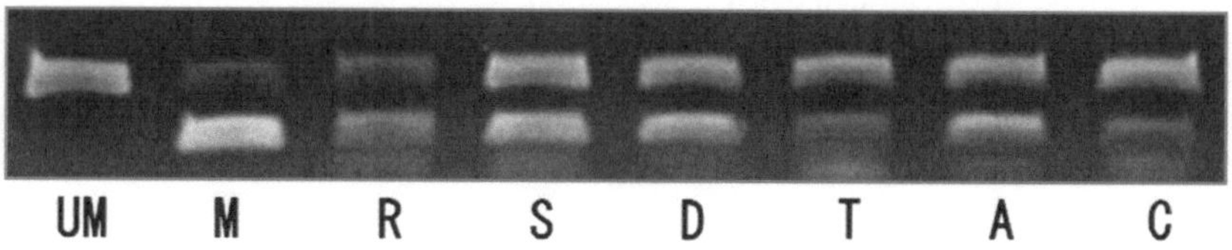

(a) Non-neoplastic colon epithelium with colitic cancer

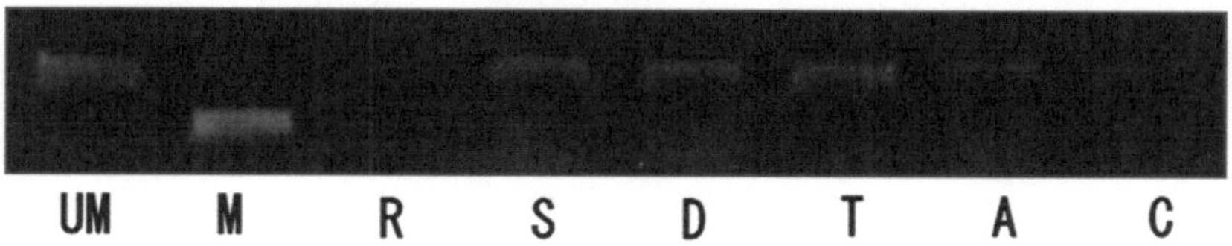

(b) Non-neoplastic colon epithelium without colitic cancer

Fig. 7. COBRA for the *ER* gene in each region of the non-neoplastic epithelium of the colorectum from patient with UC-associated neoplasia (a) and without UC-associated neoplasia (b). UM, the unmethylated breast cancer cell line MCF-7; M, the methylated colon cancer cell line DLD-1; R, rectum; S, sigmoidcolon; D, descending colon; T, transverse colon; A, ascending colon; C, cecum. A, representative samples

4. Conclusion

In this issue, we have discussed the efficacy of surveillance colonoscopy for UC associated dysplasia/neoplasia, several problems related to the diagnosis of UC–associated dysplasia/neoplasia and molecular markers that can be used to identify individuals with UC at increased risk of dysplasia/neoplasia. Current surveillance colonoscopy remains unsatisfactory, due to difficulties with endoscopic and histological diagnosis of UC-associated dysplasia/neoplasia. These difficulties may be overcome by introducing adjunctive techniques for diagnosing UC-associated dysplasia/neoplasia, analysis of *p53* gene alteration and/or new endoscopic system. However, it seems impartial for all UC patients with conventional risk factors, long-standing disease and extensive colitis to undergo close surveillance colonoscopy using such techniques. In order to realize the full potential of close surveillance colonoscopy, higher-risk groups selecting from patients with long - standing and extensive UC. Analyses of age-related methylation and expression of DNMT1 in nonneoplastic epithelium may allow identification of such higher-risk patients.

5. Acknowledgment

The authors thank Dr. S. Kameok a and Dr. M. Itabashi (Department of Surgery II, Tokyo Women's Medical College), Dr. B. Iizuka (Institute of Gastroenterology, Tokyo Women's Medical College), Dr. H. Mitooka (Division of Gastroenterology, Kobe Kaisei Hospital), Dr. T. Tanaka (Division of Gastroenterology, Shizuoka City Shizuoka Hospital) and Dr. N. Kitajima (Division of Gastroenterology, Kasai City Hospital) for kindly supplying the tissue materials. We would like to thank Dr. K. Ichikawa, Dr. J, Imura (Department of Surgical and Molecular Pathology, DOKKYO Medical University School of Medicine), Dr. H. Yamagishi (Department of Pathology, DOKKYO Medical University Koshigaya Hospital), and Dr. H. Fukui (Division of Upper Gastroenterology, Department of Internal Medicine, Hyogo College of Medicine) for their insightful comments. The authors greatly thank Ms C. Sato - Matsuyama, A. Shimizu, T. Ono, M. Katayama, N. Nagashima, (Department of Surgical and Molecular Pathology, DOKKYO Medical University School of Medicine) for technical assistance and to Ms. A. Kikuchi (Department of Surgical and Molecular Pathology, DOKKYO Medical University School of Medicine) for secretarial assistance in preparing the manuscript.

This work was partially supported by the Grant-in-Aid for Young Scientists (B: No 16790390), Grant-in-Aid for Scientific Research (C: No 18659101, 23590410) from the Ministry of Education, Culture, Sports, Science and Technology (MEXT) of Japan and Dokkyo Medical University Young Investigator Award (2009 for graduate student Dr. H. Tanaka and 2011-03-2 for graduate student Dr. K. Oono).

6. References

Baker, SJ.; et al. (1990). p53 gene mutations occur in combination with 17p allelic deletions as late events in colorectal tumorigenesis. *Cancer Research,* Vol.50, No.23, (December 1990), pp. 7717-7722, ISSN 0008-5472 (Print), 1538-7445 (Electronic)

Brentnall, TA.; et al. (1994). Mutations in the p53 gene: an early marker of neoplastic progression in ulcerative colitis. *Gastroenterology,* Vol.107, No.2 (August 1994), pp. 369-378, ISSN 0016-5085 (Print), 1528-0012 (Electronic)

East, JE,; et al.(2006). Narrow band imaging with magnification for dysplasia detection and pit pattern assessment in ulcerative colitis surveillance: a case with multiple dysplasia associated lesions or masses. *Gut,* Vol.55, No.10, (October 2006), pp. 1432-1435, ISSN 0017-5749 (Print), 1468-3288 (Electronic)

Fujii, S.; Fujimori, T. & Kashida, H. (2002). Ulcerative colitis-associated neoplasia. *Pathology International,* Vol.52, No.3, (March 2002), pp. 195-203, ISSN 1320-5463 (Print), 1440-1827 (Electronic)

Fujii, S.; Fujimori, T. & Chiba, T. (2003a). Usefulness of analysis of p53 alteration and observation of surface microstructure for diagnosis of ulcerative colitis-associated colorectal neoplasia. *Journal of Experimental & Clinical Cancer Research,* Vol.22, No.1, (March 2003), pp. 107-115, ISSN 1756-9966(Print)

Fujii, S.; et al. (2003b). Efficacy of surveillance and molecular markers for detection of ulcerative colitis-associated colorectal neoplasia. *Journal of Gastroenterology,* Vol.38,

No.12, (Decenber 2003), pp. 1117-1125, ISSN 0944-1174 (Print), 1435-5922 (Electronic)

Fujii, S.; et al. (2005a). Methylation of the oestrogen receptor gene in non-neoplastic epithelium as a marker of colorectal neoplasia risk in longstanding and extensive ulcerative colitis. *Gut,* Vol.54, No.9, (December 2005), pp. 1287-1292, ISSN 0017-5749 (Print), 1468-3288 (Electronic)

Fujii, S.; Katsumata, D. & Fujimori, T. (2008). Limits of diagnosis and molecular markers for early detection of ulcerative colitis-associated colorectal neoplasia. *Digestion,* Vol.77, No.supplement 1, (January 2008), pp. 2-12, ISSN 1421-9867 (Print), 0012-2823 (Electronic)

Fujii, S.; Katake, Y. & Tanaka, H. (2010). Increased Expression of DNA Methyltransferase-1 in Non-Neoplastic Epithelium Helps Predict Colorectal Neoplasia Risk in Ulcerative Colitis. *Digestion,* Vol.82, No.3, (June 2010), pp. 179-186, ISSN 1421-9867 (Print), 0012-2823 (Electronic)

Holzmann, K.; et al. (2001). Comparison of flow cytometry and histology with mutational screening for p53 and Ki-ras mutations in surveillance of patients with long-standing ulcerative colitis. *Scandinavian Journal of Gastroenterology,* Vol.36, No.12 (December 2001), pp. 1320-1326, ISSN 0036-5521 (Print), 0036-5521 (Electronic)

Hsieh, C.; et al. (1998). Hypermethylation of the p16INK4a promoter in colectomy specimens of patients with long-standing and extensive ulcerative colitis. *Cancer Research,* Vol.58, No.17, (September 1998), pp. 3942-3945, ISSN 0008-5472 (Print), 1538-7445 (Electronic)

Issa, JP.; et al. (1994). Methylation of the oestrogen receptor CpG island links ageing and neoplasia in human colon. *Nature Genetics,* Vol.7, No.4, (August 1994), pp. 7717-7722, ISSN 1061-4036 (Print), 1546-1718 (Electronic)

Konishi, F.: et al. (1993). Histological Classification of the Neoplastic Epithelium Arising in Ulcerative Colitis. *Annual Report (for 1992) of the Research Committee of Inflammatory Bowel Disease. Tokyo: Ministry of Health and Welfare of Japan,* 1993; pp. 153–156 (in Japanese with English abstract).

Lashner, BA.; et al. (1999). Evaluation of the usefulness of testing for p53 mutations in colorectal cancer surveillance for ulcerative colitis. *The American Journal of Gastroenterology,* Vol.94, No.2, (February 1999), pp. 456-462, ISSN 0002-9270 (Print), 1572-0241 (Electronic)

Matts, SG. (1961). The value of rectal biopsy in the diagnosis of ulcerative colitis. *The Quarterly journal of medicine,* Vol.30, No.4, (October 1961), pp. 393-407, ISSN 0033-5622 (Print), 0033-5622 (Electronic)

Okano, M.; et al. (1999). DNA methyltransferases Dnmt3a and Dnmt3b are essential for de novo methylation and mammalian development. *Cell,* Vol.99, No.3, (October 1999), pp. 247-257, ISSN 1097-4172 (Print), 0092-8674 (Electronic)

Riddel, RH.; et al.(1983). Dysplasia in inflammatory bowel disease: standardized classification with provisional clinical applications. *Human Pathology,* Vol.14, No.11, (November 1983), pp. 931-968, ISSN 0046-8177 (Print), 1532-8392 (Electronic)

Tominaga, K.; et al. (2005). Prediction of colorectal neoplasia by quantitative methylation analysis of estrogen receptor gene in nonneoplastic epithelium from patients with ulcerative colitis. *Gut,* Vol.11, No.24 Part 1, (December 2005), pp. 8880-8805, ISSN 1078-0432 (Print), 1557-3265 (Electronic)

Yamagishi, H.; et al. (2009). Pathological Approach for Surveillance of Ulcerative Colitis-associated cancer: Usefulness of Immunohistochemistry for p53. *Dokkyo Journal of Medical Science,* Vol.36, No.1, (March 2009), pp. 27-32, ISSN 0385-5023 (Print), 0385-5023 (Electronic)

10

Pathology of Staging of Early Colorectal Lesions During Surveillance Programmes

Emil Salmo[1] and Najib Haboubi[2]
[1]*Department of Histopathology, Royal Bolton NHS Foundation Trust, Bolton,*
[2]*Department of Histopathology, Clinical Sciences Building,*
University Hospital of South Manchester,
United Kingdom

1. Introduction

Colorectal carcinoma (CRC) is the second most common cancer in women after carcinoma of the breast and the third most common cancer in men after carcinoma of the prostate and lung with a lifetime risk in the UK of one in 16 for men and one in 20 for women (C-R-UK, 2011). In 2008, around 40,000 people in the UK were diagnosed with bowel cancer and approximately 16,000 died from the disease. In the same year, there were an approximately 334,000 new cases of CRC in the European Union (GLOBOCAN, 2008). The lowest rates for both men and women were in Greece and the highest rates for men were in Hungary and for women in Denmark. Rates for the UK for men and women were below the EU27 average (C-R-UK, 2011). Worldwide, every year, more than 1 million will develop CRC (Parkin et al., 2005).

Over 90% of CRC is sporadic in nature and affects 25 per 100 000 per year of individuals aged 45–55, but over 300 per 100 000 per year in individuals aged 75 and over (West et al., 2008). Internationally, the UK has an incidence of CRC close to the average for all EU countries, which is slightly lower than that for Australia, New Zealand and North America (Halloran, 2009).

Survival rates in individuals with CRC have increased substantially in the past few years, possibly as a result of early diagnosis and improved treatment. Although substantial information about risk factors exists, about 75% of diagnoses are in patients with no apparent risk factors other than old age (ACS, 2011), however, the 5-year survival is still less than 60% in most European countries (Verdecchia et al., 2007).

2. Why screen for bowel cancer?

In 1998 the NHS started to develop the Bowel Cancer Screening Programme (Hardcastle et al., 1996) and in 2006, the English CRC screening programme started a 2-yearly screening for individuals between the ages of 60 and 69 (extended to 74 years in 2010) (Halloran, 2009). The decision was based on the results of four large randomized controlled trials, including one in Nottingham (Hardcastle et al., 1996), where a 16% reduction in mortality was associated with the implementation of bowel screening. These trials showed that population screening with the faecal occult blood test (FOBT) every two years has the potential to reduce colorectal mortality between 15% to 18% in people aged 45-74 (Hardcastle et al., 1996; Kronborg et al., 1996; Lindholm et al., 2008; Mandel et al., 1993). Individuals who attend screening have a 25% reduction in their risk of dying from CRC. These studies supported similar results from trials in Nottingham (Hardcastle et al., 1996; Steele et al., 2009; UK-Colorectal-Cancer-Screening-Pilot-Group, 2004).

The use of flexible sigmoidoscopy has also been investigated as a screening tool (Atkin et al., 1993; UK-Flexible-Sigmoidoscopy-Screening-Trial-Investigators, 2002) which showed that a once-only flexible sigmoidoscopy between the ages of 55 and 64 could reduce CRC incidence by 33% and mortality from CRC by 43% (Atkin et al., 2010). The test was also found to be safe and acceptable (Atkin et al., 1993). Several randomised trials and Cochrane reviews have provided high-quality evidence that this test, if offered every 2 years, has the potential to reduce mortality rates associated with CRC by 16% (Towler et al., 1998) and reduces incidence and mortality rates of distal CRC by 60–80% (Newcomb et al., 2003; Selby et al., 1992).

In general, the NHS Bowel Cancer Screening Programme (NHS BCSP) commenced in April 2006 and invites men and women aged 60–69 to participate via submission of faecal occult blood test every 2 years; those with a positive result will be offered colonoscopy (West et al., 2008).

As a marker of the success of the programme, at colonoscopy, the proportion of Duke's stage A and B lesions is markedly higher than that diagnosed amongst the symptomatic population (Goodyear et al., 2008; Halloran, 2009).

3. Principles of screening

The aim of screening for CRC is to prevent the development of advanced disease through detection of early and premalignant adenomas, from which at least 80% of cancers are thought to arise (Cunningham et al., 2010). As outlined by Wilson and Jungner, (1968) the criteria for screening (Table 1), which have been adopted by the WHO, demonstrates that CRC is an ideal disease for screening. Population screening therefore continues to offer the best prospects for reduction in mortality rates (Cunningham et al., 2010).

WHO screening principles:

1. The condition sought should be an important health problem for the individual and community.
2. There should be an acceptable treatment or useful intervention for patients with the disease.
3. Facilities for diagnosis and treatment should be available.
4. There should be a recognizable latent or early symptomatic stage.
5. There should be a suitable screening test or examination.
6. The test should be acceptable for the population.
7. The natural history of the disease should be adequately understood.
8. There should be an agreed policy for referral for further examination and for whom to treat as patients.
9. The cost should be economically balanced in relation to possible expenditure on medical care as a whole.
10. Case finding should be a continuing process and not a once-only project.

Table 1. (Wilson and Jungner, 1968)

The programme uses faecal occult blood testing (FOBt) as the primary screening modality to select patients for colonoscopy (BCSP, 2011). Colonoscopy is the best means we have to detect CRC and it provides an opportunity for therapeutic intervention, which is not possible with virtual colonoscopy (computerized tomography colonography). CT colonography (virtual colonoscopy) is as sensitive as colonoscopy for the detection of cancers and large adenomas, but includes exposure to radiation, requires full bowel preparation, and, at the end, colonoscopy is necessary for definite treatment (Halligan et al., 2005; Whitlock et al., 2008). Whilst the morbidity and mortality associated with colonoscopy might be considered acceptable for patients with signs and symptoms of the disease, they are unacceptable as a first line population screening. Perforation and clinically significant bleeding occur after colonoscopic polypectomy in about 0.2% and 1% of cases, respectively (Bond, 2000).

Flexible sigmoidoscopy carries significantly lower risk but will miss some 30 to 40% of proximal lesions (Halloran, 2009). As a screening test, the guaiac FOBT (gFOBT) has significant limitations as it cannot detect low concentrations of blood and has a poor analytical specificity. Any blood that reaches the stool may give a positive test result such as in cases of ulcerative colitis, Crohn's disease, haemorrhoids, major dental surgery or upper gastrointestinal bleeds, as does a diet of large raw steaks and black pudding (Halloran, 2009). Evidence from randomized controlled trials designed to assess the impact of FOBt-based screening on mortality in the screened population have suggested that FOBt is more likely to detect distal colonic and sigmoid lesions rather than right-sided tumours (Thomas et al., 1992).

The sensitivity of FOBt varies but has been quoted as between 6.2% and 83.3% in a recent systematic review when considering all neoplasms (Burch et al., 2007).

Harmston et al. (2010) showed that the location of screen-detected cancers does not differ from that seen in the unscreened population which suggests that faecal occult blood test screening detects cancer irrespective of location within the colon. It should be stressed that patients with negative FOB negative should not be given the impression of being cancer free.

Hol et al. (2010) recently showed in a population-based CRC screening trial using immunochemical FOB (IFOB) randomized against guaiac-based FOB that the detection rate was far better in the former. The authors strongly suggest using the IFOB in screening programmes, however, these findings need to be validated before changing practice of screening.

As a result of bowel screening, there will be more cases of malignant polyps detected in the screening programme than in symptomatic patients. Furthermore, how should patients with positive FOB and negative colonoscopy be managed?

One review from Canada (McLoughlin and Telford, 2007) addressed the issue and showed that when there is positive FOB and the patient undergoes both upper and lower gastrointestinal endoscopy, the yield for upper tract pathology is significant. These authors, however, argue that in those patients with a positive FOB test and negative colonoscopy, it is not cost effective to perform routine upper endoscopy unless the patient is anaemic, symptomatic or has risk factors for gastric cancer.

What happens to the population outside the screening age group?

In an important study, Shellnut et al. (2010) looked at the appropriateness of restricting the screened age group and found that not screening individuals under 50 and over 75 years would miss around 49 to 50% of patients in their study. Harmston et al. (2010) looked at 100 patients with CRC in the NHSBCSP and analysed their symptoms. They found that 70% had significant symptoms such as rectal bleeding, tenesmus, change in bowel habit and abdominal pain and they argued that with proper public awareness, these symptoms would have triggered referral. The study also showed that there was a significant increase in detecting Dukes A lesions in 28.5% of cases.

Ellul et al. (2010) again showed that with screening there is earlier detection of Dukes A over a non screened population of 45.3% compared with 10.1%. This is good evidence for the benefit of screening. It is remarkable, however, that the proportion of Dukes A stage tumours varied widely from 45.3% in the study of Ellul et al. to 28.5% in that of Harmston et al. with no apparent explanation for this variation. The screening programme is likely to be an effective and practical way of reducing CRC, but it does have its limitations, which can only be reduced by further research to maximize overall patient care (Haboubi, 2010).

4. Pathology and management of early (pT1) colorectal lesions in the NHSBCSP

Colorectal polyps are extremely common in Western countries and are found in up to 30% of autopsies performed in people aged more than 60 years (Williams et al., 1982). Histologically, colorectal polyps are divided into neoplastic or nonneoplastic and it is well known that more than 95% of CRC arise from neoplastic adenomatous polyps (adenomas) (Bond, 2000; Morson, 1966) through the well documented adenoma–carcinoma sequence (Muto et al., 1975).

By definition, all adenomas show dysplasia and is divided into either low or high grade (Quirke et al., 2007; Riddell et al., 1983) and architecturally into either tubular, tubulovillous or villous types according to the WHO classification (Hamilton and Aaltonen, 2000). High grade dysplasia shows complex glandular crowding and irregularity, prominent budding, cribriform architecture with 'back to back' glands and prominent cellular atypia (Quirke et al., 2007; Riddell et al., 1983). The latter includes loss of cell polarity or nuclear stratification, markedly enlarged nuclei with a dispersed chromatin pattern and a prominent nucleolus, abundant mitotic figures with atypical mitoses and prominent apoptosis.

A malignant colorectal polyp is a lesion in which cancer has invaded through the muscularis mucosae and into the submucosa (Cooper, 1983; Cooper et al., 1995; Lipper et al., 1983; Morson et al., 1984; Volk et al., 1995) and T1 adenocarcinoma is defined as invasion into the submucosa and not into the muscularis propria (Edge et al., 2010). The incidence of malignant colonic polyps amongst all removed colonic adenomas varies between 2.6% and 9.7%, with an average incidence of 4.7% (Coverlizza et al., 1989).

Increasing dysplasia and, presumably, malignant potential correlate with increasing adenoma size, villous component, and patient age (Konishi and Morson, 1982). The likelihood of invasive carcinoma also increases with increasing polyp size (Fenoglio and Pascal, 1982). Size is perceived to be one of the most important risk factor which put an adenoma into high risk category of malignant transformation. Amongst 5137 adenomas of diameter of less than 5 mm, none demonstrated malignant transformation (Nusko et al., 1997).

Generally, malignant colorectal polyps are divided into high and low risk lesions. High risk malignant polyps were defined as having one of the following: incomplete polypectomy, an involved resection margin, lymphatic or venous invasion, or are poorly differentiated histologically (Netzer et al., 1997). Adverse outcome in a malignant colorectal polyp was defined as residual cancer in a resection specimen and local or metastatic recurrence in the

follow up period (Netzer et al., 1998). In the high risk group, surgery is recommended when either of the two independent risk factors, such as incomplete polypectomy or a positive margin is present or if there is a combination of other risk factors. As lymphovascular invasion or poorly differentiated cancer did not have an adverse outcome when studied alone, operations in such cases should be individually assessed taking the risk of surgery into consideration (Netzer et al., 1998) as the risk for death from elective colonic resection averages about 2% (from 0.2% in the young to more than 5% in the elderly) (Greenburg et al., 1981).
An analysis of published series of malignant polyps estimated that the risk of residual cancer or nodal metastases from endoscopically resected pedunculated and sessile malignant polyps with favourable criteria was 0.3% and 1.5%, respectively (Cranley et al., 1986). Another review of endoscopically resected polyps with poor prognostic factors (poorly differentiated cancer, margin involvement, or presence of lymphatic or vascular invasion) reported residual cancer in 8.5% and 14.4%, for patients with pedunculated and sessile malignant polyps, respectively (Coverlizza et al., 1989). The American College of Gastroenterologist recommends no further treatment if the polyp is considered to be completely excised by the endoscopist, the cancer is not poorly differentiated and there is no vascular or lymphatic permeation and the margin of excision is free (Bond, 2000). Invasion of the stalk of a pedunculated polyp, by itself, is not an unfavorable prognostic finding, as long as the cancer does not extend to the margin of resection (Bond, 2000). In large sessile polyps which are not resectable endoscopically or that might contain invasive carcinoma with unfavorable prognostic features, it is useful to mark the polypectomy site (Shatz et al., 1997) to aid future identification of the site if necessary.
If the polyp is removed in one piece, the area of diathermy can be used as the histological landmark for the true transected margin of resection. If the polypectomy has been performed in piecemeal, it may be impossible to determine the true margin of resection, therefore precluding an accurate reporting on the status of completeness of excision (Cooper, 2007).
The presence of multiple adenomas in the same segment as the malignant polyp might be an argument for resection, particularly if the other polyps subsequently show high grade dysplasia (Haboubi and Scott, 2000). Similarly, the presence of a malignant adenoma in association with a strong family history of large bowel cancer would also be in favour of resection (Haboubi and Scott, 2000).

4.1 Factors against resection

Surgical resection is associated with a significant risk of mortality and morbidity with the risk of diarrhea after extensive colonic resection, particularly in the elderly (Haboubi and Scott, 2000) with an overall mortality of 5% (Scott et al., 1995). In practice, any individual patient with a histologically unfavourable malignant polyp has either a 10% chance of cancer-specific treatment failure or a 3-5% risk of postoperative death (Haboubi and Scott, 2000).

4.2 Margins of excision

Cancer at or near the resection margin is a histological finding that signifies the potential for an adverse outcome (Hackelsberger et al., 1995; Hassan et al., 2005; Ueno et al., 2004a). In one study, 21.4% of cases with cancer at or near the resection margin had an adverse outcome (Cooper et al., 1995). It is also important to record completeness of excision of the deep and mucosal margins as surgery is usually an indication when the former is involved and further local excision may be tempted if the mucosal margin is believed to be involved (Quirke et al., 2007).

An involved margin has many definitions in the literature. Cancer near the margin has been variously defined as cancer cells 1mm or less from the transacted margin, (Cooper et al., 1995) cancer cells 2mm or less from the transacted margin, (Netzer et al., 1997; Volk et al., 1995) and cancer within the diathermy and/or within one high-power field of the diathermy (Morson et al., 1984; Ueno et al., 2004b). However, most studies showed that the presence of cancer near the transected margin has the same clinical significance as cancer at the actual margin (Cooper et al., 1995; Hackelsberger et al., 1995; Netzer et al., 1997).
Presently, there is no consensus on what represents a 'negative margin'. A negative margin has been defined as one in which cancer is not within the actual diathermy, (Morson et al., 1984) more than one high-power field from the diathermy, greater than 1mm from the margin (Cooper et al., 1995) and more than 2mm from the margin (Netzer et al., 1997; Seitz et al., 2004). Incomplete local excision is not a judgement based on histology alone but a decision made jointly by the endoscopist and pathologist (Cooper, 2007).

4.3 Histological grade

Poorly differentiated (grade III) cancer, which has been classified as a poor risk factor in a malignant polyp, comprise 5–10% of cases and are associated with a significantly greater incidence of poor outcome than for better differentiated tumours (Kyzer et al., 1992; Nivatvongs et al., 1991).

4.4 Vascular invasion

Many studies showed that vascular invasion has been associated with an adverse outcome (Hassan et al., 2005; Ueno et al., 2004b). Muller et al. (Muller et al., 1989) demonstrated that vascular invasion on its own predicted an adverse outcome, but other studies have not supported these findings (Cooper et al., 1995; Volk et al., 1995):

4.5 Haggitt levels

Haggitt level of invasion in a pedunculated polyp is an important risk factor. In the Haggitt system (Haggitt et al., 1985) the level of invasion in a malignant pedunculated polyp is defined as follows:
Level 1: Carcinoma invading into the submucosa, but limited to the head of the polyp.
Level 2: Carcinoma invading to the level of the neck (the junction of the head and stalk) of the adenoma.
Level 3: Carcinoma invading any part of the stalk.
Level 4: Carcinoma invading into the submucosa of the bowel wall below the level of the stalk but above the muscularis propria.
According to these criteria, invasive cancer arising in a pedunculated adenoma could be classified as level 1 to level 4, but invasive cancer arising in a sessile adenoma is by definition a level 4 lesion. Studies have shown that level 4 invasion correlates with an adverse outcome and that patients with level 1-3 cancers and grade I or II cancers, and no lymphatic or venous invasion, can be successfully treated by polypectomy alone (Haggitt et al., 1985; Pollard et al., 1992).
Follow-up surgical resection has been recommended following polypectomy showing Haggitt level 4 invasion (Haggitt et al., 1985; Kyzer et al., 1992; Nivatvongs et al., 1991) or with any level polyp with grade III cancer, (Pollard et al., 1992) and/or lymphatic invasion (Haggitt et al., 1985).

4.6 Kikuchi's levels

In pT1 tumours, the frequency of lymph node metastasis in sessile tumours that involve the superficial, middle and deep thirds of the submucosa (so-called Kikuchi levels sm1, sm2 and sm3 respectively) (Kikuchi et al., 1995) has been reported to be 2%, 8% and 23% respectively (Nascimbeni et al., 2002). Invasion to level SM1 has been reported to have a significantly lower incidence of lymph node metastasis than level SM2 or SM3 invasion (Nascimbeni et al., 2002).

However, neither the Kikuchi (for sessile tumours) nor the Haggitt (for polypoid tumours) system is easy to interpret, especially if there is fragmentation or suboptimal orientation of the polyp.

More recently, Ueno et al. (Ueno et al., 2004b) proposed that the depth of invasion measured in microns beyond the muscularis mucosae provides a more objective measure, and this system has been adopted in Japan. However, again this system is difficult to use in routine practice.

It has to be highlighted that each classification has advantages and disadvantages. The Kikuchi system cannot be used if there is no muscularis mucosa in the biopsy and the Haggitt system is of no value in sessile lesions and measurement depends on a recognisable submucosa and good orientation of the polyp (Quirke et al., 2007).

In an extensive review of the literature (31 studies involving 1900 patients), Hassan et al. (2005) reported god outcome in polyps showing favourable histological features (e.g. negative margin, grade I or II and absence of lymphovascular invasion), supporting the suggestion that endoscopic polypectomy alone is adequate treatment in these patients.

The treatment of patient with an endoscopically removed malignant colorectal polyp must be individualized for each patient, taking all factors into consideration. Guidelines endorsed by the American Gastroenterological Association (Bond, 2000) recommend no further treatment is indicated after colonoscopic resection of a malignant colorectal polyp if the following criteria are fulfilled:

- The polyp is considered by the endoscopist to have been completely excised
- The cancer is not poorly differentiated
- There is no vascular or lymphatic permeation
- The margin of excision is not involved.

The guidelines also comment that when a patient's malignant polyp has poor prognostic features, the relative risks of surgical resection should be weighed against the risk of death from metastatic cancer.

4.7 Tumour budding

Tumour budding is defined as isolated single cancer cells or small clusters (fewer than five cells) of cancer cells at the advancing edge of the tumour. Several studies have defined a tumour as positive for budding when there are five or more buds per 20 power field (Kaneko et al., 2007; Ueno et al., 2004b). Studies of T1 cancers have shown that the presence of tumour budding is significantly associated with lymph node metastasis and other adverse outcomes (Kaneko et al., 2007; Masaki et al., 2001a; Ueno et al., 2004b).

4.8 Cribriform histology

T1 CRC with a cribriform histology showed a high rate of lymph node metastasis when analyzed with multivariate analysis. In one of the studies, all the cases were all initially treated by surgical resection (Egashira et al., 2004).

4.9 Potential 'molecular' markers

Masaki et al. (Masaki et al., 2001b) showed that expression of MMP-7 (a matrix metalloproteinase) at the invasive margin of T1 cancers was significantly associated with other poor histological features and unfavourable outcome. Hirano and Minimoto (2000) reported that a high expression of p53 and a low expression of p27 were significantly associated with metastasis in cases of T1 CRC.

4.10 Pseudoinvasion/misplaced mucosa

Pseudoinvasion is misplacement of the whole mucosa into the submucosa and this herniated mucosa often mimics invasive cancer causing a diagnostic difficulty for pathologists. Even among experienced gastrointestinal pathologists, there is a lack of unanimity in differentiating invasive carcinoma from pseudoinvasion (Cooper et al., 1995; Muto et al., 1973). It is commonly seen in prolapsed polyps in the sigmoid colon and is perceived to be one of the most difficult areas in the interpretation of polyp and in the context of the bowel screening programme (Quirke et al., 2007).

In cases of pseudoinvasion, the rounded contour of the neoplastic glands and the cytological similarity of the herniated epithelium to the surface adenoma, continuity of the surface epithelium with the 'deep' epithelium and the presence of lamina propria around the submucosal are all indications of pseudoinvasion rather than invasive cancer (Cooper, 2007). The presence of haemosiderin deposits provides a clue to the presence of misplaced epithelium. The distinction between invasion and pseudoinvasion is made more difficult when the herniated epithelium is severely dysplastic (Pascal et al., 1990) and there are instances where the differentiation is difficult with 100% certainty and the pathology report should indicate this uncertainty.

4.11 Serrated lesions of the colorectum

Serrated lesions have only recently been highlighted as having distinct genetic features and a different architecture from classical adenomas. The family of serrated polyps comprises sessile serrated adenomas, also called sessile serrated polyps (SSA/Ps), traditional serrated adenomas, hyperplastic polyps, and mixed hyperplastic/adenomatous polyps or admixed polyps (Ensari et al., 2010).

It is estimated that SSA/Ps represent 8-20% of serrated polyps with a predilection for the right colon. The diagnosis is mainly based on architectural features and are usually larger than hyperplastic polyps, measuring from 5 mm to more than 10 mm. They are flat to sessile. The crypts are elongated and epithelial serration and dilatation are usually more prominent in the basal part of the crypts in a 'crescendo' fashion.

Traditional hyperplastic polyps that are large (>1 cm) and/or multiple and/or located in the proximal colon are associated with an increased risk for CRC, notably in the hyperplastic polyposis syndrome where they occur throughout the colon with a 50% risk of CRC (Leggett et al., 2001). From the management point of view they should be treated similar to conventional adenomas.

5. Conclusion

The histopathology reports on malignant colorectal specimens are of major importance regarding patient management, prognostic assessment, audit and research. It has been shown that use of proforma greatly improves the quality of such reports (Quirke et al., 2007; Quirke and Morris, 2007).

The bowel cancer screening programme will generate many early cancers (pT1) for which there is poor management protocols as opposed to pT2 tumours which they need a definite surgical excision (Haboubi, 2010; Quirke et al., 2007).

The preferred care for patients with polypectomy specimens which contain invasive carcinoma is controversial (Haboubi and Scott, 2000). Taking into considerations all factors involved, the issue of polypectomy for malignant polyps versus surgical resection is best resolved by a multidisciplinary team involving the surgeon, pathologist and endoscopist, taking the patient's condition and wishes into account (Mitchell and Haboubi, 2008).

6. References

ACS. (2011). *Americal Cancer Society: Colorectal Cancer Early Detection* [Online]. Available at: http://www.cancer.org/Cancer/ColonandRectumCancer/MoreInformation/ColonandRectumCancerEarlyDetection/colorectal-cancer-early-detection-risk-factors-for-c-r-c [Accessed 1 March 2011].

Atkin, W. S., Cuzick, J., Northover, J. M.& Whynes, D. K. (1993). Prevention of colorectal cancer by once-only sigmoidoscopy. *Lancet,* Vol. 341, No. 8847, (Mar 20), pp. 736-40. 0140-6736

Atkin, W. S., Edwards, R., Kralj-Hans, I., Wooldrage, K., Hart, A. R., Northover, J. M. A., et al. (2010). Once-only flexible sigmoidoscopy screening in prevention of colorectal cancer: a multicentre randomised controlled trial. *The Lancet,* Vol. 375, No. 9726, pp. 1624-1633. 0140-6736

BCSP. (2011). *How is the bowel cancer screening programme organised?* [Online]. Available at: http://www.cancerscreening.hns.uk/bowel/how-organised [Accessed 6 March 2011].

Bond, J. H. (2000). Polyp guideline: diagnosis, treatment, and surveillance for patients with colorectal polyps. Practice Parameters Committee of the American College of Gastroenterology. *Am J Gastroenterol,* Vol. 95, No. 11, (Nov), pp. 3053-63. 0002-9270 (Print) 0002-9270 (Linking)

Burch, J. A., Soares-Weiser, K., St John, D. J., Duffy, S., Smith, S., Kleijnen, J., et al. (2007). Diagnostic accuracy of faecal occult blood tests used in screening for colorectal cancer: a systematic review. *J Med Screen,* Vol. 14, No. 3, pp. 132-7. 0969-1413 (Print) 0969-1413 (Linking)

C-R-UK. (2011). *Cancer Research UK: Bowel cancer statistics - Key Facts* [Online]. Available at: http://info.cancerresearchuk.org/cancerstats/types/bowel/?script=true [Accessed 1 March 2011].

Cooper, H. (2007). CooperPathology of the endoscopically removed malignant colorectal polyp. *Current Diagnostic Pathology* Vol. 13, No., pp. 423-437.

Cooper, H. S. (1983). Surgical pathology of endoscopically removed malignant polyps of the colon and rectum. *Am J Surg Pathol,* Vol. 7, No. 7, (Oct), pp. 613-23. 0147-5185 (Print) 0147-5185 (Linking)

Cooper, H. S., Deppisch, L. M., Gourley, W. K., Kahn, E. I., Lev, R., Manley, P. N., et al. (1995). Endoscopically removed malignant colorectal polyps: clinicopathologic correlations. *Gastroenterology,* Vol. 108, No. 6, (Jun), pp. 1657-65. 0016-5085 (Print) 0016-5085 (Linking)

Coverlizza, S., Risio, M., Ferrari, A., Fenoglio-Preiser, C. M.& Rossini, F. P. (1989). Colorectal adenomas containing invasive carcinoma. Pathologic assessment of lymph node metastatic potential. *Cancer,* Vol. 64, No. 9, (Nov 1), pp. 1937-47. 0008-543X (Print) 0008-543X (Linking)

Cranley, J. P., Petras, R. E., Carey, W. D., Paradis, K.& Sivak, M. V. (1986). When is endoscopic polypectomy adequate therapy for colonic polyps containing invasive carcinoma? *Gastroenterology,* Vol. 91, No. 2, (Aug), pp. 419-27. 0016-5085 (Print) 0016-5085 (Linking)

Cunningham, D., Atkin, W., Lenz, H. J., Lynch, H. T., Minsky, B., Nordlinger, B., et al. (2010). Colorectal cancer. *Lancet,* Vol. 375, No. 9719, (Mar 20), pp. 1030-47. 1474-547X (Electronic) 0140-6736 (Linking)

Edge, S., Byrd, D., Compton, C., Fritz, A., Greene, F.& Trotti, A. (2010). *AJCC Cancer Staging Manual* (7th ed.), Springer-Verlag, 9780387884400, New York, NY.

Egashira, Y., Yoshida, T., Hirata, I., Hamamoto, N., Akutagawa, H., Takeshita, A., et al. (2004). Analysis of pathological risk factors for lymph node metastasis of submucosal invasive colon cancer. *Mod Pathol,* Vol. 17, No. 5, pp. 503-511. 0893-3952

Ellul, P., Fogden, E., Simpson, C. L., Nickerson, C. L., McKaig, B. C., Swarbrick, E. T., et al. (2010). Downstaging of colorectal cancer by the National Bowel Cancer Screening programme in England: first round data from the first centre. *Colorectal Dis,* Vol. 12, No. 5, (May), pp. 420-2. 1463-1318 (Electronic) 1462-8910 (Linking)

Ensari, A., Bosman, F. T.& Offerhaus, G. J. (2010). The serrated polyp: getting it right! *J Clin Pathol,* Vol. 63, No. 8, (Aug), pp. 665-8. 1472-4146 (Electronic) 0021-9746 (Linking)

Fenoglio, C. M.& Pascal, R. R. (1982). Colorectal adenomas and cancer: pathologic relationships. *Cancer,* Vol. 50, No. 11 Suppl, (Dec 1), pp. 2601-8. 0008-543X (Print) 0008-543X (Linking)

GLOBOCAN. (2008). *Cancer Incidence and Mortality Worldwide in 2008: THE GLOBOCAN PROJECT* [Online]. Available at: http://globocan.iarc.fr/ [Accessed 5 March 2011].

Goodyear, S. J., Stallard, N., Gaunt, A., Parker, R., Williams, N.& Wong, L. (2008). Local impact of the English arm of the UK Bowel Cancer Screening Pilot study. *Br J Surg,* Vol. 95, No. 9, (Sep), pp. 1172-9. 1365-2168 (Electronic) 0007-1323 (Linking)

Greenburg, A. G., Saik, R. P., Coyle, J. J.& Peskin, G. W. (1981). Mortality and gastrointestinal surgery in the aged: elective vs emergency procedures. *Arch Surg,* Vol. 116, No. 6, (Jun), pp. 788-91. 0004-0010 (Print) 0004-0010 (Linking)

Haboubi, N. (2010). Why screening and who is benefiting? *Colorectal Dis,* Vol. 12, No. 5, (May), pp. 395-6. 1463-1318 (Electronic) 1462-8910 (Linking)

Haboubi, N.& Scott, N. (2000). Clinicopathological management of the patient with a malignant colorectal adenoma. *Colorectal Disease,* Vol. 2, No. 1, pp. 2-7. 1463-1318

Hackelsberger, A., Fruhmorgen, P., Weiler, H., Heller, T., Seeliger, H.& Junghanns, K. (1995). Endoscopic polypectomy and management of colorectal adenomas with invasive carcinoma. *Endoscopy,* Vol. 27, No. 2, (Feb), pp. 153-8. 0013-726X (Print) 0013-726X (Linking)

Haggitt, R. C., Glotzbach, R. E., Soffer, E. E.& Wruble, L. D. (1985). Prognostic factors in colorectal carcinomas arising in adenomas: implications for lesions removed by endoscopic polypectomy. *Gastroenterology,* Vol. 89, No. 2, (Aug), pp. 328-36. 0016-5085 (Print) 0016-5085 (Linking)

Halligan, S., Altman, D. G., Taylor, S. A., Mallett, S., Deeks, J. J., Bartram, C. I., et al. (2005). CT colonography in the detection of colorectal polyps and cancer: systematic review, meta-analysis, and proposed minimum data set for study level reporting. *Radiology,* Vol. 237, No. 3, (Dec), pp. 893-904. 0033-8419 (Print) 0033-8419 (Linking)

Halloran, S. P. (2009). Bowel cancer screening. *Surgery,* Vol. 27, No. 9, pp. 397-400. 0263-9319

Hamilton, S. R.& Aaltonen, L. A. (2000). *Pathology and genetics of tumours of the digestive system* IARC Press ; Oxford : Oxford University Press [distributor], 9283224108 (pbk.) : No price, Lyon.

Hardcastle, J. D., Chamberlain, J. O., Robinson, M. H., Moss, S. M., Amar, S. S., Balfour, T. W., et al. (1996). Randomised controlled trial of faecal-occult-blood screening for colorectal cancer. *Lancet,* Vol. 348, No. 9040, (Nov 30), pp. 1472-7. 0140-6736 (Print) 0140-6736 (Linking)

Harmston, C., Hunter, J.& Wong, L. (2010). Does the location of screen-detected cancers differ from that seen in the unscreened population? *Colorectal Dis,* Vol. 12, No. 4, (Apr), pp. 324-6. 1463-1318 (Electronic) 1462-8910 (Linking)

Hassan, C., Zullo, A., Risio, M., Rossini, F. P.& Morini, S. (2005). Histologic risk factors and clinical outcome in colorectal malignant polyp: a pooled-data analysis. *Dis Colon Rectum,* Vol. 48, No. 8, (Aug), pp. 1588-96. 0012-3706 (Print) 0012-3706 (Linking)

Hirano, K.& Minamoto, T. (2000). Altered expression of p53 and p27 proteins, alone or combined, as a predictor of metastatic potential in early invasive carcinoma of colon and rectum--a comparative clinicopathologic and molecular analysis. *Cancer Detect Prev,* Vol. 24, No. 4, pp. 343-55. 0361-090X (Print) 0361-090X (Linking)

Hol, L., van Leerdam, M. E., van Ballegooijen, M., van Vuuren, A. J., van Dekken, H., Reijerink, J. C., et al. (2010). Screening for colorectal cancer: randomised trial comparing guaiac-based and immunochemical faecal occult blood testing and flexible sigmoidoscopy. *Gut,* Vol. 59, No. 1, (Jan), pp. 62-8. 1468-3288 (Electronic) 0017-5749 (Linking)

Kaneko, I., Tanaka, S., Oka, S., Kawamura, T., Hiyama, T., Ito, M., et al. (2007). Lymphatic vessel density at the site of deepest penetration as a predictor of lymph node metastasis in submucosal colorectal cancer. *Dis Colon Rectum,* Vol. 50, No. 1, (Jan), pp. 13-21. 0012-3706 (Print) 0012-3706 (Linking)

Kikuchi, R., Takano, M., Takagi, K., Fujimoto, N., Nozaki, R., Fujiyoshi, T., et al. (1995). Management of early invasive colorectal cancer. Risk of recurrence and clinical guidelines. *Dis Colon Rectum,* Vol. 38, No. 12, (Dec), pp. 1286-95. 0012-3706 (Print) 0012-3706 (Linking)

Konishi, F.& Morson, B. C. (1982). Pathology of colorectal adenomas: a colonoscopic survey. *J Clin Pathol,* Vol. 35, No. 8, (Aug), pp. 830-41. 0021-9746 (Print) 0021-9746 (Linking)

Kronborg, O., Fenger, C., Olsen, J., Jorgensen, O. D.& Sondergaard, O. (1996). Randomised study of screening for colorectal cancer with faecal-occult-blood test. *Lancet,* Vol. 348, No. 9040, (Nov 30), pp. 1467-71. 0140-6736 (Print) 0140-6736 (Linking)

Kyzer, S., Begin, L. R., Gordon, P. H.& Mitmaker, B. (1992). The care of patients with colorectal polyps that contain invasive adenocarcinoma. Endoscopic polypectomy or colectomy? *Cancer,* Vol. 70, No. 8, (Oct 15), pp. 2044-50. 0008-543X (Print) 0008-543X (Linking)

Leggett, B. A., Devereaux, B., Biden, K., Searle, J., Young, J.& Jass, J. (2001). Hyperplastic polyposis: association with colorectal cancer. *Am J Surg Pathol,* Vol. 25, No. 2, (Feb), pp. 177-84. 0147-5185 (Print) 0147-5185 (Linking)

Lindholm, E., Brevinge, H.& Haglind, E. (2008). Survival benefit in a randomized clinical trial of faecal occult blood screening for colorectal cancer. *Br J Surg,* Vol. 95, No. 8, (Aug), pp. 1029-36. 1365-2168 (Electronic) 0007-1323 (Linking)

Lipper, S., Kahn, L. B.& Ackerman, L. V. (1983). The significance of microscopic invasive cancer in endoscopically removed polyps of the large bowel. A clinicopathologic study of 51 cases. *Cancer,* Vol. 52, No. 9, (Nov 1), pp. 1691-9. 0008-543X (Print) 0008-543X (Linking)

Mandel, J. S., Bond, J. H., Church, T. R., Snover, D. C., Bradley, G. M., Schuman, L. M., et al. (1993). Reducing mortality from colorectal cancer by screening for fecal occult blood. Minnesota Colon Cancer Control Study. *N Engl J Med,* Vol. 328, No. 19, (May 13), pp. 1365-71. 0028-4793 (Print) 0028-4793 (Linking)

Masaki, T., Goto, A., Sugiyama, M., Matsuoka, H., Abe, N., Sakamoto, A., et al. (2001a). Possible contribution of CD44 variant 6 and nuclear beta-catenin expression to the formation of budding tumor cells in patients with T1 colorectal carcinoma. *Cancer,* Vol. 92, No. 10, (Nov 15), pp. 2539-46. 0008-543X (Print) 0008-543X (Linking)

Masaki, T., Matsuoka, H., Sugiyama, M., Abe, N., Goto, A., Sakamoto, A., et al. (2001b). Matrilysin (MMP-7) as a significant determinant of malignant potential of early invasive colorectal carcinomas. *Br J Cancer,* Vol. 84, No. 10, (May 18), pp. 1317-21. 0007-0920 (Print) 0007-0920 (Linking)

McLoughlin, M. T.& Telford, J. J. (2007). Positive occult blood and negative colonoscopy--should we perform gastroscopy? *Can J Gastroenterol,* Vol. 21, No. 10, (Oct), pp. 633-6. 0835-7900 (Print) 0835-7900 (Linking)

Mitchell, P. J.& Haboubi, N. Y. (2008). The malignant adenoma: when to operate and when to watch. *Surg Endosc,* Vol. 22, No. 7, (Jul), pp. 1563-9. 1432-2218 (Electronic) 0930-2794 (Linking)

Morson, B. C. (1966). Factors influencing the prognosis of early cancer of the rectum. *Proc R Soc Med,* Vol. 59, No. 7, (Jul), pp. 607-8. 0035-9157 (Print) 0035-9157 (Linking)

Morson, B. C., Whiteway, J. E., Jones, E. A., Macrae, F. A.& Williams, C. B. (1984). Histopathology and prognosis of malignant colorectal polyps treated by endoscopic polypectomy. *Gut,* Vol. 25, No. 5, (May), pp. 437-44. 0017-5749 (Print) 0017-5749 (Linking)

Muller, S., Chesner, I., Egan, M., Rowlands, D., Collard, M., Swarbrick, E., et al. (1989). Significance of venous and lymphatic invasion in malignant polyps of the colon and rectum. *Gut,* Vol. 30, No., pp. 1385-1391.

Muto, T., Bussey, H. J.& Morson, B. C. (1973). Pseudo-carcinomatous invasion in adenomatous polyps of the colon and rectum. *J Clin Pathol,* Vol. 26, No. 1, (Jan), pp. 25-31. 0021-9746 (Print) 0021-9746 (Linking)

Muto, T., Bussey, H. J.& Morson, B. C. (1975). The evolution of cancer of the colon and rectum. *Cancer,* Vol. 36, No. 6, (Dec), pp. 2251-70. 0008-543X (Print) 0008-543X (Linking)

Nascimbeni, R., Burgart, L. J., Nivatvongs, S.& Larson, D. R. (2002). Risk of lymph node metastasis in T1 carcinoma of the colon and rectum. *Dis Colon Rectum,* Vol. 45, No. 2, (Feb), pp. 200-6. 0012-3706 (Print) 0012-3706 (Linking)

Netzer, P., Binek, J., Hammer, B., Lange, J.& Schmassmann, A. (1997). Significance of histologic criteria for the management of patients with malignant colorectal polyps and polypectomy. *Scand J Gastroenterol,* Vol. 32, No. 9, (Sep), pp. 910-6. 0036-5521 (Print) 0036-5521 (Linking)

Netzer, P., Forster, C., Biral, R., Ruchti, C., Neuweiler, J., Stauffer, E., et al. (1998). Risk factor assessment of endoscopically removed malignant colorectal polyps. *Gut,* Vol. 43, No. 5, (Nov), pp. 669-74. 0017-5749 (Print) 0017-5749 (Linking)

Newcomb, P. A., Storer, B. E., Morimoto, L. M., Templeton, A.& Potter, J. D. (2003). Long-term efficacy of sigmoidoscopy in the reduction of colorectal cancer incidence. *J Natl Cancer Inst,* Vol. 95, No. 8, (Apr 16), pp. 622-5. 0027-8874 (Print) 0027-8874 (Linking)

Nivatvongs, S., Rojanasakul, A., Reiman, H. M., Dozois, R. R., Wolff, B. G., Pemberton, J. H., et al. (1991). The risk of lymph node metastasis in colorectal polyps with invasive adenocarcinoma. *Dis Colon Rectum,* Vol. 34, No. 4, (Apr), pp. 323-8. 0012-3706 (Print) 0012-3706 (Linking)

Nusko, G., Mansmann, U., Altendorf-Hofmann, A., Groitl, H., Wittekind, C.& Hahn, E. G. (1997). Risk of invasive carcinoma in colorectal adenomas assessed by size and site. *Int J Colorectal Dis,* Vol. 12, No. 5, pp. 267-71. 0179-1958 (Print) 0179-1958 (Linking)

Parkin, D., Bray, F., Ferlay, J.& Pisani, P. (2005). Global Cancer Statistics, 2002. *CA Cancer J Clin,* Vol. 55, No., pp. 74-108.

Pascal, R. R., Hertzler, G., Hunter, S.& Goldschmid, S. (1990). Pseudoinvasion with high-grade dysplasia in a colonic adenoma. Distinction from adenocarcinoma. *Am J Surg Pathol,* Vol. 14, No. 7, (Jul), pp. 694-7. 0147-5185 (Print) 0147-5185 (Linking)

Pollard, C. W., Nivatvongs, S., Rojanasakul, A., Reiman, H. M.& Dozois, R. R. (1992). The fate of patients following polypectomy alone for polyps containing invasive carcinoma. *Dis Colon Rectum,* Vol. 35, No. 10, (Oct), pp. 933-7. 0012-3706 (Print) 0012-3706 (Linking)

Quirke, P., Carey, F., Newbold, M., Shepherd, N., Warren, B.& Williams, G. (2007). *Reporting lesions in the NHS Bowel Cancer Screening Programme* [Online]. Sheffield: NHS BCSP publication Available at: http://www.cancerscreening.nhs.uk/bowel/publications/nhsbcsp01.pdf [Accessed 1 March 2011].

Quirke, P.& Morris, E. (2007). Reporting colorectal cancer. *Histopathology,* Vol. 50, No. 1, (Jan), pp. 103-12. 0309-0167 (Print) 0309-0167 (Linking)

Riddell, R. H., Goldman, H., Ransohoff, D. F., Appelman, H. D., Fenoglio, C. M., Haggitt, R. C., et al. (1983). Dysplasia in inflammatory bowel disease: standardized classification with provisional clinical applications. *Hum Pathol,* Vol. 14, No. 11, (Nov), pp. 931-68. 0046-8177 (Print) 0046-8177 (Linking)

Scott, N. A., Jeacock, J.& Kingston, R. D. (1995). Risk factors in patients presenting as an emergency with colorectal cancer. *Br J Surg,* Vol. 82, No. 3, (Mar), pp. 321-3. 0007-1323 (Print) 0007-1323 (Linking)

Seitz, U., Bohnacker, S., Seewald, S., Thonke, F., Brand, B., Braiutigam, T., et al. (2004). Is endoscopic polypectomy an adequate therapy for malignant colorectal adenomas? Presentation of 114 patients and review of the literature. *Dis Colon Rectum,* Vol. 47, No. 11, (Nov), pp. 1789-96; discussion 1796-7. 0012-3706 (Print) 0012-3706 (Linking)

Selby, J. V., Friedman, G. D., Quesenberry, C. P., Jr.& Weiss, N. S. (1992). A case-control study of screening sigmoidoscopy and mortality from colorectal cancer. *N Engl J Med,* Vol. 326, No. 10, (Mar 5), pp. 653-7. 0028-4793 (Print) 0028-4793 (Linking)

Shatz, B. A., Weinstock, L. B., Swanson, P. E.& Thyssen, E. P. (1997). Long-term safety of India ink tattoos in the colon. *Gastrointest Endosc,* Vol. 45, No. 2, (Feb), pp. 153-6. 0016-5107 (Print) 0016-5107 (Linking)

Shellnut, J. K., Wasvary, H. J., Grodsky, M. B., Boura, J. A.& Priest, S. G. (2010). Evaluating the age distribution of patients with colorectal cancer: are the United States Preventative Services Task Force guidelines for colorectal cancer screening appropriate? *Dis Colon Rectum,* Vol. 53, No. 1, (Jan), pp. 5-8. 1530-0358 (Electronic) 0012-3706 (Linking)

Steele, R. J., McClements, P. L., Libby, G., Black, R., Morton, C., Birrell, J., et al. (2009). Results from the first three rounds of the Scottish demonstration pilot of FOBT screening for colorectal cancer. *Gut,* Vol. 58, No. 4, (Apr), pp. 530-5. 1468-3288 (Electronic) 0017-5749 (Linking)

Thomas, W. M., Pye, G., Hardcastle, J. D.& Walker, A. R. (1992). Screening for colorectal carcinoma: an analysis of the sensitivity of haemoccult. *Br J Surg,* Vol. 79, No. 8, (Aug), pp. 833-5. 0007-1323 (Print) 0007-1323 (Linking)

Towler, B., Irwig, L., Glasziou, P., Kewenter, J., Weller, D.& Silagy, C. (1998). A systematic review of the effects of screening for colorectal cancer using the faecal occult blood test, hemoccult. *BMJ,* Vol. 317, No. 7158, (Aug 29), pp. 559-65. 0959-8138 (Print) 0959-535X (Linking)

Ueno, H., Mochizuki, H., Hashiguchi, Y., Shimazaki, H., Aida, S., Hase, K., et al. (2004a). Risk factors for an adverse outcome in early invasive colorectal carcinoma. *Gastroenterology,* Vol. 127, No. 2, (Aug), pp. 385-94. 0016-5085 (Print) 0016-5085 (Linking)

Ueno, H., Mochizuki, H., Hashiguchi, Y., Shimazaki, H., Aida, S., Hase, K., et al. (2004b). Risk factors for an adverse outcome in early invasive colorectal carcinoma. *Gastroenterology,* Vol. 127, No. 2, pp. 385-394. 0016-5085

UK-Colorectal-Cancer-Screening-Pilot-Group. (2004). Results of the first round of a demonstration pilot of screening for colorectal cancer in the United Kingdom. *BMJ,* Vol. 329, No. 7458, (July 17, 2004), p. 133.

UK-Flexible-Sigmoidoscopy-Screening-Trial-Investigators. (2002). Single flexible sigmoidoscopy screening to prevent colorectal cancer: baseline findings of a UK multicentre randomised trial. *The Lancet,* Vol. 359, No. 9314, pp. 1291-1300. 0140-6736

Verdecchia, A., Francisci, S., Brenner, H., Gatta, G., Micheli, A., Mangone, L., et al. (2007). Recent cancer survival in Europe: a 2000-02 period analysis of EUROCARE-4 data. *Lancet Oncol,* Vol. 8, No. 9, (Sep), pp. 784-96. 1470-2045 (Print) 1470-2045 (Linking)

Volk, E. E., Goldblum, J. R., Petras, R. E., Carey, W. D.& Fazio, V. W. (1995). Management and outcome of patients with invasive carcinoma arising in colorectal polyps. *Gastroenterology,* Vol. 109, No. 6, (Dec), pp. 1801-7. 0016-5085 (Print) 0016-5085 (Linking)

West, N. J., Poullis, A. P.& Leicester, R. J. (2008). The NHS Bowel Cancer Screening Programme--a realistic approach with additional benefits. *Colorectal Dis,* Vol. 10, No. 7, (Sep), pp. 708-14. 1463-1318 (Electronic) 1462-8910 (Linking)

Whitlock, E. P., Lin, J. S., Liles, E., Beil, T. L.& Fu, R. (2008). Screening for colorectal cancer: a targeted, updated systematic review for the U.S. Preventive Services Task Force. *Ann Intern Med,* Vol. 149, No. 9, (Nov 4), pp. 638-58. 1539-3704 (Electronic) 0003-4819 (Linking)

Williams, A. R., Balasooriya, B. A.& Day, D. W. (1982). Polyps and cancer of the large bowel: a necropsy study in Liverpool. *Gut,* Vol. 23, No. 10, (Oct), pp. 835-42. 0017-5749 (Print) 0017-5749 (Linking)

Wilson, J.& Jungner, Y. (1968). Principles and practice of screening for disease. *Chron World Health Organ* Vol. 22, No., p. 473.

11

Endoscopic Submucosal Dissection for Colorectal Lesions

Takashi Shida
Department of Surgery, Funabashi Central Social Insurance Hospital, Funabashi, Chiba, Japan

1. Introduction

Recently in Japan, Endoscopic submucosal dissection (ESD) is beginning to become widely performed for the treatment of colorectal lesions. However, ESD is a very difficult technique which may lead to perforation of the colonic wall and also time consuming compared to Endoscopic mucosal resection (EMR). In this article, I would like to introduce the indications and the practical procedure of colorectal ESD.

Since Endoscopic mucosal resection (EMR) is widely and safely performed throughout the world, the indications for colorectal ESD are as follows: 1) lesions which are difficult to remove en block with a snare EMR due to size, such as those in the LST-NG category, lesions exhibiting V_I pit patterns, shallow submucosal invasive carcinoma, large depressed type tumors and large protruded type lesions suspected to be carcinoma. 2) lesions with fibrosis due to biopsy or peristalsis. 3) sporadic localized lesions in chronic inflammation, such as ulcerative colitis. 4) local residual carcinoma after EMR. This indication was proposed by Tanaka S et al and is widely applied in Japan.[1] Since, most early colorectal lesions can be treated by EMR or Endoscopic piecemeal mucosal resection (EPMR), indications for ESD is relatively limited. The most beneficial point of ESD is the accuracy of en block resection of the lesion without regard to the specimen size.

Needle knife, IT (Insulated Tipped) knife, Hook knife, Flex knife and Dual knife are representative knives for ESD.[1] For colorectal ESD, Flex knife, Dual knife and Hook knife are mainly used. Also transparent hood is essential for colorectal ESD. Glycerol or sodium hyaluronate solution is necessary for submucosal injection.[2] A good quality high-frequency power supplies like VIO300D, ICC200 (ERBE, Germany), or ESG-100 (Olympus, Japan) is also required. To decrease patient's discomfort, the Carbon dioxide insulation system (UCR system, Olympus, Japan) is useful. Carbon dioxide can be absorbed into the human tissue more than 100 times faster than room air. The use of this system can decrease the distention of the colon. [3]

In order to perform colorectal ESD, the most important point is to place the lesion opposite toward the gravity. You have to change the patient's position to check this point before starting ESD. General anesthesia is not necessary because it becomes difficult to change the patient's position during the ESD procedure. In Japan, colorectal ESD is mainly performed under conscious sedation.

After locating the lesion in the appropriate position, submucosal injection is performed. You have to inject enough amount of solution to elevate the lesion completely (Glycerol or sodium hyaluronate solution). ESD requires larger volume of submucosal injection compared to EMR. Usually, we dilute the sodium hyaluronate solution by glycerol 4 ~5 folds containing a small amount of indigo carmine and epinephrine hydrochloride. Indigo carmine is useful for a better visualization of the submucosal layer.

After submucosal injection, mucosal incision is performed. For mucosal incision, Flex knife or Dual knife is used. It is important to fix the knife gently to the colonic wall and not to press it strongly. Colonic wall is very thin, and there is no need to press the knife strongly towards the wall. When using the Flex knife, appropriate length of the knife may be about 2mm or less. If the lesion is larger than 40mm, it is important not to complete the circular mucosal incision before the submucosal dissection. This is because the submucosal solution leaks out from the mucosal incision space, and the observation of the submucosal space becomes poor. For submucosal dissection, the important point is to slide into the submucosal space by using the transparent hood as soon as possible. Flex knife or Dual knife is mainly used, but in difficult situation, Hook knife is useful. Hook knife is safe because it allows submucosal dissection by hooking and pulling the tissue towards the luminal side.[4)] During this procedure, vessels are usually seen and sometimes it requires hemostasis. Since the colonic wall is extremely thin, a special hemostatic forceps with a small cup is used (50~60W, soft coagulation). To prevent delayed perforation, excess coagulation must be avoided. Post ESD bleeding is a rare event in colorectal ESD, so there is no need for excess coagulation.

Figure 1 shows a case treated by ESD. This is a granular-type laterally spreading tumor (LST-G) with a scar, 35mm in diameter in the sigmoid colon. As shown in **figure1**, you can see that the lesion is positive for non-lifting sign. It is impossible to perform en-block resection by conventional EMR method in a case like this. The lesion had severe fibrosis in the center but it was successfully removed by ESD. The procedure time was 70 minutes.

The most hazardous and dangerous complication in colorectal ESD is the perforation of the bowel wall. This must be managed with extreme caution because it will easily lead to peritonitis and may sometimes be life threatening. When the perforation is admitted during the ESD procedure, the perforation site must be closed by an endoscopic clip immediately.[5)] To continue the ESD procedure or not depends on the condition of the patient. In my opinion, you should stop the ESD and manage the lesion later (ie; laparoscopic operation). Leading the patient to a life threatening situation should be avoided as much as possible. The most important point is that colorectal ESD is a very difficult technique and is still a clinical research procedure. Colorectal ESD should be performed only by a well experienced colonoscopist.

Colorectal ESD is now beginning to be performed in many hospitals in Japan, but is still at a clinical research level. More devices and safe procedures are warranted for the establishment of standard safe colorectal ESD. I hope that all colorectal lesions will be properly treated by a treatment method appropriately selected from among EMR, ESD and surgical resection (including laparoscopic operation) after precise preoperative diagnosis.

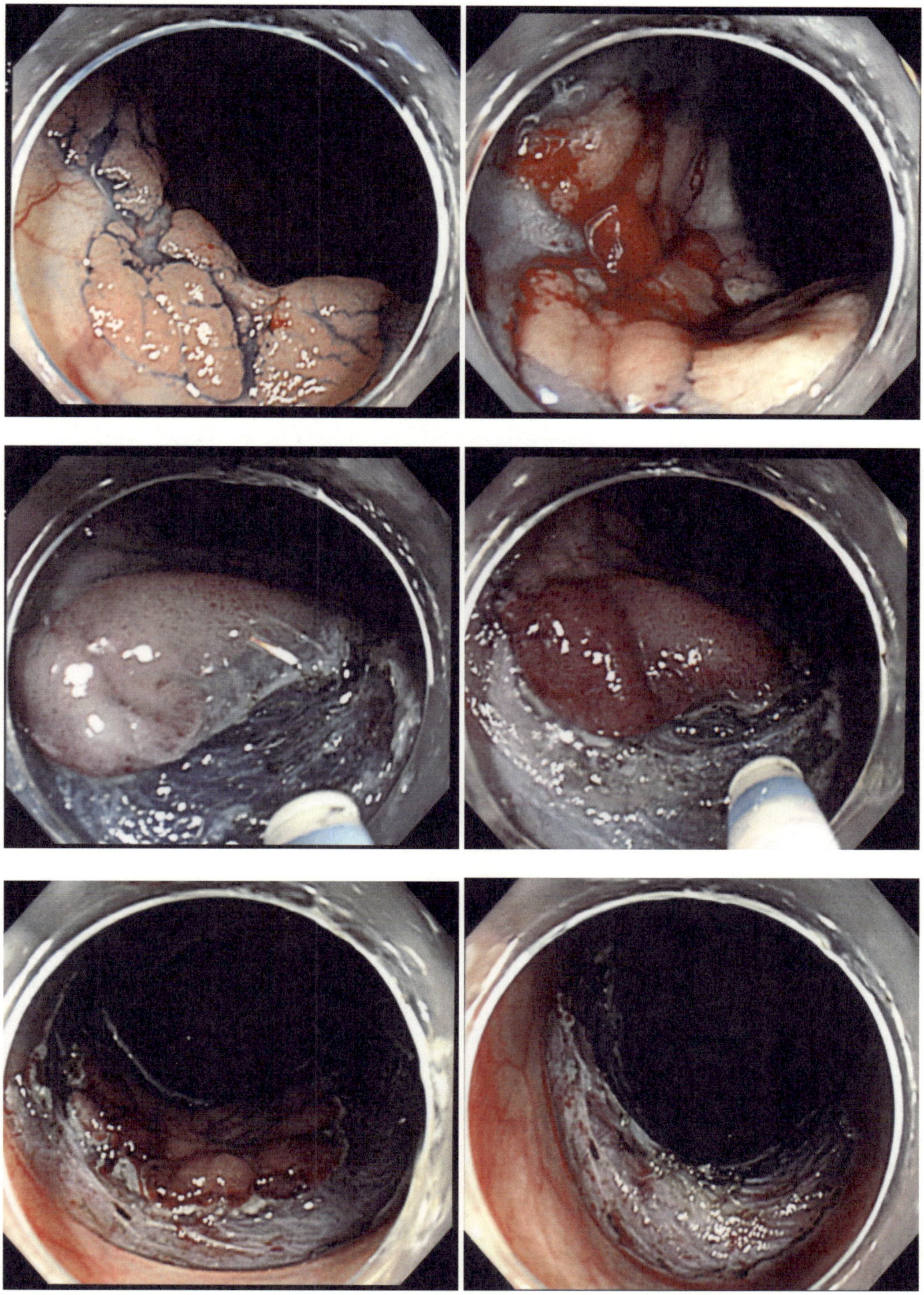

Fig. 1.

2. Reference

[1] Tanaka S, Oka S, Chayama K: Colorectal endoscopic submucosal dissection: present status and future perspective, including its differentiation from endoscopic mucosal resection. J Gastroenterol 2008;43:641-651

[2] Fujishiro M, Yahagi N, Nakamura M, et al. Successful outcomes of a novel endoscopic treatment for GI tumors: endoscopic submucosal dissection with a mixture of high-molecular-weight hyaluronic acid, glycerin, and sugar. Gastrointest Endosc 2006;63:243-249

[3] Saito Y, Uraoka T, Matsuda T, et al. A pilot study to assess the safety and efficacy of carbon dioxide insufflation during colorectal endoscopic submucosal dissection with the patient under conscious sedation. Gastrointest Endosc 2007;65:537-542

[4] Tamegai Y, Saito Y, Masaki N, et al. Endoscopic submucosal dissection: a safe technique for colorectal tumors. Endoscopy 2007;39:418-422

[5] Tanaka S, Oka S, Kaneko I, et al. Endoscopic submucosal dissection for colorectal neoplasia: possibility of standardization. Gastrointest Endosc 2007;66:100-107

12

Portal Hypertensive Colopathy

Vatsala Misra, Vishal Dhingra, S P Misra and Manisha Dwivedi
MLN Medical College, Allahabad,
India

1. Introduction

The portal vein drains blood from the small and large intestines, stomach, spleen, pancreas, and gallbladder. The superior mesenteric vein and the splenic vein unite behind the neck of the pancreas to form the portal vein. Normal portal pressure is generally defined between 5 and 10 mm Hg. An increase in the blood pressure to 12 mm Hg or greater, within a system of veins is called portal hypertension (PHT). The most common cause of portal hypertension is cirrhosis of the liver. Other causes include portal vein thrombosis and a parasitic infection by Schistosomiasis. Sometimes the cause is unknown.

Portal hypertension leads to hemodynamic disturbances throughout the gastrointestinal tract. McCormack et al (1985) coined the term congestive gastropathy to represent the mucosal changes in gastric mucosa of patients with portal hypertension and distinguished it histologically from inflammatory gastritis. (McCormack et al., 1985) The entity was attributed to alteration in gastric microcirculation.(Sarfeh et al., 1987 & Tarnawaski et al., 1988).Initial reports mainly focused on portal hypertensive gastropathy which demonstrated endoscopic and histologic changes seen in the gastric mucosa.(Baxter & Dobbs, 1988; Corbishley et al.,1988; Foster et al.,1989; SP Misra et al., 1990; Papazian et al., 1986 & Triger & Hosking,1989)The entity was renamed as 'portal hypertensive intestinal vasculopathy' with the evidence of small intestinal and colonic involvement. (Kozarek et al., 1991; Thiruvengadam & Gostout, 1989 & Viggiano & Gostout, 1992). The term portal hypertensive colopathy was initially described in the 1990, as a poorly defined entity by Naveau et al. (1991)

In patients with liver cirrhosis and portal hypertension, vascular changes in upper gastrointestinal tract in the form of varices of the esophagus, stomach and portal hypertensive gastropathy and enteropathy are well described. (V Misra et al., 1997, 1998 & SP Misra et al., 1990). In present chapter various aspects of changes in colonic mucosa of the patients with portal hypertension are described in detail.

2. Colonoscopy

Initially some authors have described hemorrhoids and colorectal hypervascularity in patients with portal hypertension (Britton,1963; Hosking et al., 1989 & Jacobs, 1980) followed by hemorrhage from lower G.I. tract (Herman et al., 1993;Izsak & Finlay,1980; Weinshel et al., 1986). The reported prevalence of hemorrhoid and anorectal varices varied from 25.2% to 63 %(Britton, 1963;Hosking et al., 1989 & Jacobs, 1980) and 0% to 89.3%(Chawala & Dilawari, 1991 & Rabinovitz et al., 1990).

None of these studies were planned or had control population. We planned a study (SP Misra et al., 1996) to find out the prevalence and factor influencing hemorrhoid, anorectal varices and colopathy. The study included 70 patients with cirrhosis and portal hypertension and 70 controls. A full length colonoscopy was carried out in all cases and presence of hemorrhoids, anorectal varices and colopathy was noted. Hemorrhoids and anorectal varices were noted in 36% and 40% patients as compared to 40% and 0% in controls respectively. The difference was statistically significant for anorectal varices($P < 0.001$). No correlation to severity of cirrhosis (Child's grade), oesophageal varices, presence or absence of gastric varices, gastropathy or sclerotherapy treatment was observed. Colopathy was seen in 48.5% and 3% of patients and controls respectively and it was seen more frequently in patients with large oesophageal varices as compared to smaller varices(87% vs 28.5%, $P<0.001$) and more often in those with gastric varices than without it (71%vs28.5%, $P< 0.001$).

Ghoshal et al.(2001) reported haemorrhoids in 21.9% patients with PHT and 16% controls (p = ns). Colorectal varices were seen in 31.7% patients with PHT and none of the controls ($p = 0.005$). Portal colopathy was present in 36.6% patients with PHT and none of the controls ($p = 0.0005$). None of the parameters (e.g. aetiology of PHT, Child's class, oesophageal variceal eradication by Endoscopic Sclerotherapy with or without Endoscopic variceal ligation, history of variceal bleeding, grade of oesophageal varices, presence of portal hypertensive gastropathy or gastric varices) predicted the occurrence of colorectal varices and portal hypertensive colopathy. Detection of colorectal varices but not portal hypertensive colopathy was associated with occurrence of hematochezia.

Assuming that PHT may cause the changes all over the gastrointestinal (GI) tract, a number of colonoscopic studies were performed. (Chen et al., 1996; Scandalis et al., 1994 & Sharma et al., 1995).The colonoscopy revealed vascular ectasias, vascular irregularity, vascular dilatation, solitary red spots, diffuse red spots and hemorrhoids. Portal hypertension produces changes in the colorectal mucosa similar to those seen in the mucosa of upper gastrointestinal tract. Other endoscopic abnormalities mentioned in this setting are anorectal and recto-sigmoid varices, hemorrhoids, multiple vascular ectasia like lesions, and nonspecific inflammatory changes. These changes were classified into four types. Solitary vascular ectasias were found predominantly in the transverse and ascending colon (55%). Diffuse vascular ectasias were found predominantly in the right side colon (45%). Redness was found in the overall colon and blue vein in the rectum. (Ito et al., 2005). They observed portal hypertensive colopathy in 23% of patients in rectosigmoid colon, 11% in the descending colon, 24%in the transverse colon, 23% in the ascending colon and16% in the cecum. These complications are a common cause of lower gastrointestinal hemorrhage.

Bresci et al(2006). also studied the colonoscopic changes in patients with portal hypertension. They found colonic varices in 31 % of the patients, portal hypertensive colopathy (PHC; defined as diffuse hyperemia, edema, spider angiomas, and spontaneous bleeding of the colonic mucosa) in 54 %, and normal colonic findings in 18 %. Colonic varices and PHC were present simultaneously in 27 % of the patients. They concluded that colonic lesions are frequent in cirrhotic patients, but statistical analysis showed that these lesions are not specific for the disease and do not correlate with the etiology and degree of cirrhosis, with the endoscopic treatment of esophageal varices, or with the risk of bleeding from the lower gastrointestinal tract.

3. Histopathological changes

Portal hypertension leads to hemodynamic disturbances throughout the GI tract. Despite several studies describing endoscopic changes, histological changes in gastric mucosa were not studied in detail. In earlier studies the congestion of the mucosal capillaries was described as the common change seen in gastric mucosa of the patients with portal hypertension. (Corbishley et al., 1988; Foster et al., 1989 & SP Misra et al, 1990). Studies of biopsies from the upper GI tract (stomach, duodenum and jejunum) have recorded predominant changes in the mucosal vessels (venules and capillaries). (Kozarek et al., 1991; Thiruvengadam & Gostout, 1989 & Viggiano & Gostout, 1992). Later on a detailed histomorphometric study of mucosal vascular changes seen in gastric, duodenal and jejunal mucosa showed that irregularity and thickening of the mucosal capillary wall is more specific than only congestion(V Misra et al., 1997, 1998) that can be seen due to artifactual factors also. (Corbishley et al.,1988).Despite well documented colonoscopic features very few studies were there describing histopathological changes, that too in brief.(Eleftheriadis et al., 1993;Naveau et al., 1991 & Scandalis et al 1994). S P Misra et al (1996) found dilated and congested mucosal capillaries in 42% of colonic biopsies whereas dilated and thick walled capillaries were seen in 49%.

We did a detailed histomorphometric study of changes in mucosal capillaries in colonic biopsies from 55 patients with portal hypertension and 25 controls. (Misra V et al., 2003). After full length colonoscopy biopsies were taken from caecum, ascending colon, transverse colon, descending colon and rectum. Morphometric assessment of diameter of the capillaries and thickness of the capillary wall was done. Presence and absence of the congestion was also noted. Dilated and congested capillaries, as well as, capillaries with irregular thickening of the wall were seen in significantly higher number of sections from patients than controls. Morphometric assessment also showed a significantly higher diameter and thickness of the capillary wall in sections from patients with portal hypertension than controls. A peculiar feature observed was thick walled dilated capillaries without red blood cells in the lumen that were seen in 46.5% biopsies (irrespective of site) from patients with portal hypertension as compared to 12% in controls ($P < 0.025$). The histological changes had no correlation with the clinical or endoscopic findings except that the thickness of the capillary wall was higher in patients who had undergone endoscopic sclerotherapy as opposed to those who had not received sclerotherapy. Besides vascular changes, other important histological features seen in the biopsies are edema, increased mononuclear cell infiltration and fibromuscular proliferation in lamina propria.

It is very important to differentiate the vascular changes of colopathy with angiodysplasia of the colon which may sometimes lead to massive lower GI bleeding. (Sharma et al., 1995) Lesions of angiodysplasia are fewer, smaller, and less widely distributed as compared to those of portal hypertension, (Naveau et al., 1995) because they are usually formed due to degenerative changes (V Misra et al., 2003) in contrast to PHT where increased venous pressure seems to be the main cause. Besides, the age of the patient (angiodysplasia usually occurs in the elderly), association with cirrhosis and endoscopic appearance may also help in differentiation. Histopathology examination of rectal mucosal lesions in patients with portal hypertension shows dilatation of blood vessels in the mucosa, increased lymphocytes and plasma cells in the lamina propria and edema of the mucosa.

4. Prognosis and treatment

Lower gastrointestinal bleeding, is the major complication of portal hypertensive colopathy. These patients may have occult blood loss or overt hematochezia. In patients with liver cirrhosis as the Child-Pugh class worsens and platelet count decreases, the prevalence of portal hypertensive colopathy increases. A colonoscopic examination in patients with liver cirrhosis is indicated, especially those with worsening Child-Pugh class and/or decreasing platelet count, to prevent complications such as lower gastrointestinal bleeding (Ito et al., 2005). Octreotide is a safe and effective treatment for severe acute bleeding from PHC, especially if the patient is not a candidate for transjugular intrahepatic portosystemic shunt (TIPS) or treatment with a beta-blocker due to the severity of liver disease or haemodynamic instability. Aydede H et al (2003) studied the effects of octreotide and propranolol on colonic mucosa in rats with portal hypertensive colopathy and showed that the mucosal changes in portal hypertensive colopathy could be corrected by drugs modifying portal blood flow.However, a sufficient reduction of portal pressure by propranolol or other medical treatment may be needed in order to discontinue octreotide infusion without the recurrence of bleeding. (Yoshie et al., 2001) Significant relationship between colorectal varices and liver disease has been reported and colorectal varices is highly appeared in patients with extrahepatic portal obstruction. Such patients have revealed arteriovenous communications at angiogram. In general, colonic resection or transanal ligation should be the first option for treatment of bleeding colonic varices and colonic mucosal lesions. Oesophageal variceal band ligation (SP Misra et al., 2002) or sclerotherapy (SP Misra et al., 1999) does not affect the anorectal varices or portal hypertensive colopathy.

5. Conclusion

Thus, portal hypertension is an important factor in the etiology of a relatively new entity portal hypertensive colopathy, and these need to be evaluated as they can be the cause of lower gastrointestinal bleeding, in these patients. Major histopathological changes seen in colonic biopsies of patients with PHT are dilated tortuous mucosal capillaries with irregular wall-thickening, edema of lamina propria and mild chronic inflammatory infiltrate, which does not show any association with clinical and endoscopic features. However, these mucosal changes, if present, should not be overlooked and a report on colonic biopsies from patients with PHT should include comments on these parameters.

6. References

Aydede H, Sakarya A, Erhan Y, Kara E, Ilkgul O, Ozdemir N.(2003). Effects of octreotide and propranolol on colonic mucosa in rats with portal hypertensive colopathy. *Hepatogastroenterology,* Vol. 50, Sept-Oct, pp.1352-1355, (ISSN: 0172-6390).

Baxter, J & Dobbs, B. (1988). Portal hypertensive gastropathy. *J.Gastroenterol. Hepatol.,* Vol. 3, pp.635-644. (ISSN: 0815-9319).

Bresci, G; Parisi, G & Capria.(2006) A Clinical relevance of colonic lesions in cirrhotic patients with portal hypertension *Endoscopy,* Aug., Vol.38, Nos.8, pp.830-835.(ISSN 0013-726X)

Britton, RC. (1963). Influence of portal-systemic collateral patterns and distribution of varices on results of surgical treatment of bleeding esophageal varices. *Surgery,* May *Vol.*53, pp.567-574 (ISSN 0039-6060)

Chawla, Y & Dilawari, JB.(1991).Anorectal varices--their frequency in cirrhotic and non-cirrhotic portal hypertension.*Gut,* Mar, Vol.32, Nos.3, pp.309-311. (ISSN 0017-5749)

Chen, LS; Lin, HC; Lee, FY; Hou, MC & Lee SD. (1996). Portal hypertensive colopathy in patients with cirrhosis. *Scand. J.Gastroenterol.,* May, Vol. 31, Nos.5, pp.490–494. (ISSN0036-5521)

Corbishley, CM; Saverymuttu, S& Maxwell, JD. (1988). Use of endoscopic biopsy for diagnosing congestive gastropathy.*J. Clin. Pathol.,* Nov., Vol. 41, Nos.11, pp.1187–1190. (ISSN 0021-9746)

Eleftheriadis, E; Kotazampassi, K; Karakavelas, G; Tzioufa, V & Papadimitriou, K.(1993) Portal hypertensive colopathy: endoscopic, hemodynamic and morphometric study. *Digestive Endoscopy,* Vol.5, pp.224-230.(ISSN 0915-5635)

Foster, PN; Wyatt, JI; Bullimore, DW& Losowsky, MS. (1989). Gastric mucosa in patients with portal hypertension: prevalence of capillary dilatation and Campylobacter pylori.*J. Clin. Pathol.,* Sept., Vol. 42, Nos.9, pp.919–921. (ISSN 0021-9746)

Ghoshal, UC; Biswas, PK; Roy, G; Pal, BB; Dhar, K & Banerjee, PK.(2001). Colonic mucosal changes in portal hypertension. *Trop Gastroenterol,* Jan-Mar, Vol.22, Nos.1, pp.25-27.(ISSN 0250-626X)

Herman, BE; Baum, S; Denobile, J& Volpe, RJ.(1993). Massive bleeding from rectal varices. *Am J Gastroenterol.,* Jun, Vol.88, Nos.6, pp.939-942.(ISSN 0002-9270)

Hosking, SW; Smart, HL; Johnson, AG& Triger, DR.(1989) Anorectal varices, haemorrhoids, and portal hypertension. *Lancet,* Feb, Vol.18, Nos.1(8634), pp.249-352.(ISSN 0140-6736)

Ito, K; Shiraki, K; Sakai T; Yoshimura, H & Nakano T.(2005) Portal hypertensive colopathy in patients with liver cirrhosis. *World J Gastroenterol.,* May, Vol.11, Nos.20, pp.3127-3130.(ISSN 1007-9327)

Izsak, EM & Finlay, JM. (1980).Colonic varices. Three case reports and review of the literature. *Am J Gastroenterol.*; Feb, Vol.73, Nos.2, pp.131-136. (ISSN 0002-9270)

Jacobs, DM; Bubrick, MP; Onstad, GR & Hitchcock, CR. (1980).The relationship of hemorrhoids to portal hypertension. *Dis Colon Rectum,* Nov-Dec, Vol.23, Nos.8, pp.567-569.(ISSN 1530-0358)

Kozarek, RA; Botoman, VA; Bredfeldt, JE;Roach, JM; Patterson, DJ & Ball, TJ. (1991). Portal colopathy: prospective study in patients with portal hypertension. *Gastroenterology,* Nov, Vol. 101, Nos. 5, pp.1192–1197.(ISSN 0016-5085)

McCormack, TT; Sims, J; Eyre-Brook, I. et al. (1985). Lesions in Portal hypertension: Inflammatory gastritis or congestive gastropathy?. *Gut,* Nov, Vol. 26, Nos 11, pp. 1226–1232. (ISSN *0017-5749)*

Misra, SP; Dwivedi, M; Misra, V; Agarwal, SK; Gupta, R; Gupta, SC & Mittal, VP. (1990). Endoscopic and histological appearance of gastric mucosa in patients with portal hypertension. *Gastrointestinal Endoscopy,* Nov-Dec, Vol. 36, Nos 6, pp. 575-579.(ISSN 0016 5107)

Misra, SP; Dwivedi, M & Misra, V. (1996). Prevalence and factors influencing hemorrhoids, anorectal varices and colopathy in patients with portal hypertension. *Endoscopy,* May, Vol. 28, Nos.4, pp.340 -345. .(ISSN 0013-726X)

Misra, SP; Misra, V & Dwivedi, M. (1999). Effect of oesophageal variceal sclerotherapy on hemorrhoids, anorectal varices and portal colopathy. *Endoscopy, Nov.*, Vol.31, Nos 9, pp.741-744. .(ISSN0013-726X)

Misra, SP; Misra, V & Dwivedi, M.(2002). Effect of esophageal band ligation on hemorrhoids, anorectal varices and portal hypertensive colopathy. *Endoscopy*, Mar., Vol.34, Nos.3, pp.195-198. .(ISSN 0013-726X)

Misra, V; Misra, SP;Dwivedi, M & Gupta, SC. (1997). Histomorphometric study of portal hypertensive enteropathy. *American Journal of Clinical Pathology*, Dec, Vol. 108, Nos 6, pp. 652-7.(ISSN 0002- 9173)

Misra, V; Misra, SP& Dwivedi, M. (1998). Thickened gastric mucosal capillary wall: a histological marker for portal hypertension. *Pathology*, Feb, Vol.30, Nos 1, pp. 10-13.(ISSN 0031-2025)

Misra, V; Misra, SP; Dwivedi, M; Singh, PA & Kumar, V. (2003) Colonic mucosa in patients with portal hypertension. *J Gastroenterol Hepatol*, MarVol.18, Nos 3, pp.302-8. (ISSN: 0815-9319).

Naveau, S; Leger-Ravet, MB; Houdayer, C; et al.(1995) . Nonhereditary colonic angiodysplasias. *Dig. Dis. Sci.* Apr, Vol. 40, Nos 4, pp. 839–842.(ISSN 0163 2116)

Papazian, A; Braillon, A; Dupas, JL; Sevvent, F& Capron, JP. (1986) .Portal hypertensive gastric mucosa: an endoscopic study. *Gut*, Oct, Vol. 27, Nos10, pp. 1199–1203. (ISSN *0017-5749)*

Rabinovitz, M; Zajko, AB; et al.(1990). Diagnostic value of brush cytology in the diagnosis of bile duct carcinoma: a study in 65 patients with bile duct strictures .*Hepatology*, Oct, Vol.12, Nos.4, pp.747-752.(ISSN 1527 3350)

Sarfeh, IJ & Tarnawaski, A. (1987) .Gastric mucosal vasculopathy in portal hypertension. *Gastroenterology*, Nov, Vol.93, Nos 5, pp. 1129–1131.(ISSN 0016-5085)

Scandalis, N; Archimandritis, A; et al., (1994). Colon findings in cirrhotics with portal hypertension. A prospective colonoscopic and histological study. *J. Clin. Gastroenterol*. Jun, Vol. 18(4), pp.325–328. (ISSN 0192-0970)

Sharma, R & Gorbein, MJ. (1995) .Angiodysplasia and lower gastrointestinal tract bleeding in elderly patients. *Arch.Intern. Med*, April24, Vol. 155(8), pp.807–812.(ISSN 0003-9926)

Tarnawski, A; Sarfeh, IJ; Stachura, J et al. (1988). Microvascular abnormalities of the portal hypertensive gastric mucosa. *Hepatology, Nov-Dec*, Vol.8(6), pp. 1488–1494. (ISSN 1527 3350)

Triger, D; Hosking, S. (1989) .The gastric mucosa in portal hypertension.*J. Hepatol.*, Mar, Vol. 8(2), pp.267–272. (ISSN 1527 3350)

Thiruvengadam, R & Gostout, CJ. (1989) . Congestive gastroenteropathy: An extension of nonvariceal upper gastrointestinal bleeding in portal hypertension. *Gastrointest Endosc.*, Vol. 35(6), pp, 504–507. (ISSN 0016 5107)

Viggiano, TR & Gostout, CJ. (1992). Portal hypertensive intestinal vasculopathy: a review of the clinical, endoscopic andhistopathological features. *Am. J. Gastroenterol.*, Vol. 87(8), pp.944–954.(ISSN 0002-9270)

Weinshel, E; Chen, W; Falkenstein, DB; Kessler, R & Raicht, RF. (1986) Hemorrhoids or rectal varices: defining the cause of massive rectal hemorrhage in patients with portal hypertension. *Gastroenterology.*, Vol.90, Nos.3, pp.744-747 .(ISSN 0016-5085)

Yoshie K, Fujita Y, Moriya A, Kawana I, Miyamoto K, Umemura S. (2001)Octreotide for severe acute bleeding from portal hypertensive colopathy: a case report. *Eur J Gastroenterol Hepatol, Vo.*13, Nos.9, pp.1111-1113. (ISSN 0954 691X)

Part 3

The Future?

13

Research and Therapeutic Innovation: Tissue Resonance InterferoMeter Probe in Early Detection-Screening for Rectal Cancer

Alberto Vannelli and Luigi Battaglia
Fondazione IRCCS "Istituto Nazionale Tumori", Milan, Italy

1. Introduction

Clarke's Second Law is: "The only way of discovering the limits of the possible is to venture a little way past them into the impossible" (Clarke, 1962). Tissue Resonance InterferoMeter Probe (trimprob) issues this challenge.

Cancer is a major health problem in developed countries, in many of which it is the second most common cause of death for all ages combined. At the beginning of the 21st century 10 million people in the world develop cancer each year (Blackledge, 2003).

In the Globocan 2002 database of the International Agency for Research on Cancer (IARC), the worldwide burden of colorectal cancer (CRC) is estimated as 550,000 incident new cases and 278,000 deaths for men, and 473,000 incident new cases and 255,000 deaths for women. In 2002, CRC comprised 9.4% of the global cancer burden in both sexes and was most frequent in North America, Australia, New Zealand, and parts of Europe. This has led to colorectal cancer being considered as a disease of the Western lifestyle (Winawer, 2007). The advent of molecularly targeted drugs promised to change survival. Within 20 years CRC will be considered a chronic disease, joining conditions such as diabetes, heart disease and asthma. Although very successfully used in combination, chemotherapy results in metastatic CRC have been disappointing with little more than palliative benefit. For example chemotherapy for advanced CRC cured with a low complete response and most patients relapsed with resistant disease (Vincenzi et al., 2004). These conditions impact on the way people live but will not inexorably lead to death. Individual cancer risk assessment will lead to tailored prevention messages and a specific screening programme to pick up early cancer and have far reaching public health consequences. Therefore, improving screening shows the challenges that need to be addressed in order to deliver most health benefit. But cancer prevention absorbs only 2 per cent of the total funding of cancer care and research in the world. Information regarding resources allocated to cancer is particularly scarce, even more so for CRC (Kanavos et al., 2008). CRC is rapidly increasing in Asia, but screening guidelines are lacking (Sung et al., 2005). Data regarding resources allocated to CRC in Latin America or Africa are absent. CRC expenditure adjusted for cancer population burden in the few countries collecting cancer expenditure, found large variations between countries (high of €85,116 per total cancer death in Sweden to a low of €9,528 in Russia). This continued with CRC expenditure, where the range was from €10,288 per CRC mortality

(Hungary) to €122,828 (France). Approximately half of surveyed countries had formal resource allocation mechanisms; fewer had disease-specific resource allocation, and only Australia reported cancer-specific resource allocation. The majority of countries perceived insufficient resources were allocated to cancer care and CRC care. Eastern European countries reported significant problems with cancer-specific funds, with persistent shortcomings and insufficient funding. Many of the countries that have formal screening activities, be it for CRC or other cancers, have formal screening resource allocation. Australia, some European countries and the USA all have governmental funding for their CRC screening programmes, ranging from €8-25 million. These values are half of what these countries allocate to their breast cancer screening programmes. It appears that cancer spending displays significant variation between countries, along with the majority of countries not accounting for cancer in its resource allocation mechanisms. As cancer accounts for significant morbidity and mortality after cardiovascular disease, this seems to be an important omission. Cancer care is a significant part of health care expenditure, and should be accounted and planned for appropriately.

All these data reinforce the opinion on which the CRC is one on the most important problem in Healthcare. What's the solution? The current opinion suggests to spread screening programmes.

But what is a screening? Screening programmes would be developed on a national basis if they are simple, robust and cheap. Patients would expect the screening to take place at a convenient venue for them – in shopping malls and not be painful or overly time-consuming. Health professionals would demand that any programme is accurate and does not give misleading results, and governments would demand that its costs would lead to more effective use of other resources. Novel providers of risk assessment services are likely to emerge. (Sikora, 2007). According to Mayo Clinic staff: "Colon cancer is cancer of the large intestine (colon), the lower part of your digestive system. Rectal cancer is cancer of the last several inches of the colon. Together, they're often referred to as colorectal cancers. Most cases of colon cancer begin as small, noncancerous (benign) clumps of cells called adenomatous polyps. Over time some of these polyps become colon cancers. Polyps may be small and produce few, if any, symptoms". For this reason, doctors recommend regular screening tests to help prevent colon cancer by identifying polyps before they become colon cancer.

Therefore it's correct to assume that most CRCs arise from sporadic adenomas, and a few from genetic polyposis syndromes or inflammatory bowel disease (IBD). Because of high prevalence, as well as a long asymptomatic phase and treatability of precancerous lesions, colorectal cancer is an ideal target for screening. But these axioms cast doubts about the efficacy of CRC screening.

The term "polyp" refers to a discrete mass that protrudes into the intestinal lumen, but the reported prevalence of adenomatous polyps, on the basis of screening colonoscopy data, is only in the range of 18–36%. Moreover the risk for CRC varies from country to country and even within countries. The risk also varies among individual people based on diet, lifestyle, and hereditary factors. Current guidelines are directed to test asymptomatic men and women who are likely to have adenomatous polyps or cancer but current CRC screening are efficacy only on symptomatic population. This screening always needs to be applied within the framework of a program that includes: primary prevention (diet, lifestyle), timely diagnostic work-up with colonoscopy (where available and consistent with the cascade) overall in those screened positive, and timely treatment (polypectomy, surgery). CRC screening is particularly challenging, as reflected in current low screening rates in most countries where there is a high risk for CRC. CRC screening is complex, as there are multiple options, it requires considerable patient effort (fecal occult blood test slides, colonoscopy preparation, etc.), and it requires sedation and a health-care partner for some tests (colonoscopy). For a screening program to be successful, multiple events have to occur, beginning with awareness and recommendation from the primary-care physician, patient acceptance, financial coverage, risk stratification, screening test, timely diagnosis, timely treatment, and appropriate follow-up. If any one of these steps is faulty or is not of high quality, the screening will fail.

Previous studies have investigated the cost-effectiveness of colonoscopy, flexible sigmoidoscopy, and fecal occult blood testing as screening alternatives (Sonnemberg et al, 2000). Flexible sigmoidoscopy was less cost-effective than fecal occult blood testing and colonoscopy. Fecal occult blood testing is a simple, low-cost screening method, but colonoscopy was more effective in saving lives. All standard options for CRC screening are not convincing because are cost-effective only in average-risk individuals. They are more cost-effective than other forms of medical screening: cholesterol in hypertension.

Screening tests	Evidence		
	Sensitivity	Specificity	
Occult blood tests	50-60%	95.2%	Fecal occult blood testing using the guaiac smear is currently being replaced in many countries by fecal immunochemical tests.
Fecal DNA tests	52%	94.4%	the optimal set of molecular markers remains to be determined, and the feasibility of such tests when applied to the general population is as yet unknown.
Flexible sigmoidoscopy	35-70%,	98–100%	the sensitivity is low due to the significant number of right-sided adenomas that occur in the absence of distal tumors and are therefore missed on flexible sigmoidoscopy.
Colonoscopy	at least 95% for large polyps	at least 95% for large polyps	There are no prospective randomized studies that have examined the impact of colonoscopy on incidence or mortality.
Double-contrast barium enema	48%	50%	It's more likely than colonoscopy to yield false-positives.
Computed-tomographic colonography	93% for polyps 10 mm or larger	97% for polyps 10 mm or larger	When polyps of all sizes were included, the studies were too heterogeneous in sensitivity (range 45–97%) and specificity (range 26–97%).

Table 1. Screening tests and evidence.

Systematic screening colonoscopy in first-degree relatives of patients with CRC, starting at the age of 40, demonstrates an economic benefit only in comparison with multiple-drug intensive chemotherapy for advanced cancer, screening is cost-saving (Table 1). However, high costs and low compliance rates for colonoscopy have encouraged a search for different methods. It has been proposed that cancer exposed to a low level of electromagnetic incident waves may behave differently than healthy tissue. The phenomenon of "nonlinear resonance interaction," which is produced when the oscillations of an electromagnetic probe are coupled with those from biological tissue, can be used to test for differences between healthy and cancerous tissues (Vedruccio et al., 2004).

2. Electro-medical device for non invasive diagnostics

2.1.1 Historical background

Diagnosis of cancer in humans is mainly based on microscopic observation of morphological changes in cells and irregularities in tissues through the use of cytological and histological methods (Bibbo, 1997). All these processes are the manifestation of hidden processes of biochemical as well as physical nature. One of the most important as well as misleading effect is the Mitochondrial Warburg Effect. For a long time, disturbances in physical processes in cancer development were not adequately taken into consideration. To understand what does it mean, it's necessary to start by the end of this process. Therapeutic selectivity, or preferential killing of cancer cells without significant toxicity to normal cells, is one of the most important considerations in cancer chemotherapy (Pelicano et al., 2006). Understanding the biological differences between normal and cancer cells is essential for the design and development of anticancer drugs with selective anticancer activity. Cancer is a family of diseases that involve uncontrolled cell division and tissue invasiveness (metastasis). In the recent years, tremendous progress has been made in our understanding of the molecular mechanisms of cancer, in identification of specific genes and signalling pathways involved in carcinogenesis and cancer progression, and in developing chemical compounds or specific antibodies that specifically target the oncogenic molecules.

Cancers result from a series (progression) of gene mutations that typically involve two categories of function: promotion of cell division and inactivation of cell cycle suppression. Proto-oncogenes are normal genes that promote cell growth and mitosis, whereas tumor suppressor genes discourage cell growth. Proto-oncogenes can be mutated by carcinogenic agents to become oncogenes. Oncogenes produce excessive levels of growth promoting proteins. Tumor suppressor gene products typified by p53 are frequently transcription factors that suppress mitosis and cell growth to allow for DNA repair. Nearly half of all cancers involve altered p53 genes. Other suppressor genes include Rb (retinoblastoma family), APC (adenomatous polyposis coli), SMAD4, TP53, p16/CDKN2A and BRCA (breast cancer susceptibility protein) types 1 and 2. Cancer results from cumulative mutations of proto-oncogenes and suppressor genes which together allow the unregulated growth of cells. Oncogenes are typically dominant because they provide gain-of-function, whereas suppressor genes are recessive. They contain loss-of function mutations. Both copies of a suppressor gene need to mutate to cause loss-of-suppressor function. Only one copy of a proto-oncogene needs to mutate for gain-of-function. Mutations of tumor suppressor genes can be inherited. Over time malignant cells can self-select for characteristics that make them more malignant: ability to avoid apoptosis; immortalization due to over expression of telomerase; growth-factor self-sufficiency and resistance to anti-growth factors; increased cell division; altered differentiation; loss of contact inhibition, become metastatic; and able to promote angiogenesis. The target-specific agents have major advantages over the traditional chemotherapeutic compounds in that the targeting agents specifically interact with the key molecular players in cancer cells and have low toxicity to the normal cells. In the past researchers assumed that cancer cells and normal cells had much in common in terms of the internal machinery that allows them to carryout the many activities necessary to stay alive. Chemotherapy drugs effectively target processes that cancer cells need to grow and divide, such as the ability of the cancer cells to replicate their DNA. However, many normal cells, like the cells that line the digestive tract, also need to replicate. In short, though chemotherapy drugs are particularly toxic to cancer cells, they also damage healthy cells. The use of standard chemotherapy therefore produces many, and often severe, side effects. Furthermore, these side effects sometimes prevent patients from being able to take high enough doses to fight the cancer most effectively. While chemotherapy drugs are quite effective treatments for many forms of cancer, researchers have been working diligently to produce drugs that target the processes of cancer cells specifically so as to leave healthy cells unharmed. The accumulation of knowledge about the specific differences between normal and cancerous cells has allowed for the development of treatments targeted at cancer-specific activities.

One of the most fundamental changes found in cancer cells is the presence of mutations in the genes that are responsible for causing cell growth (oncogenes). The defective proteins produced by these altered genes are prime candidates for targeted therapy. As an example, some cancers are caused in part by mutant proteins that send constant signals into the cell causing cell division. Drugs that block only the mutant form of the protein but do not interfere with the activity of the normal version would only affect cancer cells, and would leave healthy cells untouched. Alternatively, many cancers result when genes that normally prevent cell growth (tumor suppressors) are inactivated or turned off. Drugs that "fix" the activity of these proteins would repair the damaged cancer cells, but theoretically have no effect on normal cells.

New agents with a high degree of target specificity and clinical therapeutic activity, exemplified by Gleevec (imatinib), Iressa (gefitinib), herceptin (trastuzumab), and rituximab, represent an exciting direction for cancer drug development. However, the mechanisms underlying cancer development and the disease progression are extremely complex, and it is now recognized that in many types of cancers there are multiple genetic and epigenetic alterations. Even within a specific cancer type, the malignant cell populations are heterogeneous and contain diverse genetic changes, which further alter over time because of genetic instability as the disease progresses. As such, it would be difficult to specifically kill these cancer cells by targeting a single gene. Proper combination of multiple target-specific agents may be required to effectively eliminate the entire cancer cell population.

An alternative strategy to achieve both therapeutic selectivity and efficiency is to take advantage of the fundamental difference between cancer cells and normal cells in their biochemical metabolism. Cell proliferation requires the conversion of nutrients into biomass. One of the first differences noted between cancer cells and normal cells was a difference in metabolism (Vander Heiden et al., 2009). One of the most prominent metabolic alterations in cancer cells is the increase in aerobic glycolysis and the dependency on glycolytic pathway for ATP generation as showed in Figure 1 (Erickson & Cerione , 2010).

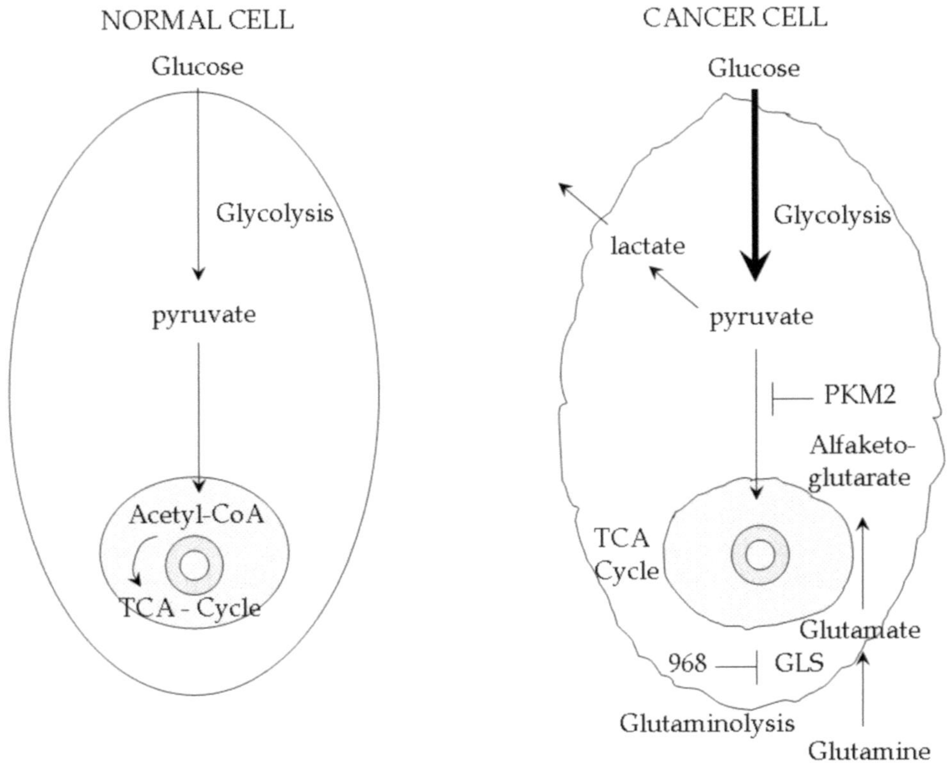

Fig. 1. Different metabolic pathway

This is the Warburg effect (Warburg et al., 1924; Warburg, 1930, 1956). As this metabolic alteration is frequently seen in cancer cells of various tissue origins, targeting the glycolytic pathway may preferentially kill the malignant cells and therefore have broad therapeutic implications. Although cancer cell energy generation is mainly dependent on reactive anaerobic glycolysis, most malignant tumors still breathe, in part by an uncoupling protein-mediated mitochondrial pathway. Uncoupling proteins help import fatty acids and are over expressed in various types of chemo-resistant cancer cells (Mayevsky, 2009). New technologies will help accomplish this systematic work.

2.1.2 Warburg effect

Otto Heinrich Warburg (October 8th, 1883, Freiburg im Breisgau - August 1st, 1970, Berlin), was a German physiologist, medical doctor and Nobel laureate. "Warburg effect" is used for two unrelated observations in biochemical, one in plant physiology and the other in oncology, As early as 1924 he demonstrated that tumor cells exhibit an altered sugar metabolism as they are metabolizing up to 20 times more glucose compared to healthy cells (Warburg et al., 1924). These cancer cells produce lactate in large amounts not only under anaerobic conditions (like their healthy counterparts) but also in the presence of oxygen. This so called “Warburg effect” or “aerobic glycolysis”. This is remarkable, since glucose metabolism under aerobic conditions via Embden-Meyerhof pathway (EMP), citrate cycle and respiratory chain yields 38 ATP per molecule glucose, while glycolysis to lactate leads to only 2 ATP. In the presence of oxygen and glucose, healthy cells generate a vast majority of energy in form of ATP by complete combustion of glucose to CO2, while tumor cells metabolize the majority of glucose via pentose phosphate pathway (PPP) to lactate. According to standard textbooks the PPP provides cells with reduction equivalents in form of NADPH and moreover with ribose- 5-P, a key metabolite for DNA/RNA biosynthesis. The non-oxidative part of PPP is controlled by transketolase. Ever since the pioneering observation that aerobic glycolysis in cancer is preferred over oxidative phosphorylation as a mechanism to generate ATP from glucose, numerous experiments have supported and extended the significant role that metabolisms have on transformation, proliferation, angiogenesis and metastasis in cancer. Thus, scanning human tumors with positron emission tomography (PET) has verified that a high uptake rate of glucose constitutes a hallmark in cancer cells, presumably required to confer adaptive advantages when facing acidic and hypoxic environments.

Normal cells use glycolysis prior to respiration in the mitochondria and complete breakdown of glucose by the tricarboxylic acid (TCA) cycle (Figure 1). In cancer cells, glycolysis becomes the primary mode of glucose metabolism resulting in lactate and its secretion. The M2 isoform of pyruvate kinase (PKM2) becomes tyrosine phosphorylated and attenuates pyruvate acetyl-CoA conversion while glutaminolysis provides the cancer cell with an alternate source of biosynthetic precursors, fueling the TCA cycle with glutamine-derived α-keto-glutarate. The anti-tumor drug 968 inhibits glutamine metabolism by inhibiting the enzyme glutaminase (GLS).

Cancer cells have a high glycolysis rate even in the presence of oxygen (Figure 1). Otto Warburg, assumed that because of mitochondrial malfunction, cancer cells had to depend on anaerobic glycolysis to generate ATP (Warburg, 1956). This hypothesis was later disproved. It was demonstrated, however, that cancer cells with intact mitochondria also showed evidence of the Warburg effect. This effect provides a marker for detecting tumor cells. With positron emission tomography using a glucose radioisotope (18fluorodeoxyglucose), cancer cells can be visualized owing to their significantly higher than normal glucose uptake.

Thus, an alternative explanation was proposed: the Warburg effect helps cancer cells harness additional ATP to meet the high energy demand required for their extraordinary growth while providing a basic building block of metabolites for their proliferation. A third view suggests that the Warburg effect is a defense mechanism, protecting cancer cells from the higher than usual oxidative environment in which they survive. Interestingly, the latter view does not conflict with the high-energy production view, as increased glucose metabolism enables cancer cells to produce larger amounts of both antioxidants to fight oxidative stress and ATP and metabolites for growth. It may be related to the surprising fact that although aerobic respiration produces 18 times the ATP per mole of glucose compared with anaerobic glycolysis, the rate of anaerobic glycolysis is 100 times that of aerobic respiration. According to a population biology model developed at the Max Delbrück Center for Molecular Medicine in Germany, ATP production at a higher rate but lower yield may confer a selective advantage in competing for shared energy resources. Lactate, also a product of glycolysis, induces several oncogenes. In addition, lactate surrounds cancer cells, providing an acidic environment that protects cancer cells from the immune system. A key enzyme of the pentose phosphate pathway, transketolase, was shown to play an important role in cancer proliferation and malignancy. Among colon and uroepithelial cancer patients, the expression level of transketolase-like gene 1 (one of the transketolase genes) was strongly related to the patients' survival rate. Autopsy results confirmed the correlation between increased expression of transketolase-like gene 1 and a higher mortality rate (Langbein et al, 2006). Several factors contribute to cellular oxidative stress, which occurs when the balance between oxidants and antioxidants is disrupted, resulting in an overall increase in reactive oxygen species (ROS). ROS are produced as a result of various metabolic events; for example, in the formation of water molecules during mitochondrial respiration. Molecular oxygen (O2) is the terminal electron acceptor in the electron transport system of mitochondria and is converted to water (H2O). In some cases, O2 receives just one electron, becoming a superoxide anion. It is estimated that 4-5% of O2 molecules are normally converted to superoxide anions (Spitz et al, 2000). Superoxides are then converted to peroxides by an enzyme called superoxide dismutase. Subesquent, pyruvate scavenges the peroxides and converts them into water. Thus, an increased glycolysis rate that leads to increased pyruvate production may reduce oxidative stress.

There are two more ways in which the Warburg effect may reduce oxidative stress. Mitochondrial dysfunction may result in reduced oxidative stress, given that mitochondria are a main source of ROS generation (Orrenius, 2007). Alternatively, the antioxidant production associated with the Warburg effect may protect cancer cells from the negative effects of their explosive glycolysis.

Network modeling of the interconnections among the crucial factors involved in metabolic flow and signaling pathways is a necessary future undertaking. In addition, the mitochondrial uncoupling effect should not be overlooked. Although cancer cell energy generation is mainly dependent on reactive anaerobic glycolysis, most malignant tumors still breathe, in part by an uncoupling protein-mediated mitochondrial pathway (Samudio et al., 2007). Uncoupling proteins help import fatty acids and are over expressed in various types of chemo-resistant cancer cells. This may increase an apoptotic threshold level. On the one hand a better understanding of metabolism in cancer cells may lead to the development of novel therapeutic strategies exploiting their uniqueness.

On the other current technologies may help accomplish this systematic work. In addition to PET and magnetic resonance, the next-generation scans is needed to precisely study cancer cell biochemical. As evidenced by current proteomics and biomarker studies, detection limits should be less than femto- to ato- mole levels, considering that significant proteins or small peptides secreted from a tiny tumor cell may represent only 1% of the total protein and are extensively diluted throughout the human body.

2.1.3 Metabolomics

After the pioneered study of Warburg, current research findings confirm that a major difference between healthy and malignant cells is the supply of energy within the cell by oxidative phosphorylation in the mitochondria and glycolysis in the cytoplasm. This biochemical assumption let to develop another innovative consideration in oncology. Traditional Chinese Medicine, Ayuvedic Medicine and the Ancient Greek and Roman Doctors all incorporated 'types' into their healing methods the idea that biological fluids reflect the health of an individual; with the introduction of Warburg effect it has been possible to think a further step: metabolic effect. During the 1940's and 50's Dr. Roger Williams developed the concept of 'biochemical individuality' and determined that "metabolic profiles" were needed to effectively evaluate and treat patients with nutrition. First time was born the concept that individuals might have a “metabolic profile” that could be reflected in the makeup of their biological fluids. The work of Williams and his group, however, was apparently not duplicated by others, to whom his task must have seem rather herculean, with but few promises of tangible results. Hence, his ideas about the utility of metabolic pattern analysis remained essentially dormant until the late 1960s, when gas chromatography and liquid chromatography was advanced sufficiently to permit such studies to be carried out with considerably less effort. In this way it became feasible to quantitatively (as opposed to qualitatively) measure metabolic profiles. The term "metabolic profile" was introduced at the beginning 1970s after they demonstrated that gas chromatography, especially when interfaced with mass spectrometry could be used to measure compounds present in human urine and tissue extracts, defining the patterns of biochemically related metabolites (Horning, et. al. 1971). Moreover it demonstrated the utility of using nuclear magnetic resonance spectroscopy to detect metabolites in unmodified biological samples.

In general terms the systematic study of the unique chemical fingerprints that specific cellular processes leave behind - specifically, the study of their small-molecule metabolite profiles is metabolomics. Such approach has found applications in many topics: for example oncology. Metabolomics have led to several successes in the field of cancer biology, such as the identification of new tumour subtypes, as well as transcriptional and protein biomarkers for certain types of cancer. Metabolic activity can also be quantified, as various analytical tools have been developed to measure concentrations of low-molecular-weight metabolites. This is a particularly challenging task as low-molecular-weight metabolites represent a diverse range of chemicals.

Metabolomics has also been used to differentiate between different cancer cell lines and to monitor metabolic processes that occur in cancer cells during events such as apoptosis. Despite the successful use of metabolomics to investigate phenotypes of transgenic animals and plants, and its use in the pharmaceutical industry, most functional genomic studies of cancer have focused on transcriptomics and proteomics. Global metabolic prowling analysis holds the promise to permit simultaneous monitoring of precursors, intermediates and products of metabolic pathways. It is a research tool that can detect and monitor unidentified compounds as well as identified metabolites that play important roles in metabolism and physiology (Kaplan et al., 2004). For example metabolite profiling was used to characterize stress responses of potato tissue subjected to reversible electroporation, providing insights on how potato tissue responds to a physical stimulus such as pulsed electric fields (PEF), which is an artificial stress (Galindo et al, 2009).

2.1.4 Vedruccio theory

Today the study of biochemical interactions becomes the prevailing paradigm used to explain cellular functions and disease progression in oncology. Yet many biological questions cannot be answered with biochemical explanations alone such as the role of endogenously created electromagnetic fields and electrical currents in the body. In the past century, a great number of researchers have given their contribution to the study of the interactions between biological matter and electromagnetic fields. Electromagnetic fields are waves that transport energy through space. They are characterized by wavelength and frequency, the two of which are inversely correlated. Electromagnetic fields include the following (in order of decreasing wavelength and increasing frequency): electromagnetic fields of extremely low frequency (from electric sources), electromagnetic fields of low frequency, electromagnetic fields of radiofrequency and microwaves (from mobile telephones, television antennas etc), ultrasounds, infrared rays, ultraviolet rays, X rays and gamma rays. Since the 1970s the non thermal effects of electromagnetic fields on living organisms have been well known and also the non thermal mechanisms have been investigated. In the case of a biochemical system we assume that each molecule can be labelled with a mean velocity energy which, in turn, defines an average energy associated with each degree of freedom of the molecule itself. In such a picture a perturbation is termed "thermal" if it is able to change the average kinetic energy associated to each degree of freedom, in such a way that the average of the energies on the ensemble is changed. The rotating motion of water molecules induced by microwaves is the most evident achievement of such a thermal effect. Electromagnetic fields and life identified several significant effects of the interaction of electromagnetic fields with living organisms. If living organisms possess the ability to utilize electromagnetic fields and electricity there must exist physical structures within the cells that facilitate the sensing, transducing, storing and transmitting of this form of energy.

Normal cells possess the ability to communicate information inside themselves and between other cells. The coordination of information by the cells of the body is involved in the regulation and integration of cellular functions and cell growth. When cancer arises cancer cells are no longer regulated by the normal control mechanisms. Measurements on biological materials were based on resistivity or impedance and instruments such as the Wheatstone bridge (Presman, 1970). After the second world conflict, investigations on biological materials were extended into the microwave bands (Messen, 2000). In the 1920s Some authors discovered that both proliferating cells and cancer cells had cell membrane potentials that have been lower than the cell membrane potential of healthy adult cells (Fricke, 1926). They reported that "malignant tumors have a greater polarizability than normal breast tissues or benign tumors". They carried out their experiments at low frequencies around 20 kHz. In cancerous tissue the electrical potential of cell membranes is maintained at a lower level than that of healthy cells and electrical connections are disrupted (Cone, 1975).

Electric fields induce or a cause alignment in dipole movements. Most of the molecules in the body are electrical dipoles (Beal, 1996). These dipoles electronically function like transducers in that they are able to turn acoustic waves into electrical waves and electrical waves into acoustic waves. The natural properties of biomolecular structures enables cell components and whole cells to oscillate and interact resonantly with other cells. According to Smith and Best, the cells of the body and cellular components possess the ability to function as electrical resonators. A dipole movement is a function of polarization processes and the strength of the electric field. When biological tissue is exposed to an electric field in the right frequency and amplitude windows a preferential alignment of dipoles becomes established. Since the cell membrane contains many dipole molecules, an electric field will cause preferential alignment of the dipoles. This may be one mechanism that electrical fields alter membrane permeability and membrane functions.

Theoretically we assume two type of electric capacity, the first is the "static capacity" that is independent to the frequency of the alternating current, the second is the "polarization" type that depends upon the interphases in the tissues and suggest that capacity might have a considerable biologic significance. The "polarization" capacity is related to the alternating current applied or irradiated to the tissue under test. Activation of cell membrane receptors that act as antennas for certain windows of frequency and amplitude leading to the concepts of electromagnetic reception, transduction. Biological organisms use weak electromagnetic fields (electric and photonic) to communicate with all parts of themselves. The major charge carriers of biological organisms are negatively charged electrons, positively charged hydrogen protons, positively charged sodium, potassium, calcium and magnesium ions and negatively charged anions particularly phosphate ions.

For a long time, disturbances in physical processes in cancer development were not adequately taken into consideration despite Warburg's experimental discovery of deteriorated oxygen metabolism. Renewed interest in the Warburg effect has led to research on physical mechanisms in living cells. The role of mitochondrial dysfunction and cytoskeleton disintegration in cancer diagnostics has been recently restyling with the metabolic effect in metabolomics.

There is no doubt that the pathological physical alterations express essential changes in cancer development. Any diagnostic method has to detect important parameters disturbed by cancer process. A new diagnostic method developed by Vedruccio utilizes frequency selective (resonant) absorption of electromagnetic waves in malignant tumors (Bellorofonte et al. 2005). In malignant tumors, therefore, we should expect to find structures oscillating at the frequencies of the emitted signals, whose dissipation is different from that of healthy tissue. As the measurement results do not depend on the tumor size, the electromagnetic resonant interactions might be assumed to take place in cancer cells. The damping of oscillations is significantly It has been proposed that cancer exposed to a low level of electromagnetic incident waves may behave differently than healthy tissue (Vedruccio et al., 2004). The phenomenon of ''nonlinear resonance interaction,'' which is produced when the oscillations of an electromagnetic probe are coupled with those from biological tissue, can be used to test for differences between healthy and cancerous tissues. increased during cancer development.

2.2 Tissue resonance interferoMeter probe

In the 1920s the pioneers in the field of radio frequency reported that "malignant tumours have a greater polarizability than normal breast tissues or benign tumours". The authors moreover declared that "It seems probable that the measurement of the capacity may provide a very practical method for diagnosing the malignancy of a tumor". In the 1930s, some authors extended the frequency range of the dielectric properties of biological materials up to 600 MHz, by exploring the propagation of the electromagnetic waves on Lecher wires of variable length and which were terminated by a wire surrounding the biological material. The technological advances in electronic engineering following the second world war made possible the first work on complex permittivity measurements on blood cells and other biological tissues up to 30 GHz. Several years after a method which allowed dielectric measurements on living tissue ('in vivo' measurements) has been presented. The real time determination of complex permittivity is possible over a large frequency band (100 MHz - 10 GHz) by a rapid and continuous frequency scan. One such method is based on an antenna modeling theorem and on the application of microprocessor controlled microwave measurement instrumentation. A short monopole antenna is used as the in vivo probe. A network analyzer combined with error-correction routines and a semi-automated data acquisition/processing system (microcomputer) is used to determine the real part aof the permittivity and the conductivity s of the biological tissue being analyzed. A non-destructive method for measuring the dielectric properties of materials by means of an open transmission line resonator was developed in last 1970s. In the 1980s an open-ended coaxial probe used to measure and compare the fractional power absorption for malignant tumors relative to normal adjacent tissue in rats between 30 MHz and 2 GHz. It found that "tumors have a greater absorption, with a broad peak, centered in the 300 – 400 MHz region".

The majority of the studies cited herein refer to measurements and assessments of passive biophysical parameters of the tissues investigated. Measurements were of capacitance, resistance, complex dielectric constant.

In 1992, while conducting research on the back coupling effects of the damping of the near zone electromagnetic fields on transmitter-tuned circuits, Vedruccio discovered the possibility of noninvasive cancer detection. The author analyzed the perturbation of the electromagnetic field at the open end of a transmission line due to the dielectric material of unknown properties.

In the practical application of this effect, the author first constructed some prototype pieces of apparatus then, proceeded to the international patent application n. WO 01/07909A1 and the licensing of this technology to Galileo Avionica[1]. The final stage is an apparatus devoted to medical diagnostic analysis which is CE certified with the commercial name of Trimprob . This method is fast and accurate up to 4 GHz. The open end of the coaxial line must be in direct contact with the surface of the dielectric material being investigated which has to be smooth and flat.

To avoid any air gap effect, and it is necessary to apply a pressure to the material under test. Measurements on the human skin were given as an example because of the low penetration depth but, the aim was primarily therapeutic.

Preliminary results confirmed that it was possible to observe a stimulated response in altered agglomerates of cells (Vedruccio, 2004). Furthermore, it offered the possibility of detecting responses from biological tissues. When stimulated by the particular pattern of electromagnetic oscillations these tissues responded in a very selective way and quite distinct from the previously investigated Debye and Maxwell-Wagner resonances which extend over decades of frequency. The principle of detection lies in the resonance between the coupled active nonlinear oscillator (the probe) and the passive oscillator (the tissue) in the radiofrequency range of the electromagnetic spectrum. The fundamental frequency of emitted waves is about 465 MHz. The first (930 MHz) and the second (1,395 MHz) harmonics are transmitted too. The probe consists of a linear oscillator fed from the nonlinear element T (Figure 2), together forming a nonlinear active oscillator.

In the equivalent circuit, the oscillator is capacitively coupled to the passive one, the tissue, via the near field of the antenna. The tumor tissue represents a dissipative medium for the energy stored in the field near to source. The near field energy periodically flows out of the probe (the source) and returns to it.

The frequency of the emitted signal is adjusted and locked at the point of the highest absorption. The receiver antenna is located beyond the immediate neighborhood of the source (Figure 3). In comparison with electromagnetic wave propagation without interaction with a tumor, the received signal at the fundamental frequency decreases about fivefold due to damping effects of the cancerous tissue.

The transmitter probe with a resonant cavity incorporates a transmission line tuned to the frequency of oscillation, which is in the 65 cm wavelength band (465 MHz). At the open end

---

[1] Galileo Avionica S.p.A., a Finmeccanica Company, is the Italian avionics leader. It focuses on the design, development and production of avionics and electro-optical equipment, space equipment for platform and payloads. through its Company FIAR it is a national leader in airborne radars, with METEOR company in tactical and training UAVs, training simulator. Galileo Avionica offers cooperative programs (Eurofighter, NH-90, EH-101). in 2001 Galileo Avionica had registred a revenue of more than Euro millions 452.

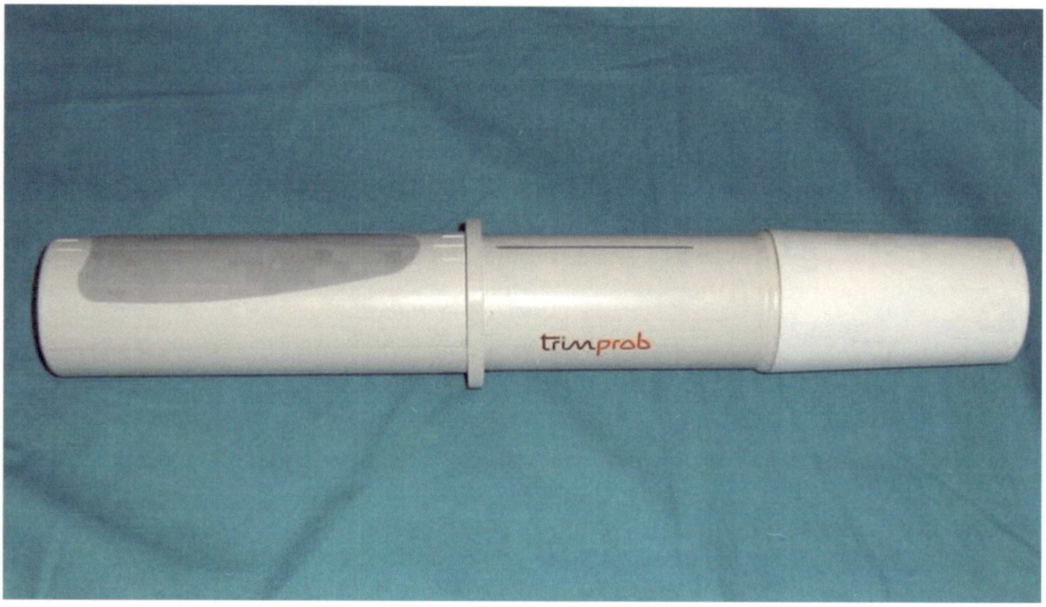

Fig. 2. Hand-held, battery-operated detection probe.

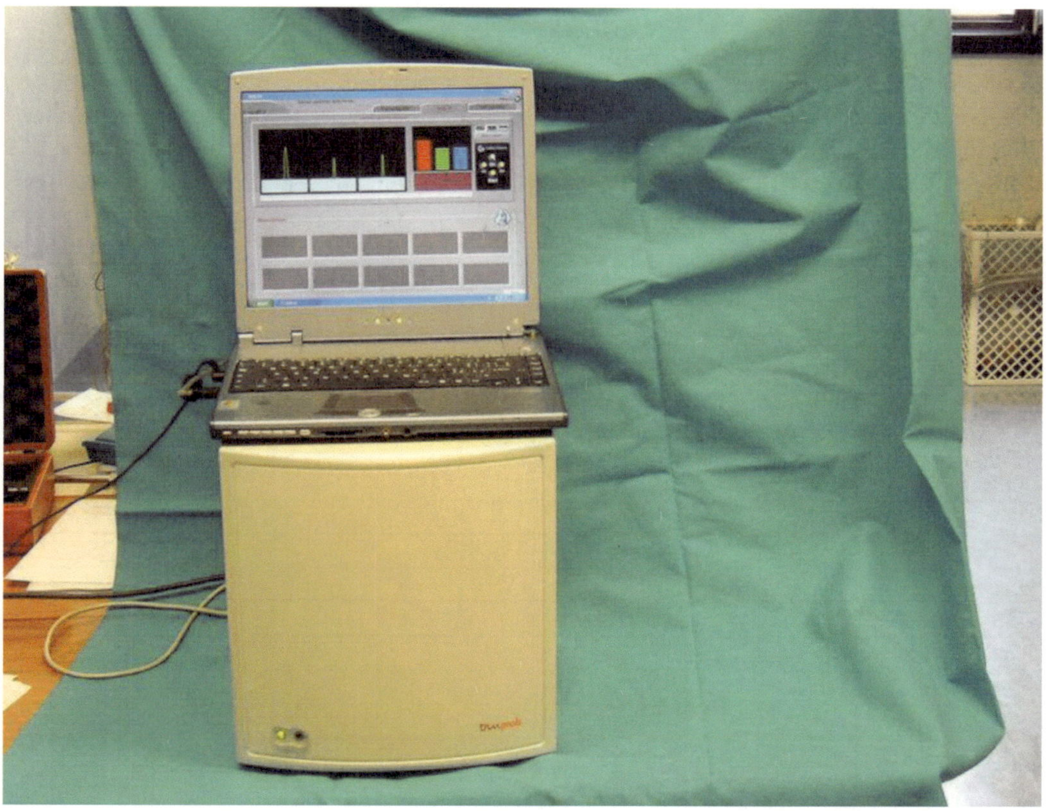

Fig. 3. Receiver, and computer display.

of this line, there is a semiconductor element with nonlinear characteristics that is activated by a nanosecond electromagnetic pulse.
This transient provides an injection of electromagnetic energy into the tuned line, which performs a damped oscillation. This particular tunable amplifier-oscillator represents the core of the Bioscanner trimprob diagnostic device.
It possesses lock-in or synchronization characteristics, and because of its particular construction, it produces a harmonically related group of coherent electromagnetic waves.
These oscillations are radiated as a beam through the beam window of the oscillator dome at the end of the probe. After geometrical focusing, the beam is used to irradiate the investigated tissues. The probe is brought close to the investigated region. Nonlinear resonance interaction between the nonlinear oscillator and the tissue reduces the energy of the emitted wave at distinct frequencies depending on the pathological state of the tested tissue. This energy is measured by the spectrum analyzer, which is fed by an antenna situated about 2 m away from the probe.

2.3 Clinical application

The device is user friendly and analyses the patient fully dressed and with no discomfort. Diagnostic accuracy of the Bioscanner was evaluated in several clinical studies. (Bellorofonte et al., 2005; Da Pozzo et al., 2007; Tubaro et al., 2008; and Gokce et al., 2009) performed studies focused on the diagnosis of prostate cancer at 465 MHz. Trimprob diagnostic findings were compared to those resulting from the standard prostate cancer diagnostic methods including digital rectal examination, biopsy, and prostate-specific antigen (PSA) level. Resulting values are shown in Table 2. Data presented are consistent across studies. Diagnostic methods are classified by the proportion of positives and negatives correctly identified, i.e., by sensitivity and specificity, respectively. Prostate cancer diagnosis using trimprob is characterized by high sensitivity; however, the specificity is rather low. Bellorofonte moreover reported a significant difference between patients with benign

Organ	Sensibility	Specificity	V.P.P.	V.P.N.	Accuracy
Prostate					
Tubaro (2008) Trimp	86	63	60	88	72
Tubaro (2008) Trimp+DRE	96	57	59	95	72
Bellorofonte (2005)	95	43	94	90	--
Bladder					
Leucci (2007)	87,5	90,5	83,3	91,1	89,5
Breast					
Paganelli-De Cicco (2006)	84	75	--	80	72
Thyroid					
Sacco (2007)	100	100	--	--	100
Stomach-duodenum					
Mascia (2005)	93	93	95	92	--
Sacco (2007)	100	100	--	--	--

Table 2. Clinical application

prostatic hyperplasia and patients with prostate cancer (Bellorofonte et al., 2005). Trimprob was also tested for detection of breast cancer (De Cicco et al. 2006), bladder cancer (Gervino et al. 2007), rectal malignant lesions (Vannelli et al. 2009), carcinomas in patients with multinodular goiter (Sacco et al. 2007a), and gastric cancer (Sacco et al. 2007b). According to the clinical experience, the trimprob seems to be a simple and reliable investigation method with good diagnostic results.

The first experiments, carried out by the author in the early days of the Bioscanner invention and development, as well as several clinical trials during the last years, have scientifically validated the efficacy of the described low level e.m.f. cancer detector in several body organs like breast, prostate, bladder, stomach-duodenum, thyroid (Vedruccio, 2010).

3. TRIMprob and rectal cancer

3.1 Test principle

The device is made of a thin probe about 30 cm long, powered by batteries and of a receiver. A specific software entirely elaborated by Galileo Avionica acquires, reads and manages the diagnostic data. The TRIMprob emits a beam of coherent electromagnetic waves at very low power which tunes on the specific frequencies of the examined structures. When the electromagnetic field hits a biologically altered tissue, a phenomenon of interference with the analysed structure takes place. The trimprob system (Galileo Avionica, Turin, Italy), also called a Tissue Resonance InterferoMeter Probe, consists of a hand-held, battery-operated detection probe, a receiver, and a computer display. The probe, which is about 30 cm long, contains a nonlinear oscillator that generates a complex electromagnetic wave of low intensity with three frequency components (465, 930, and 1395 MHz) and a high degree of spatial and temporal coherence. Malignant and normal tissues may differ in the way they interact with such electromagnetic waves because proteins acquire more surface charges in malignant tumours, and the attraction of these charges for water molecules results in the presence of more "bound water" (Bellerofonte et al., 2005) Furthermore, dramatic changes in metabolism, intercellular communication, and adhesion properties of cancer cells result in modification of the number and nature of membrane proteins. The dipolar parts of the membrane proteins, which protrude from the membrane, can be reoriented by an oscillating electric field. The electromagnetic field produced by the nonlinear oscillator of the trimprob stimulates oscillations inside the tissue. When these oscillations begin to resonate, an energy transfer can be detected in the wave emitted by the probe. The receiver situated a short distance from the probe detects the change and acts as a spectrum analyzer. When the probe is brought near cancerous tissue, interaction with the oscillating electric field causes a negative amplitude change in one or more of the spectral lines. The reduction in signal amplitude indicates the presence of abnormal tissues and structures. The frequencies 465, 930, and 1395 MHz were previously determined to be optimal because they appeared to respond in the appropriate way to the resonances of the system.

3.2 Test procedure

The test was performed for each individual patient according to the procedure shown in Figure 4. The patient stood between the operator and the receiver, at a distance of 120 cm from the receiver. There was a single operator, who was not blinded to the results of the colonoscopy, because the endpoint was the feasibility of this device. The patient was dressed normally, but no metallic objects were allowed on his or her person, and no electronic devices were admitted in the test area. The pelvic area was scanned by moving the detector at close contact over the pelvic surface through six planes, first in three directions (axial, left, and right) with the patient facing the receiver and then repeating the process with the patient turned to face the operator. The test was performed for each individual patient according to the procedure. The detector was kept in close contact with the pelvic surface and was moved through six planes: A1, posterior right lateral; A2, posterior median; A3, posterior left lateral; B1, anterior right lateral; B2, anterior median; B3, anterior left lateral. There was a single operator, who was not blinded to the results of the colonoscopy, because the endpoint was the feasibility of this device. The patient was dressed normally, but no metallic objects were allowed on his or her person, and no electronic devices were admitted in the test area. In this way, a scan of the whole pelvis volume was obtained with signal acquisition at six positions: posterior median, left lateral, and right lateral; and anterior median, left lateral, and right lateral. Each change in amplitude of the emitted signals at the established frequencies was recorded and stored in an electronic file as a value of the corresponding spectral line expressed in arbitrary units between 255 and 0. Thus, three numeric values, corresponding to the signal amplitude of the spectral lines for the frequencies 465, 930, and 1395 MHz, were obtained for each position.

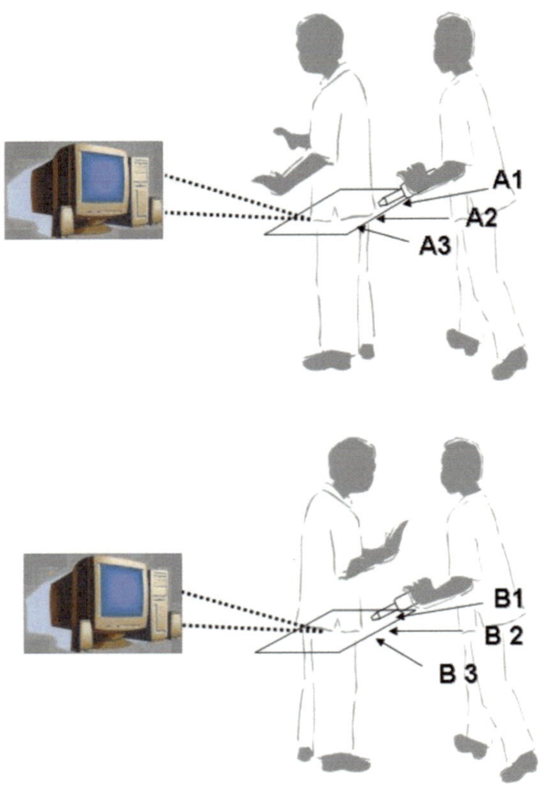

Fig. 4. Trimprob procedures. The detector was kept in close contact with the pelvic surface and was moved through six planes: A1, posterior right lateral; A2, posterior median; A3, posterior left lateral; B1, anterior right lateral; B2, anterior median; B3, anterior left lateral.

The test was performed for each individual patient according to the procedure. The detector was kept in close contact with the pelvic surface and was moved through six planes: A1, posterior right lateral; A2, posterior median; A3, posterior left lateral; B1, anterior right lateral; B2, anterior median; B3, anterior left lateral. The patient stood between the operator and the receiver, at a distance of 120 cm from the receiver. There was a single operator, who was not blinded to the results of the colonoscopy, because the endpoint was the feasibility of this device.

The patient was dressed normally, but no metallic objects were allowed on his or her person, and no electronic devices were admitted in the test area.

4. Remarkable experiments

4.1 Introduction

Population screening programs for the early diagnosis of CRC have the potential to reduce the incidence and mortality from this disease. Most of these programs are based on stool tests or structural exams (Vannelli et al., 2010). The main purpose of the screening should be to detect 90% of the sporadic cases of CRC. In a health care system with unlimited financial resources the choice of the type of screening and the suitable population for this examination does not represent a problem. Everywhere, even though there are different health care systems, financial resources are limited and the rectal screening with the current methods could be applied only to a selected population. On the other hand, the majority of adults are not receiving regular age- and risk-appropriate screenings or have never been screened at all (Zampino et al., 2009). Despite the fact that the primary barriers to screening are lack of health insurance, lack of physician recommendation, and lack of awareness of the importance of RC screening, the historical evidence shows that adults have different preferences and patterns of use among the available CRC screening tests. Thus, a less expensive, faster, and less invasive RC screening procedure with a similar or better efficacy, as compared to available methods, would provide a significant advantage for RC prevention in the general population. We recently carried out a pilot study for the identification of RC by electromagnetic detection, a method that is rapid, non-invasive, and inexpensive. As compared to the results of colonoscopy, electromagnetic detection of rectal cancer was highly specific (85%) and highly sensitive (94%) (Vannelli et al., 2009). Herein, by a prospective study we evaluated the prediction accuracy of CRC by electromagnetic detection. A pilot study has been carried out for the identification of CRC by electromagnetic detection, a method that is rapid, non-invasive, and inexpensive (Vannelli et al., 2009). A subesquent study protocol was approved by the Institutional Review Board and Ethics Committee of the Fondazione IRCCS "Istituto Nazionale Tumori" Milano. The ClinicalTtrials.gov ID of the study is: NCT00963794. This study was carried out using a blind and a prospective design, with patients undergoing electromagnetic detection followed by colonoscopy.

4.2 Preliminary results

We hypothesized to adapt trimprobe in early detection-screening for rectal cancer. Of 1,792 patients admitted to our outpatient clinic from March to September 2006 because of gastrointestinal disease, 756 patients underwent colonoscopy and were evaluated for possible participation in the Trimprob study. Exclusion criteria consisted of age younger than 18 years, history of psychiatric illness, and preoperative radiotherapy. To rule out possible interference with the electromagnetic field, we also excluded patients with active phlogistic processes, such as inflammatory bowel disease, anal abscess, or fistulas. To rule out possible interference from other types of altered tissues, we included only the rectum, with a cut-off 15 centimetres from the anal verge. A total of 228 patients (113 females and 115 males) were selected for participation in the study: 114 patients with negative colonoscopy results and 114 patients with colonoscopy positive for rectal cancer. Written informed consent was obtained from all subjects. The study protocol was approved by the Institutional Review Board of the Fondazione IRCCS "Istituto Nazionale dei Tumori" Milano.

4.3 Clinical trials

After the encouraging results we decide to prepare a prospective randomized clinical trial. 442 patients have been admitted to our outpatient's Department from January to August 2008 because of gastrointestinal disease or clinical symptoms related to colorectal risk. Exclusion criteria consisted of age younger than 18 years, history of psychiatric illness, and preoperative radiotherapy: 27 patients. Under written informed consent, 415 subjects were recruited consecutively (10 patients refused the protocol). All subjects underwent electromagnetic detection of RC, followed by colonoscopy. The patients completed the examination with computed tomography (positive colonoscopy) or abdominal sonography (negative colonoscopy). The device lets the examination limited to the pelvis and we regarded the rectum cutoff within 15 cm from the anal verge. Biopsy of suspected neoplastic lesions and histopathological exam of the eventual lesions were performed (209 patients), showing that 108 patients carried a rectal cancer whereas 101 patients carried a cancer in the upper gastrointestinal tract (right or left colon); these latter patients were excluded from this study (Table 1). The study protocol was approved by the Institutional Review Board and Ethics Committee of the Fondazione IRCCS "Istituto Nazionale dei Tumori" Milano. The ClinicalTtrials.gov ID of the study is: NCT00963794.

5. Phenomenon interpretation

No adverse effects of the Trimprob procedure were observed in the two trials. The procedure was performed in a short time (approximately 10 minutes) and was well accepted by all patients. In first trial, only the first spectral line, at the 465-MHz frequency, differentiated the group with positive colonoscopy from that with negative colonoscopy in all six probe positions ($P < 0.001$). At 930 MHz, the two groups differed significantly only in the posterior right, posterior median, posterior left, and anterior left positions; no significant differences were seen at 1395 MHz. To evaluate the applicability of trimprob electromagnetic signal as a marker for distinguishing between CRC and non-CRC disease groups, we performed Receiver Operating Characteristic (ROC) curve analysis. Figure 5 shows the curves ROC calculated for each frequency. Only the 465-MHz frequency had an AUC-ROC value close to 1 (0.94), indicating good discrimination between positive and negative colonoscopy at this frequency. In contrast, 930 MHz and 1395 MHz had AUC-ROC values close to 0.5, indicating poor discrimination. ROC curve showed the diagnostic ability of trimprob electromagnetic signal in the differentiation of RC patients versus non-cancer subjects (AUC = 0.96, 95% confidence interval (CI) 0.94 - 0.98; $P < 2.2e\text{-}16$). In our cohort, the sensitivity of the trimprob device for RC was 0.94, specificity was 0.84, negative predictive value was 0.88, positive predictive value was 0.92, and accuracy was 0.90 for the electromagnetic signal cut-off value of 50 U. Indeed, an electromagnetic signal < 50 arbitrary units (U) was significantly associated with detection of RC by colonoscopy ($p < 2.2e-16$). Analysis of accuracy by cut-off value indicated that ~50-55 U represent the best cut-off values for detection of RC. Second trial of 442 subjects enrolled at our Institute due to signs of CRC risk was carried out using a blind and a prospective design, with patients undergoing electromagnetic detection followed by colonoscopy. Histopathologic analysis of biopsies revealed that all CRC cases were of the adenocarcinoma histotype. Data from 196 patients with negative colonoscopy results and 108 patients with rectal cancer by colonoscopy were available for analysis. The median patient age was 65 (range, 24-84) years for the negative colonoscopy group and 65 (range, 22-85) years for the positive colonoscopy group. All patients with a CRC diagnosis have been subjected to computed tomography, which revealed 9 liver metastasis and no other primitive cancer types. All patients with positive colonoscopy were admitted to the hospital with a diagnosis of rectal adenocarcinoma and submitted to surgery. Patients not carrying a CRC, (exception of 13 subjects), have been subjected to abdominal sonography, which revealed no cancer pathology. However, 10 patients revealed active phlogistic processes: 6 inflammatory bowel disease, 1 anal abscess and 3 fistulas. Since PSA levels were not measured as a screening for prostate cancer, this may be a possible limitation to the study results.

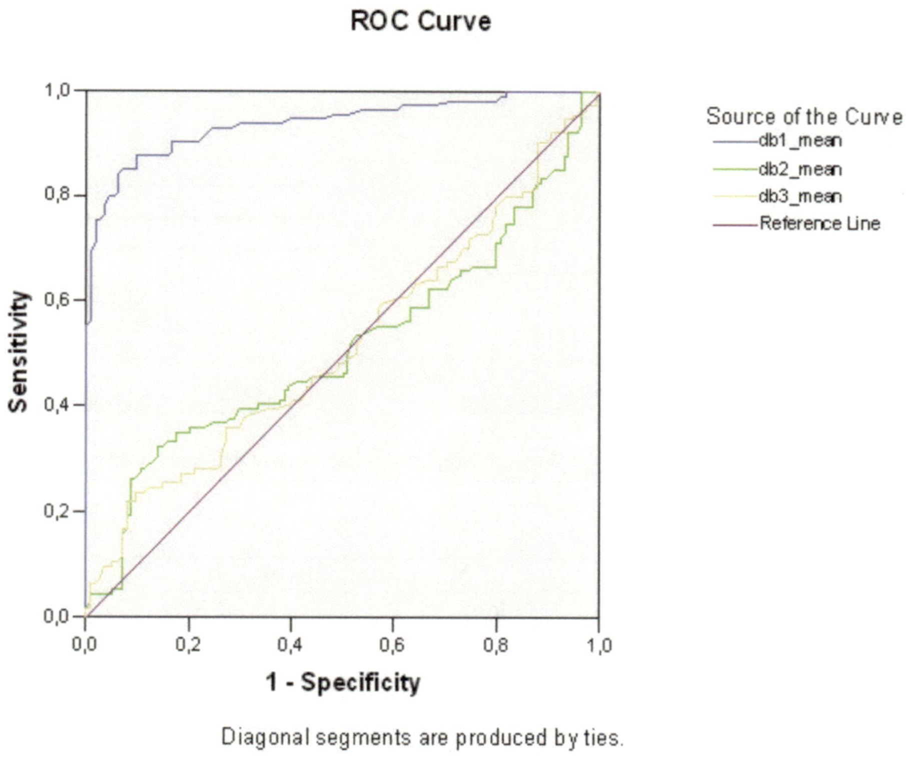

Fig. 5. ROC curve

CRC patients classified by colonoscopy showed a significantly lower electromagnetic signal than did non-CRC subjects, i.e., 40.9 ± 0.9 U (mean ± S.E.) versus 79.2 ± 1.4 U (Figure 6). To evaluate the applicability of Trimprob electromagnetic signal as a marker for distinguishing between RC and non-RC disease groups, we performed ROC (Receiver Operating

Characteristic) curve analysis. ROC curve showed the diagnostic ability of trimprob electromagnetic signal in the differentiation of RC patients versus non-cancer subjects (AUC = 0.96, 95% confidence interval (CI) 0.94 - 0.98; $P < 2.2e-16$). In our cohort, the sensitivity of the trimprob device for RC was 0.94, specificity was 0.84, negative predictive value was 0.88, positive predictive value was 0.92, and accuracy was 0.90 for the electromagnetic signal cut-off value of 50 U. Indeed, an electromagnetic signal < 50 U was significantly associated with detection of RC by colonoscopy ($p< 2.2e-16$, Table 3). Analysis of accuracy by cut-off value

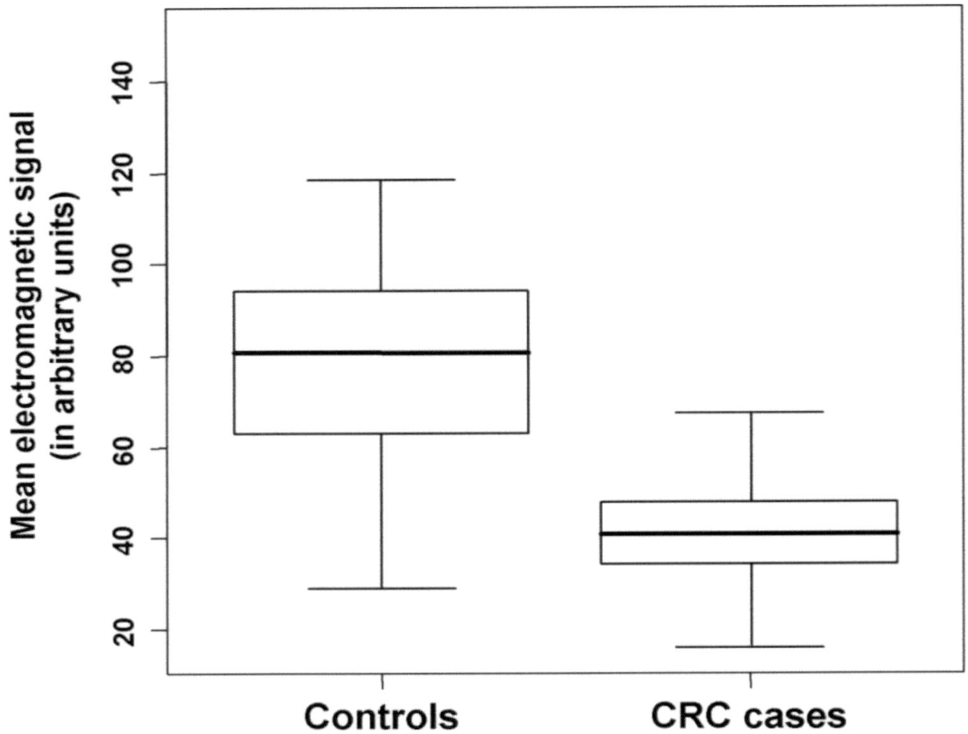

Fig. 6. Lower electromagnetic signal associated with rectal cancer carrier status. $P < 2.2e-16$, Kruskal-Wallis test.

Electromagnetic signal score	Number of subjects with		*P* [b]
	Non-CRC [a]	CRC [a]	
≥50	184	17	
<50	12	91	<1.0e-16
≥70	134	0	
<70	62	108	<1.0e-16

[a] By colonoscopy analysis. [b] Fisher's exact test.

Table 3. Association between electromagnetic score settled out at different thresholds and the CRC disease status defined by colonoscopy.

indicated that 50-55 U represent the best cut-off values for detection of RC. Since a major goal in screening tests is the minimization of false-negative rates, we identified an electromagnetic threshold, i.e., < 70 U, at which no RC was missed (Table 3). However, at this threshold, 62 (31.6%) of the non-RC subjects were false-positive (Table 3), whose disease or healthy status would have required clarification by colonoscopy. No association between nodal involvement (N0 versus N ≥ 1) and the value of the electromagnetic signal was observed. A significant inverse correlation was observed between the size of the neoplastic lesions and the value of the electromagnetic signal (Spearman's rho = -0.290, P = 0.002), whereas a significant positive correlation was found between increasing distance from anal verge and the value of the electromagnetic signal (Spearman's rho = 0.362, P = 0.0001).

6. Discussion

Since up to 10% of the general population might carry a RC, depending on the age of the population undergoing screening, new easy and non-expensive methods for population screening for RC may be helpful for early detection of such disease. The most frequently used screening methods for RC include two general categories: stool tests (tests for occult blood or exfoliated DNA) and structural exams [endoscopy, double-contrast barium enema and computed tomographic colonography (CTC)]. The popular occult blood test is characterized by simplicity, non-invasiveness, and demonstrated mortality benefit but suffers from poor sensitivity, low population compliance, and high costs of follow-up for false-positives. Indeed, in a large study of asymptomatic patients who underwent occult blood testing followed by endoscopy, the sensitivity of the occult blood test for identifying advanced neoplasia was only 24% . Compared to the occult blood test, CTC is much more expensive, whereas this technique has some clear advantages when compared to endoscopy since it is non-invasive, less time-intensive and is associated with a lower risk of complications. However, CTC requires the use of ionizing radiations, a high level of expertise in reading, and has shown wide variations in sensitivity in the various clinical trials (Vannelli et al., 2010). Endoscopy is an invasive, lengthy and expensive procedure requiring adequate clinical infrastructure and medical expertise, and is not without complications. Thus, it represents even a relatively "poor screening" method for RC at the general population level, especially as compared with screening methods, such as the PAP test, for other types of cancer. The ageing of the general population in the Western world, with the consequent increase of people at risk of RC, further makes large screening programs based on colonoscopy unfeasible. Still, early detection of RC can save lives and can also decrease the cost of the patient's clinical management, since patients with early neoplastic lesions require simpler surgical resections and treatments than those with advanced disease. Although endoscopy is generally safe, it is still an invasive procedure with several-fold higher rates of serious complications than for any other commonly used cancer screening test. Repeated examinations over time may incur a substantial cumulative rate of complications. In addition, a relatively small risk (2 to 6%) of RC remains 6 to 36 months after negative colonoscopy, especially when internists and family practice physicians rather than gastroenterologists perform endoscopies. However, in the near term, even greater incidence and mortality reductions could be achieved if a greater proportion of adults received regular screening. Although prospective randomized trials and observational studies have demonstrated mortality reductions associated with early detection of invasive disease, as well as removal of adenomatous polyps, a majority of adults are not receiving regular age and risk-appropriate screening or have never been screened at all. Recent interest has focused on use of trimprob for diagnosis of disease as new screening strategy. This technique is characterized by simplicity, efficacy, and good patient compliance. In the present prospective study, patients with CRC diagnosed by colonoscopy and histopathologic analysis showed significantly lower values of the electromagnetic signal as compared to non-CRC patients. At a signal threshold of 50 U, defined by our previous study as the optimal threshold in discriminating CRC from non-CRC patients, the electromagnetic detection showed a highly significant association with the CRC status, thus confirming in an independent cohort our previous findings. This technology has also been investigated on other cancers, in particular prostate cancers with favourable outcomes. The observed inverse correlation between the size of the neoplastic lesions and the value of the electromagnetic signal is consistent with the association between low electromagnetic signal values and high probability of CRC, and raises the possibility that CRC size represents a factor affecting the sensitivity of CRC electromagnetic detection. The positive correlation observed between increasing distance from anal verge and the value of the electromagnetic signal may reflect a decreasing detection power of the device with distance of the lesion or, alternatively, with interference of anatomical structures in the anal region. Further studies are needed to clarify the existence of a dimensional threshold or of a minimal distance from anal verge of CRC to be detected by electromagnetic signal. Notwithstanding the highly significant association between electromagnetic detection and CRC status observed using the 50 U signal threshold, the frequency of false-negative results at this threshold was relatively high (15.7%,) and, although much less than the frequency of missing CRCs by the fecal occult blood test, too high for population-based CRC screening. By increasing the signal threshold value to 70 U, we can avoid all false-negative findings in our cohort, thus we can correctly identified all CRC cases but increased the frequency of false-positives to about 30% of the non-CRC subjects. Thus, follow-up colonoscopy in real- and false positive subjects would be necessary to characterize the subject's disease status. We are aware of the limitations of our study, since the relatively small size of our series and the consequent low detection power. Also, trimprob was never tested in a multicentric study for the detection of CRC and control subjects from general population, without any gastrointestinal symptoms related to CRC risk, have not been tested. Other possible limitations that have not been addressed in the present study include operator dependence and the effects of other gastrointestinal diseases.

7. Conclusion

Our present findings point to the promise of electromagnetic detection as a simple, accurate, and inexpensive tool for early detection of CRC in cancer prevention programs at the general population level. However, the present results represent only a first step and studies in large cohorts and in different populations are needed to further compare the usefulness of this method with other CRC screening methods, especially colonoscopy. In addition, the description of benefits is complicated by different performance characteristics of the variants tests. Moreover, test performances in research settings and in clinical practice may vary. Therefore, we can imagine in the future the possibility to support the common screening tests with electromagnetic detection.

8. Acknowledgments

The authors thank Mrs. Roberta Aceto for her assistance with data collection and MD. Patrizia Gasparini for scientific consulting.

9. References

Beal, JB. (1996). Biosystems liquid crystals & potential effects of natural & artificial electromagnetic fields (EMFs), In: *Second Annual Advanced Water Sciences Symposium,* March 4 2011, Available from <http://frontpage.simnet.is/vgv/jim1.htm>

Bellorofonte, C.; Vedruccio, C.; Tombolini, P.; Ruoppolo, M. & Tubaro, A. (2005). Non-invasive detection of prostate cancer by electromagnetic interaction. *Eur Urol,* Vol. 47, No. 1, (January 2005), pp. 29-37. ISSN 1569-9056.

Bibbo, M. (1997). *Comprehensive cytopathology* (2nd edition) WB Saunders, ISBN 1-56238-380-9, Philadelphia

Blackledge, G. (2003) Cancer Drugs: The next ten years. *European Journal of Cancer,* Vol. 39, No. 3, (February 2003), pp. 273, ISSN: 0959-8049

Clarke, AC.; (1962) *Hazards of prophecy :The failure of imagination* in Profiles of the Future, Harper & Row, ISBN 0-445-04061-0, New York

Cone, C.D. (1975). The role of surface electrical transmembrane potential in normal and malignant mitogenesis. *Ann NY Acad Sci.* Vol. 238, (1975), pp. 420-35 ISSN: 1749-6632

Da Pozzo, L.; Scattoni, V.; Mazzoccoli, B.; Rigatti, P.; Manferrari, F.; Martorana. G.; Pietropaolo, F.; Belgrano, E.; Prezioso, D.; Lotti, T.; Villari, D. & Nicita, G. (2007). Tissue-resonance interaction method for the noninvasive diagnosis of prostate cancer: analysis of a multicentre clinical evaluation. *BJU Int,* Vol. 100, No. 5, (November 2007), pp. 1055-9. ISSN: 1464-410X.

De Cicco, C.; Mariani, L.; Vedruccio, C.; Ricci, C.; Balma, M.; Rotmensz, N.; Ferrari, M.E.; Autino, E.; Trifirò, G.; Sacchini, V.; Viale, G. & Paganelli, G. Clinical application of spectral electromagnetic interaction in breast cancer: diagnostic results of a pilot study. *Tumori,* Vol. 92, No 3, (May-June 2006), pp. 207-12. ISSN: 0300-8916.

Di Viccaro, D.; Perugia, G.; Cerulli, C.; Olivieri, V.; Bova, J.; Zanza, C.; Teodonio, S. & Liberti, M. (2009).The accuracy of tissue resonance interaction method probe (Trimprob tm) in non-invasive diagnosis of prostatic cancer. Analysis of the results of 782 patient. *Urologia,* Vol. 76, Suppl. 15, (2009), pp. 1-3. ISSN: 0004-0614

Erickson, J.W. & Cerione, R.A. (2010). Glutaminase: a hot spot for regulation of cancer cell metabolism? *Oncotarget* Vol.1, No. 8, (December 2010), pp. 734-40. ISSN: 1949-2553

Fricke, H. & Morse, A. (1926). The electric capacity of tumors of the breast. *J Cancer Res.* Vol. 10, (1926), pp. 340-76. ISSN: 1538-7445

Galindo, F.G.; Dejmek, P.; Lundgren, K.; Rasmusson, A.G.; Vicente, A. & Moritz, T. (2009). Metabolomic evaluation of pulsed electric field-induced stress on potato tissue. *Planta.* Vol. 230, No. 3, (august 2009), pp. 469-479. ISSN: 1432-2048

Gervino, G.; Autino, E.; Kolomoets, E.; Leucci, G. & Balma, M. Diagnosis of bladder cancer at 465 MHz. *Electromagn Biol Med,* Vol. 26, No. 2, (2007), pp. 119-34. ISSN: 1536-8386.

Gokce, O.; Sanli, O.; Salmaslioglu, A.; Tunaci, A.; Ozsoy, C. & Ozcan, F. (2009). Tissue Resonance Interaction Method (TRIMprob) has the potential to be used alongside the recognized tests in the screening protocols for prostate cancer. *Int J Urol*, Vol. 16, No. 6, (June 2009), pp. 580-3. ISSN: 1573-2584

Horning, E.C. & Horning, M.G. (1971). Metabolic profiles: gas-phase methods for analysis of metabolites. *Clin Chem*. Vol. 17, No. 8, (August 1971), pp. 802-9. ISSN:0009-9147

Kanavos, P.; Schurer, W.; Owusuapenten, C. & Sullivan, R. (2008) Colorectal cancer in Europe and Australia: challenges and opportunities for the future, In: *LSE Health*, date of access 2011, available in: <http://www2.lse.ac.uk/LSEHealthAndSocialCare/LSEHealth/pdf/colorectal/ColorectalCancerReport%2025JUNE2008.pdf>

Kaplan, F.; Kopka, J.; Haskell, D.W.; Zhao, W.; Schiller, K.C.; Gatzke, N.; Sung, D.Y. & Guy, C.L. (2004). Exploring the temperature-stress metabolome of Arabidopsis. *Plant Physiol.* Vol. 136, No. 4 (Dicember 2004), pp. 4159–4168. ISSN: 1532-2548

Kurzweil, R. & Grossman, T. (2004). *Fantastic Voyage: Live Long Enough to Live Forever*, Rodale Books (eds.) ISBN 1-57954-954-3. USA.

Lance, P. (2008). Colorectal cancer screening: confusion reigns. *Cancer Epidemiol Biomarkers Prev*, Vol 17, (September 2008), pp. 2205-7. ISSN 1538-7755

Langbein, S.; Zerilli, M.; Zur Hausen, A.; Staiger, W.; Rensch-Boschert, K.; Lukan, N.; Popa, J.; Ternullo, M.P.; Steidler, A. & Weiss, C. (2006). Expression of transketolase TKTL1 predicts colon and urothelial cancer patient survival: Warburg effect reinterpreted. *Br J Cancer*. Vol. 94, No. 4, (Februar 2006), pp. 578-585. ISSN 0007-0920

Mayevsky, A. (2009). Mitochondrial function and energy metabolism in cancer cells: past overview and future perspectives. *Mitochondrion Vol.* 9, No. 3, (Jun 2009), pp. 165-179. ISSN: 1567-7249

Meessen, A. (2000). Institut de Physique, Université Catholique de Louvain, Louvain-la-Neuvre, In : *Working Principle of an EM Cancer Detector,* March 2 2011, Available from<http://www.meessnen.net/AMeessnen/EMcancerDet2.pdf> 2000

Orrenius, S. (2007). Reactive oxygen species in mitochondria-mediated cell death. *Drug Metab Rev*. Vol. 39, No. 2-3, (2000), pp. 443-455. ISSN 1097-9883

Pelicano, H.; Martin, DS.; Xu, R.H. & Huang, P. (2006) Glycolysis inhibition for anticancer treatment. *Oncogene*. Vol. 7, No. 25, (Aug 2006), pp. 4633-46. ISSN: 0950-9232

Pokorný, J.; Vedruccio, C.; Cifra, M. & Kučera, O. (2011) Cancer physics: diagnostics based on damped cellular elastoelectrical vibrations in microtubules. *Eur Biophys J*. 2011 Mar 11. [Epub ahead of print] ISSN 0175-7571

Presman, A.S. (1970). *Electromagnetic Fields and Life* (1st edition), NY: Plenum Press, ISBN 0-688-00123-8, New York

Sacco R, Sammarco G, De Vinci R, Vescio G, Scarpelli A, Lucisano AM, Pata F, Mascia E, Martines V. (2007). Relief of gastric cancer with an electromagnetic interaction system (TRIMprob) in outpatients. *Chir Ital*, Vol. 59, No. 6, (Nov-Dec 2007), pp. 823-8. ISSN: 0009 – 4773

Sacco, R.; Innaro, N.; Pata, F.; Lucisano, A.M.; Talarico, C. & Aversa, S. (2007). Preoperative diagnosis of incidental carcinoma in multinodular goitre by means of electromagnetic interactions. *Chir Ital,* Vol. 59, No.2, (Mar-Apr 2007) pp. 247-51. ISSN: 0009 – 4773

Samudio, I.; Fiegl, M. & Andreeff, M. (2009). Mitochondrial uncoupling and the Warburg effect: molecular basis for the reprogramming of cancer cell metabolism. *Cancer Res.* Vol. 69, No. 6, (March 2009), pp. 2163-2166. ISSN: 1538-7445

Sikora, K. (2007). Personalized medicine for cancer: from molecular signature to therapeutic choice, In: *Adv Cancer Res*, Vande & Woude, pp. 345-69, Elevier, Retrieved from <http://www.sciencedirect.com/science?_ob=ArticleURL&_udi=B7CT1-4MHNPP7-F&_user=5422747&_coverDate=12%2F31%2F2006&_rdoc=1&_fmt=high&_orig=gateway&_origin=gateway&_sort=d&_docanchor=&view=c&_acct=C000067215&_version=1&_urlVersion=0&_userid=5422747&md5=62364b5c4a356341fcc62806bb8149dd&searchtype=a>

Sonnenberg, A.; Delco, F. & Inadomi, J.M. (2000). Cost-effectiveness of colonoscopy in screening for colorectal cancer. *Ann Intern Med,* Vol. 133, No. 8, (October 2000), pp. 573-84. ISSN: 1539-3704

Spitz, D.R.; Sim, J.E.; Ridnour, L.A.; Galoforo, S.S. & Lee, Y.J. (2000). Glucose deprivation-induced oxidative stress in human tumor cells. A fundamental defect in metabolism? *Ann N Y Acad Sci.* Vol. 899, (2000), pp. 349-362. ISSN: 1749-6632

Sung, J.J.; Lau, J.Y.; Goh, K.L. & Leung, W.K. (2005). Asia Pacific Working Group on Colorectal Cancer. Increasing incidence of colorectal cancer in Asia: implications for screening. *Lancet Oncol*, Vol. 6, No. 11, (November 2005), pp. 871-6. ISSN: 1470-2045

Tubaro, A.; De Nunzio, C.; Trucchi, A.; Stoppacciaro, A. & Miano, L. (2008) The electromagnetic detection of prostatic cancer: evaluation of diagnostic accuracy. *Urology.*;Vol. 72, No. 2, (August 2008), pp. 340-4. ISSN:1747-8049

Vander Heiden, M.G., Cantley, L.C., Thompson, C.B. (2009) Understanding the Warburg Effect: The Metabolic Requirements of Cell Proliferation. *Science* Vol. 324, No. 324, (May 2009), 1029-1033. ISSN 1095-9203

Vannelli, A.; Battaglia, L.; Poiasina, E. & Leo, E. (2010). Diagnosis of rectal cancer by Tissue Resonance Interaction Method. *BMC Gastroenterol,* Vol. 10, No. 45, (May 2010), pp. 1-6. ISSN 1471-230X

Vannelli, A.; Leo, E.; Battaglia, L. & Poiasina, E. (2009). Diagnosis of rectal cancer by electromagnetic interactions: preliminary results. *Dis Colon Rectum,* Vol 52, 2009, pp.162-166. ISSN, 0012-3706

Vedruccio, C. & Meessen, A. (2004). EM cancer detection by means of nonlinear resonance interaction. In: Research Symposium, Pisa Italy March 28-31 2004. *Extended Paper Book of PIERS2004- Progress in Electromagnetics,* pp. 909-12, Pisa, Italy

Vedruccio, C. (2010). Polarizability of normal and cancerous tissues, a Radiofrequency Nonlinear Resonance Interaction non invasive diagnostic Bioscanner Trimprob detector. *Eur J Oncol – Library,* Vol. 5, (2010), pp. 177-86 ISBN 978-88-6261-166-4

Vincenzi, B.; Cesa, A.L.; Santini, D.; Schiavon, G.; Grilli, C.; Graziano, F. & Tonini, G. (2004). Predictive factors for response to chemotherapy in colorectal cancer patients. *Crit Rev Oncol Hematol,* Vol. 52, No. 1, (October 2004), pp. 45-60, ISSN: 1040-8428

Warburg, O. (1956) On the origin of cancer cells. *Science.* Vol. 123, No. 3191 (Februar 1956), pp. 309–314. ISSN 1095-9203

Warburg, O.; Posener, K. & Negelein, E. (1924). U¨ ber den Stoffwechsel der Carcinomzelle. *Biochem Z,* Vol. 152, (1294), pp. 309–344

Winawer, S. (2007) Colorectal cancer screening, In: *World Gastroenterology Organisation/International Digestive Cancer Alliance Practice Guidelines,* date of access 2011, available in:
<http://www.worldgastroenterology.org/assets/downloads/en/pdf/guidelines/06_colorectal_cancer_screening.pdf>

Zampino, M.G.; Labianca, R.; Beretta, G.D.; Magni, E.; Gatta, G.; Leonardi, M.C.; Chiappa, A.; Biffi, R.; de Braud, F. & Wils, J. (2009). Rectal cancer. *Crit Rev Oncol Hematol,* Vol. 70, No. 2, (May 2009), pp.160-182. ISSN: 1040-8428

14

Autofluorescence Imaging for Diagnosing Intestinal Disorders

Mikihiro Fujiya[1], Kentaro Moriichi[1], Nobuhiro Ueno[1], Yusuke Saitoh[2] and Yutaka Kohgo[1]
[1]*Division of Gastroenterology and Hematology/Oncology, Department of Medicine, Asahikawa Medical University, Asahikawa,*
[2]*Digestive Disease Center, Asahikawa City Hospital, Asahikawa*
Japan

1. Introduction

Image enhanced endoscopies, such as narrow band imaging (NBI) and autofluorescence imaging (AFI), were recently developed and clinically applied for the diagnosis of gastrointestinal diseases. From the results of recent clinical studies, these novel technologies appear to be useful for detecting, as well as evaluating, gastrointestinal disorders. While NBI can emboss the vessel structure, AFI can capture fluorescence emitted from intestinal tissues and also describe the area in which the fluorescence intensity is reduced as a magenta color on the monitor. This device produces an excitation light source of 390-470 nm and delivers it to the tissue surface through an endoscope. The low light level autofluorescence emitted from the tissue and white light reflection are detected and amplified by two high sensitivity CCDs. The fluorescence image is then transformed into a green hue, while the reflection image is transformed into red and blue hues. Thereafter, the images are displayed on a monitor as color images in real-time **(Figure 1) (Nakashima A, et al. 2001)**.

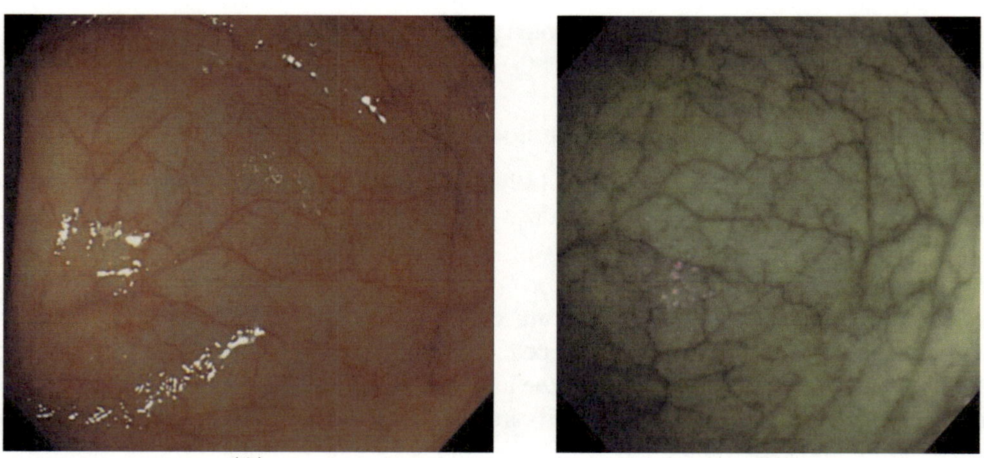

(A) (B)

Fig. 1. High resolution endoscopy (HRE) (A) and AFI (B) in the normal colon.

AFI is characterized as a tool for simply describing the abnormal findings as color changes, whereas the diagnosis of conventional endoscopy, NBI and other technologies are based on the empirical judgment of morphological features. Moreover, the characteristics that AFI provides are based on the strength of fluorescence, so the quantification of the fluorescence intensity (proposed as the "F index") using an analytical image software program can provide an objective diagnosis for intestinal disorders **(Figure 2)**.

This chapter focuses on the efficacy of AFI for the detection and differentiation of colon neoplasms, as well as the evaluation and surveillance of ulcerative colitis, and reviews the likely future progression of this technology in the diagnosis of intestinal disorders.

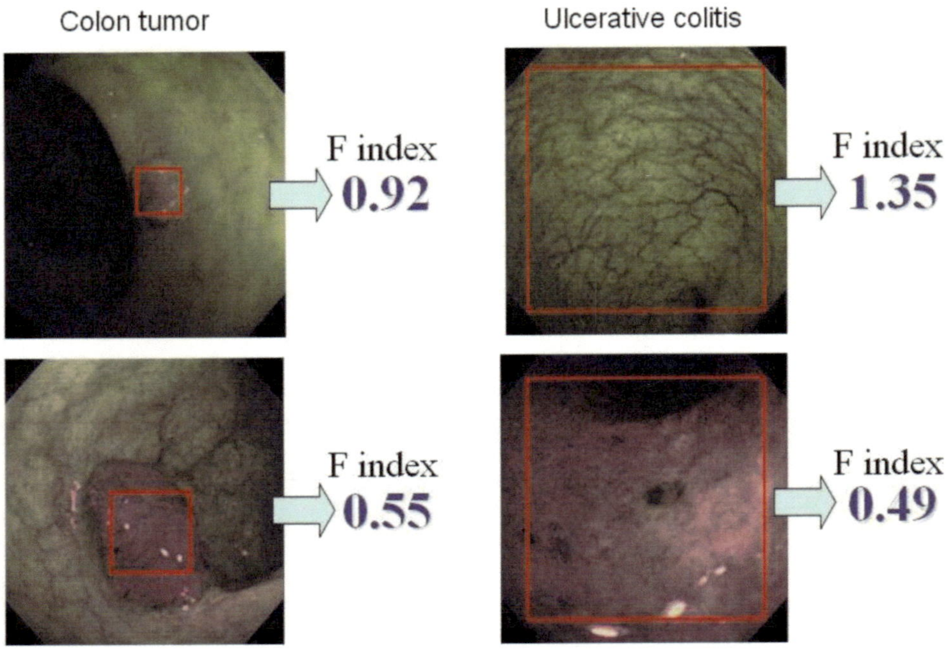

Fig. 2. Lesions are traced and measured to determine the strength of the red and green areas. The ratio of the reverse gamma value of green (fluorescence) divided by that of red (reflex) is defined as the fluorescence index (F index).

2. Endoscopic features of colonic lesions obtained by AFI

The typical images of intestinal disorders including neoplasms, inflammatory bowel disease, other types of colitis, Behcet disease, amyloidosis and other diseases are described in this section.

2.1 Colon cancer and adenoma

Almost all colon cancers and adenomas are described as magenta in AFI **(Figure 3)**. The invasion depth of the cancer does not appear to influence the intensity of the fluorescence captured by AFI **(Figure 4)**. The margin of the tumor is clear in AFI, even for flat and depressed types of tumors **(Figure 5)**. Interestingly, AFI can detect only the tumor area, but not the reactive changes surrounding the tumor **(Figure 6)**. This suggests that AFI detects some histological component of the tumor. The intensity of the fluorescence captured by AFI appears to be inversely proportional to the dysplastic grade of adenoma (Moriichi, et al. in submission).

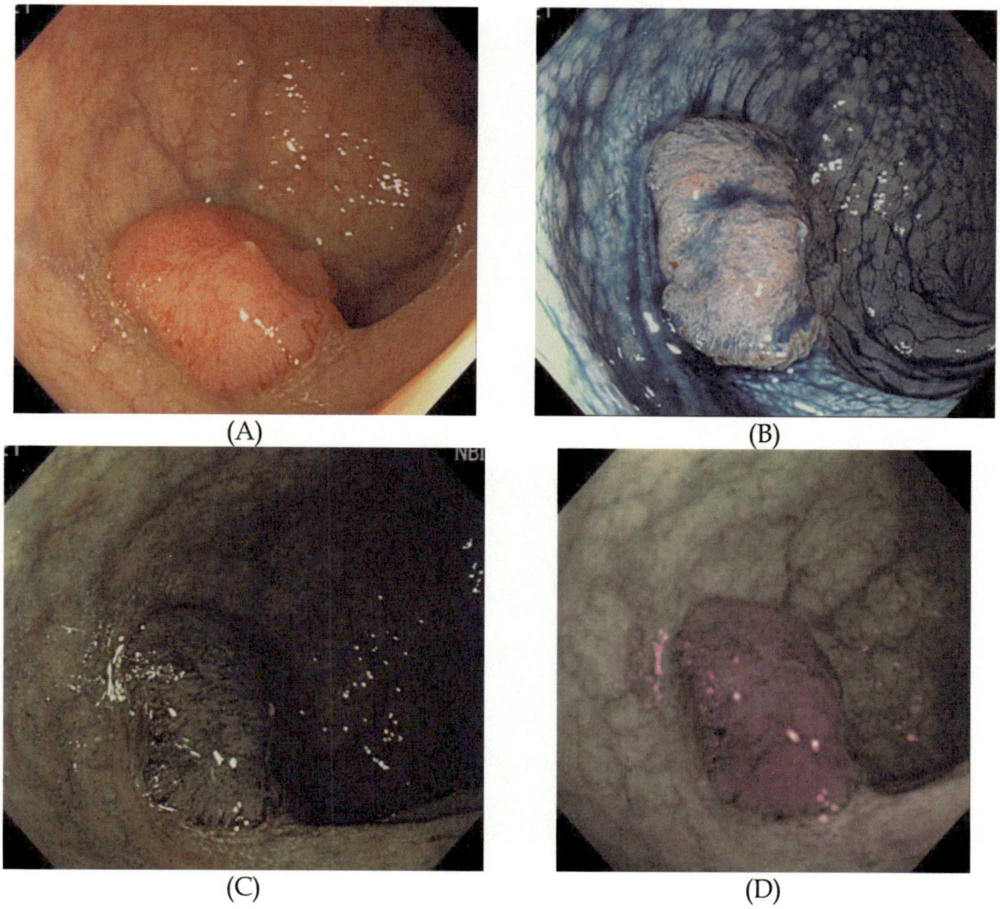

Fig. 3. HRE (A), indigocarmine-spraying image (B), narrow band imaging (C) and AFI (B) of the colon cancer with submucosal invasion.

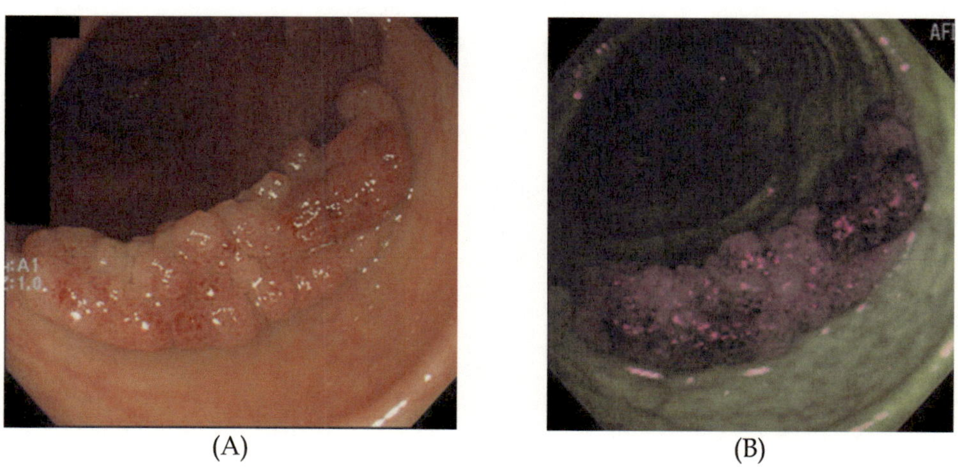

Fig. 4. HRE (A) and AFI (B) of colon cancer limited to the mucosal layer.

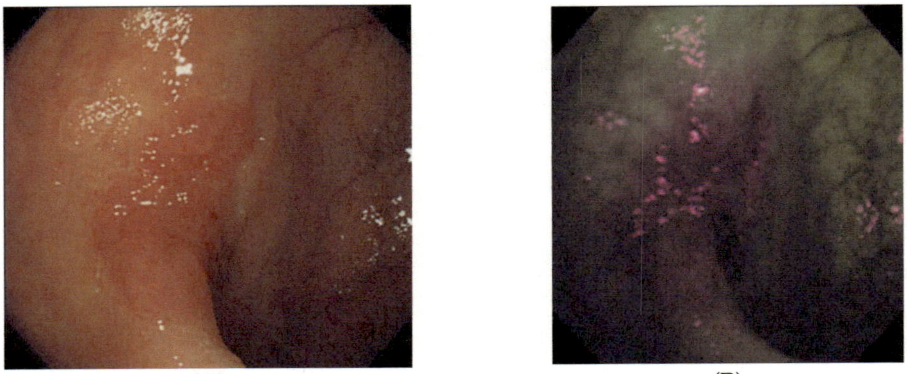

(A) (B)

Fig. 5. HRE (A) and AFI (B) of a flat and depressed type of colon cancer with submucosal invasion.

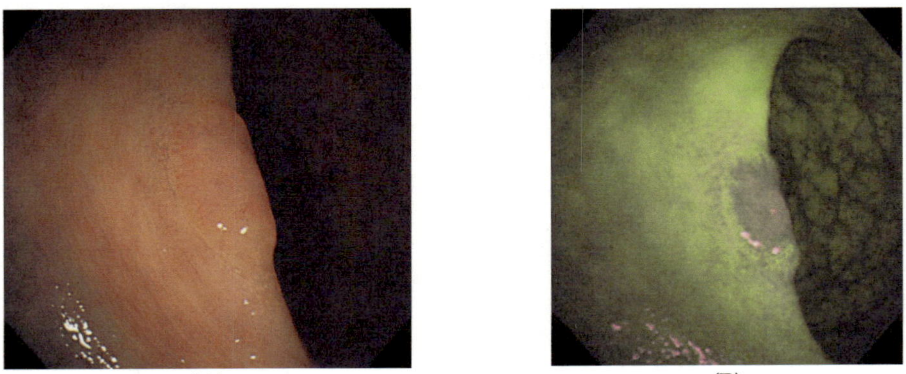

(A) (B)

Fig. 6. HRE revealed a flat and depressed type of tumor (A). AFI detected only the depressed area as magenta (B), thus suggesting that the tumor cells are limited to the depression area.

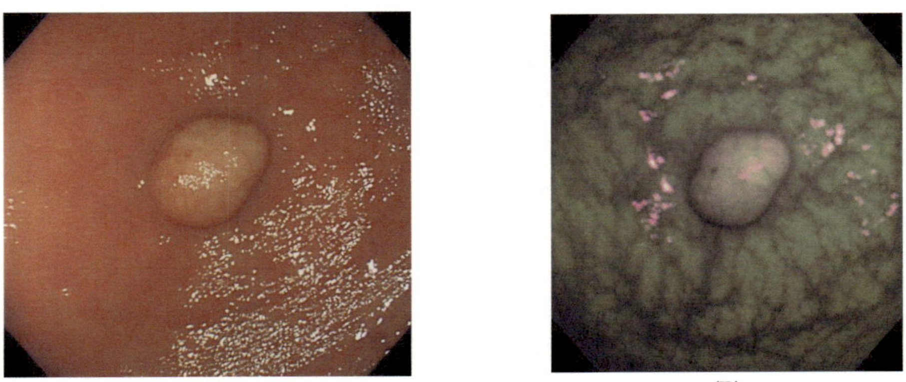

(A) (B)

Fig. 7. HRE reveals a smooth yellowish elevation (A). AFI describes the tumor as a slight magenta area. Sometimes, the surface of a carcinoid shows heterogenous magenta and green (B).

2.2 Carcinoid tumors

Carcinoid tumors form in the neuroendocrine system. This type of tumor is thought to initiate from the deep portion of the intestinal epithelia **(Modlin IM, et al. 2003)**. The tumor is therefore likely to be a submucosal tumor in the early stage. A typical finding of carcinoid tumors by white light endoscopy is a yellowish elevation with a smooth surface. AFI detects the tumor as a slight magenta area, but not strong magenta as is seen for typical colon cancer **(Figure 7)**.

2.3 Lymphoma

The intestinal tract is a major organ presenting with extranodal lymphoma lesions **(Groves FD, et al. 2000)(Gurney KA, et al. 2002)(Morton LM, et al. 2006)**. The most frequently observed types of lymphoma are non-Hodgkin's, B cell lymphomas including diffuse large B cell lymphoma, follicular lymphoma and mucosa-associated lymphoid tissue (MALT) lymphoma. Diffuse large B cell lymphoma frequently forms a submucosal tumor which is detected as a magenta area by AFI **(Figure 8)**. Conversely, Follicular, MALT and T cell lymphomas are sometimes detected as diffusely spread magenta spots or areas by AFI **(Figures 9, 10 and 11)**.

2.4 Ulcerative colitis

Ulcerative colitis is a chronic refractory colitis. While clinical symptoms are essential to assess the activity of ulcerative colitis, endoscopic assessment helps to predict the relapse or evaluate the grade of mucosal healing **(Fujiya M, et al. 2002)**. Typical endoscopic features of ulcerative colitis are an absence of vessel permeation, multiple erosions and ulcers, and hemorrhage which diffusely appears from the rectum to the oral side of colon. We previously reported that the activity of ulcerative colitis is inversely proportional to the intensity of fluorescence captured by AFI **(Figures 12 and 13) (Fujiya M, et al., 2007)**.

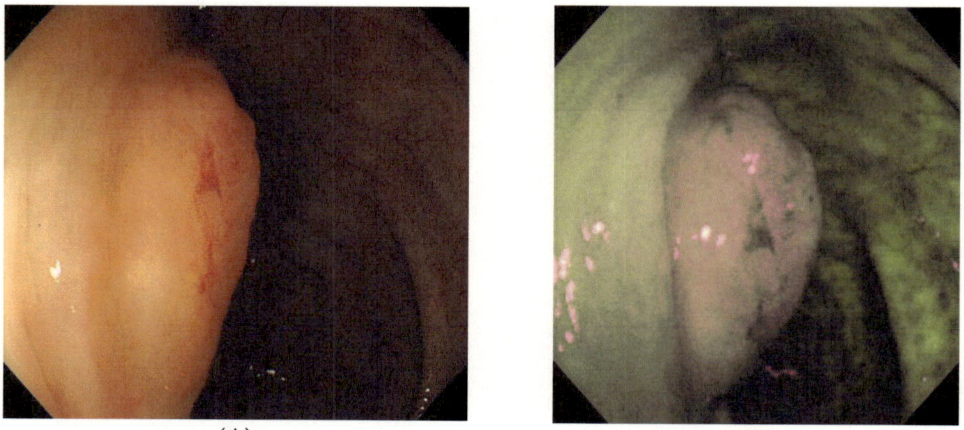

(A) (B)

Fig. 8. HRE (A) and an AFI image (B) of a diffuse large B cell lymphoma at the ileocecal valve.

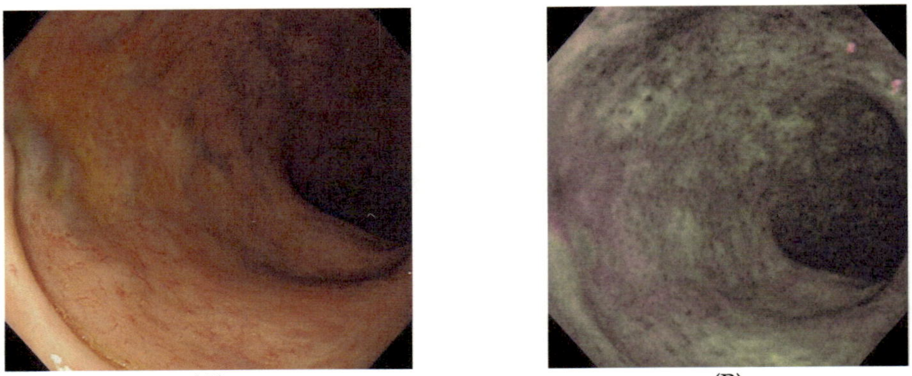

(A) (B)

Fig. 9. HRE describes many abnormal vessels in the rectum (A). AFI can detect mosaic magenta spots which correspond to the invasion of follicular lymphoma (B).

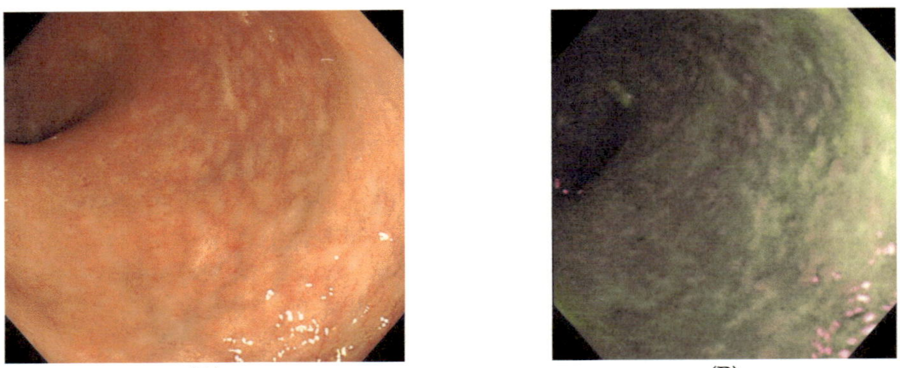

(A) (B)

Fig. 10. HRE describes a mosaic of red and white mucosa in the rectum (A). AFI detects diffusely spread magenta spots which correspond to the invasion of MALT lymphoma (B).

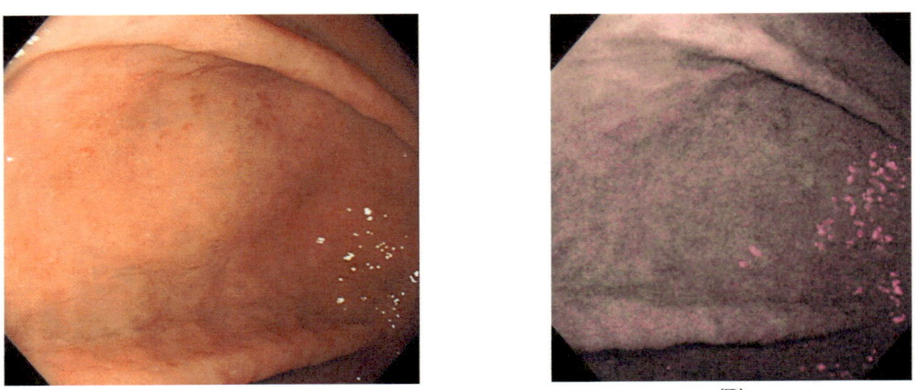

(A) (B)

Fig. 11. HRE describes an edematous mucosa with no vessel permeation (A). AFI detects a diffuse and strong magenta area which corresponds to the invasion of T cell lymphoma originating from the tonsil (B).

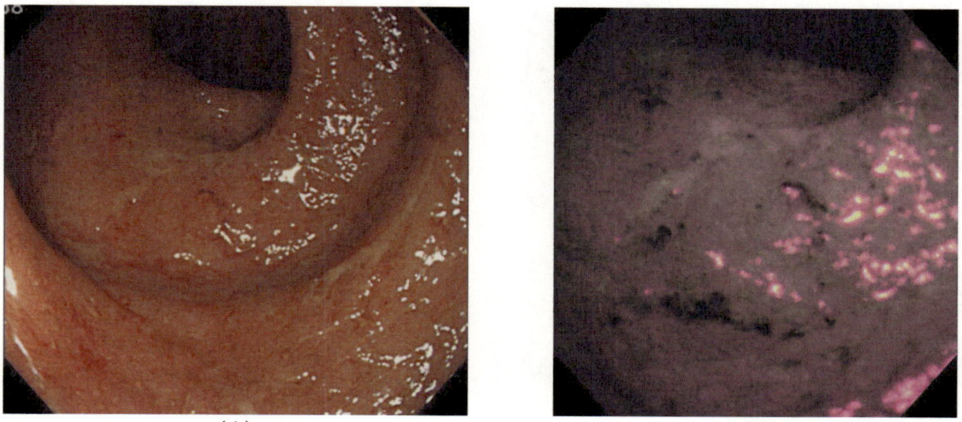

(A) (B)

Fig. 12. HRE indicates the presence of an edematous mucosa with small ulcers and bleeding in a patient with active ulcerative colitis (A). AFI demonstrated diffuse strong magenta areas with some deep green spots, which reflect the presence of histologically active inflammation (B).

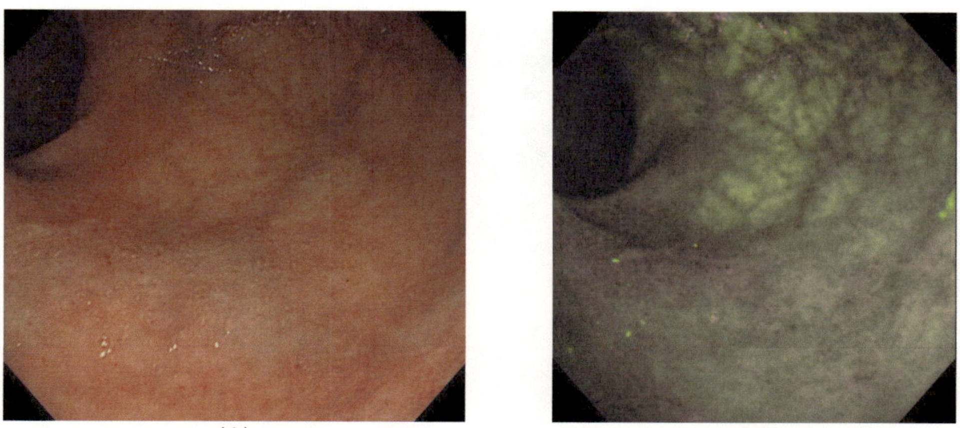

(A) (B)

Fig. 13. HRE describes the edematous mucosa and an area with vessel permeation (A). AFI demonstrated a slight magenta area and a green area with vessel permeation, which corresponds to an active lesion and a quiescent area, respectively (B).

2.5 Enterocolitis

Enterocolitis is an inflammatory disease of the digestive tract caused by various microbes, parasites and chemicals. While most cases can be diagnosed without the need for endoscopy, some enteritis that persists in spite of antibiotic treatments require endoscopic evaluation. The presence of edematous mucosa with multiple erosions, ulcers and bleeding are typically observed. These findings are enhanced as magenta areas by AFI **(Figure 14)**.

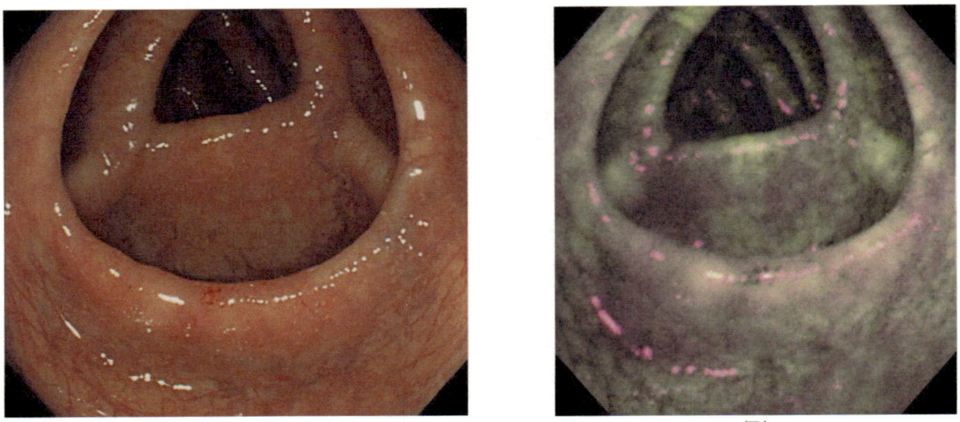

(A) (B)

Fig. 14. HRE shows the edematous mucosa with minute erosions (A). AFI enhanced the lesions as magenta areas (B).

2.6 Aphthoid colitis

Aphthoid colitis is a form of intestinal inflammation which cannot be categorized into any other category of intestinal diseases. Sometimes, aphtoid colitis is an early step in the process of developing Crohn's disease, Behcet disease or other inflammatory disorders. In AFI, aphtoid ulcers exhibit a clear magenta area surrounded by a blurred magenta area that reflects edema and the infiltration of immune cells **(Figure 15)**.

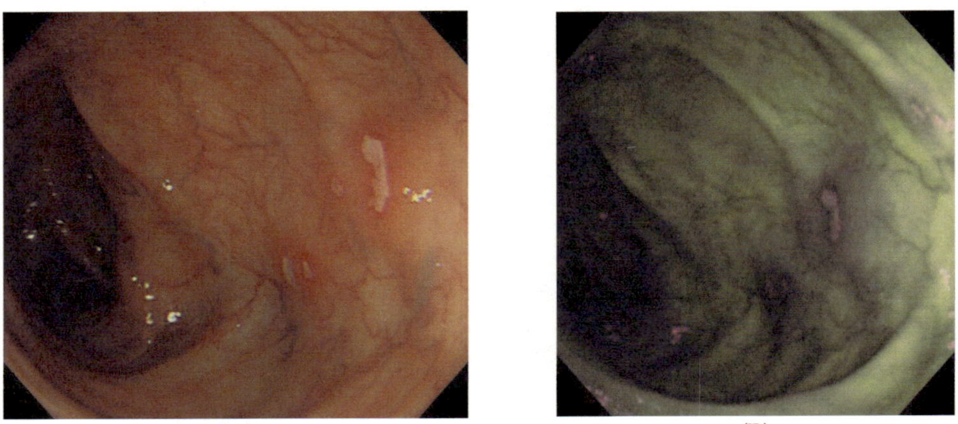

(A) (B)

Fig. 15. Aphthoid ulcers surrounded by edematous mucosa are observed by HRE (A). AFI reveals the ulcer bed as a strong magenta area with surrounding edema presented as a faint magenta area (B).

2.7 Behcet disease

Behcet disease is a systemic vasculitis that frequently presents with mucosal injury and ocular involvement **(International Study Group for Behçet's Disease, 1990)**. The small intestine, particularly the ileocecal valve, is a frequently involved site. Punched-out ulcers and aphtha are typical lesions in the intestinal tract **(Figure 16)**.

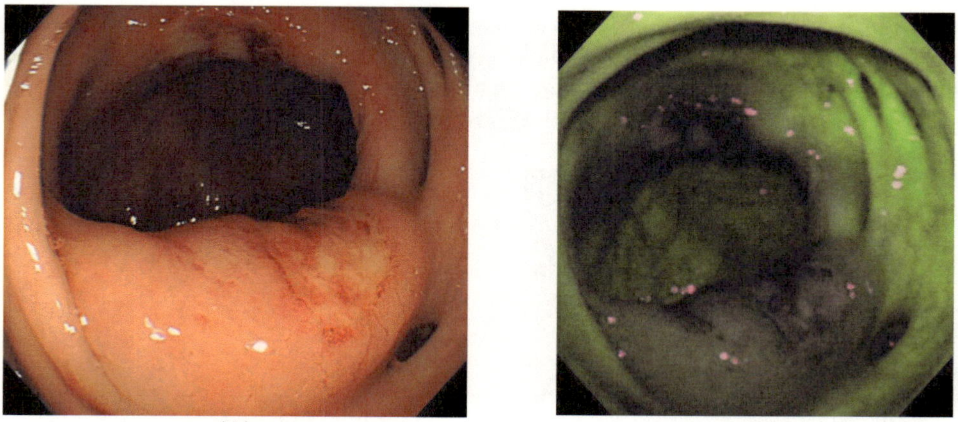

(A) (B)

Fig. 16. HRE reveals a large ulcer on the ileocecal valve with an edematous mucosa and another large ulcer on the opposite site (A). AFI describes both ulcers as slight magenta areas, and the edematous mucosa surrounding the ulcers as faint magenta areas (B).

2.8 Amyloidosis

Amyloidosis is defined as an extracellular deposit of fibril proteins, P-components, or other glycoproteins in organs and tissues, causing mild to severe pathophysiological changes **(Westermark P. 2005)**. The intestinal tract is a frequently involved site of amyloid deposition **(Koppelman RN, et al. 2000)**. The endoscopic features of intestinal amyloidosis include elevated lesions, ulcerations, nodules, petechial mucosal hemorrhage. AFI enhances these changes as magenta areas **(Figure 17)**.

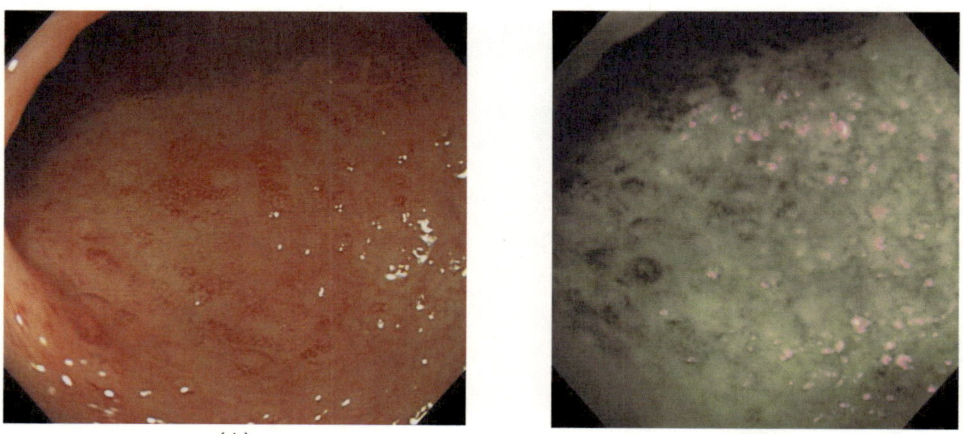

(A) (B)

Fig. 17. HRE reveals a diffuse edematous mucosa with dilated vessels (A). AFI describes the edematous mucosa as a magenta area and the dilated vessels as deep green (B).

2.9 Phlebosclerotic colitis

Phelebosclerotic colitis is characterized as the presence of sclerosis with calcification in the tributaries of the superior mesenteric vein **(Arimura Y, et al. 1998)**. This leads to chronic venous insufficiency and congestion, causing abdominal pain, diarrhea and intestinal obstruction. The endoscopic feature of pheleboscierotic colitis is a dark purple mucosa with a marked thickness and absence of the haustra at the right side colon. AFI typically reveals a strong green area with magenta spots at the corresponding site **(Figure 18)**.

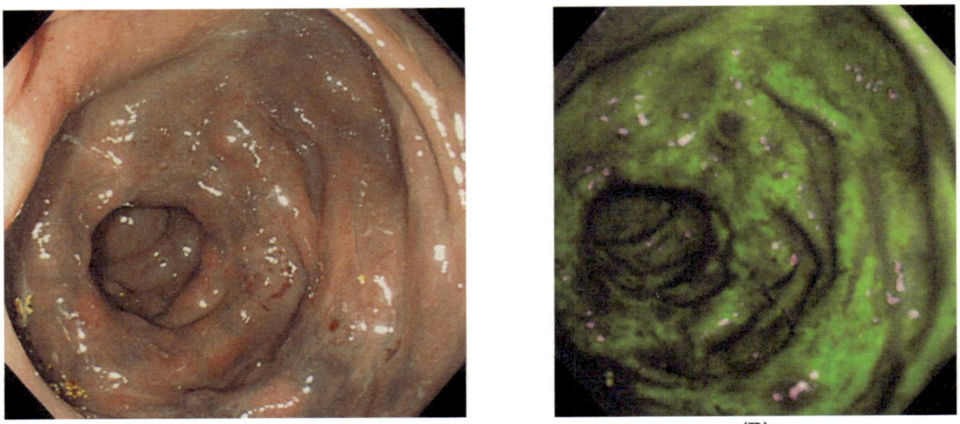

(A) (B)

Fig. 18. HRE reveals a dark purple mucosa with edematous changes and an absence of the haustra. (A). AFI exhibits a strong green area with magenta spots (B).

2.10 Disuse atrophy

When the intestinal tract does not function for a long time due to a bowel rest or an intestinal operation with a stoma, disuse atrophy of the intestine develops. The typical endoscopic features are an edematous mucosa with easy bleeding. AFI detects magenta areas in the corresponding site **(Figure 19)**.

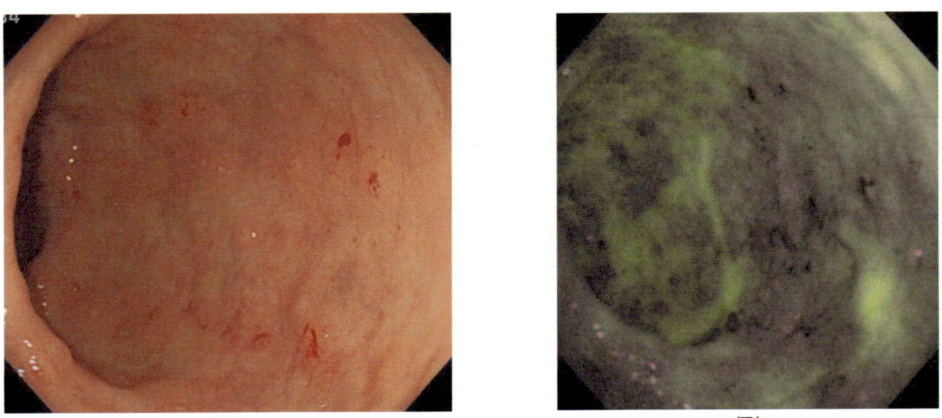

(A) (B)

Fig. 19. HRE reveals the presence of an edematous mucosa with small erosions and spotty bleeding (A). AFI enhances the erosions as magenta and the bleeding as deep green areas (B).

3. The diagnostic efficacy of AFI for colon disorders

The significance of AFI for diagnosing intestinal disorders, including colon cancer, lymphoma and ulcerative colitis are reviewed in this section.

3.1 Adenoma and cancer

During the process of colon carcinogenesis, normal epithelia are thought to initially turn into benign adenomas, accumulate gene alterations, and then transform into advanced adenocarcinomas **(Fearon ER, et al. 1990) (Lengauer C, et al. 1998)**. All adenomas are thus considered to be premalignant lesions. Indeed, several trials on endoscopic resection for colon adenoma successfully decreased the mortality of colon cancer **(Winawer SJ, et al. 1993)**. However, some patients under close colonoscopic surveillance still develop colorectal cancer **(Robertson DJ, et al. 2005.)**. This discrepancy may be caused by the rapid progression of adenomas, as well as the overlooking of colorectal adenoma by endoscopists with different levels of experience. Indeed, systematic reviews of back-to-back colonoscopies showed that 15% to 32% of colorectal adenomas were possibly missed by colonoscopy **(van Rijn JC, et al. 2006)**, particularly flat and depressed adenomas **(Rembacken BJ, et al. 2000)(Saitoh Y, et al. 2001)**.

Several studies have been conducted to assess the efficacy of AFI for detecting colon adenoma. Matsuda et al. investigated the detection rate of colon polyps at the proximal colon by AFI using a modified back-to-back method. They showed a higher detection rate of colon neoplasms by AFI than that by white light endoscopy **(Matsuda T, et al. 2008)**. In contrast, van den Broek et al. compared the detection rate of AFI with that of HRE using a procedure to inspect the entire colon twice during withdrawal: once with AFI and once with HRE by the same endoscopist. They concluded that AFI showed no significant effect on reducing the adenoma miss-rate in comparison to HRE **(van den Broek FJ, et al. 2009)**. We previously investigated the efficacy of AFI for the detection of colon adenoma by either less-experienced physicians or endoscopic experts, and found that AFI improved the detection rate of colon adenoma, particularly by less-experienced physicians. The effectiveness of AFI for detecting colon adenoma thus appears to depend on the endoscopist and his/her level of experience.

Of interest, AFI does not detect hyperplastic polyps as a clear magenta area **(Figure 20)**. Based on this property, AFI is expected to be used for discriminating colon neoplasms from non-neoplasms. However, the practical usefulness of AFI in the differential diagnosis of colon adenoma remains controversial **(van den Broek FJ, et al. 2009)(Boparai KS, et al. 2009)(van den Broek FJ, et al. 2009)**. We recently investigated the effectiveness of HRE, NBI, AFI and chromoendoscopy for differentiating colon adenoma from hyperplastic polyps. From the numerical analysis of the intensity of fluorescence captured by AFI, the strength of the fluorescence was significantly lower for colon adenoma than that in hyperplastic polyp. Furthermore, our prospective study indicated that AFI improved the diagnostic accuracy to distinguish colon adenoma from hyperplastic polyps, particularly in the resident group **(Satoh R, et al. in press)**. Therefore, it is suggested that AFI captures a lower intensity of fluorescence from colon adenoma in comparison to that from hyperplastic polyps, and AFI can therefore contribute to the differential diagnosis of colon polyps if endoscopists accurately assess the intensity of fluorescence.

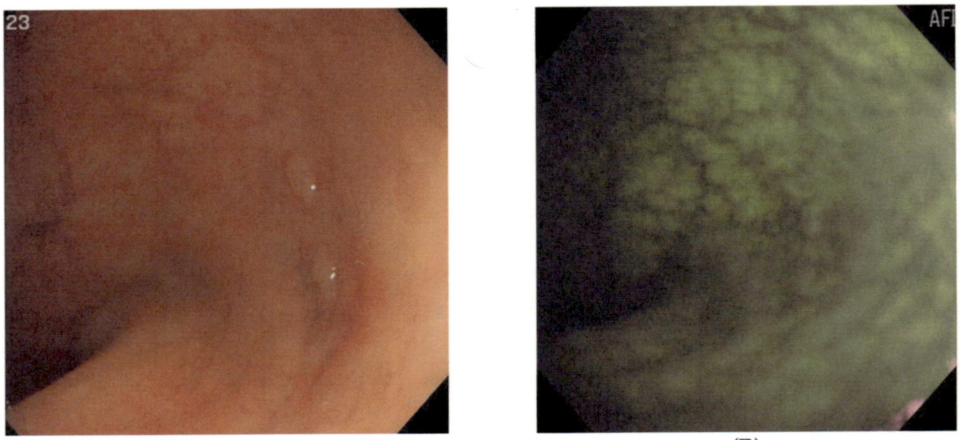

(A) (B)

Fig. 20. HRE reveals two whitish polyps (A). AFI does not enhance the polyps (B).

3.2 Lymphoma

While the intestinal involvement of lymphoma cells is enhanced as magenta by AFI as mentioned above, the efficacy of AFI for diagnosing lymphoma has not been thoroughly investigated. Our study concerning the capacity of AFI **(Ueno et al. 2010)** for diagnosing intestinal lymphoma demonstrated the usefulness of AFI **(Figure 21)**. A numerical analysis of the fluorescence intensity showed that AFI captured a stronger fluorescence from lymphoma than lymphoid hyperplasia (LH) **(Figure 22)**. A histological analysis of intestinal lymphoma and LH revealed that the cell density, but not the histological type, is a significant factor that is inversely proportional to the intensity. Consequently, AFI is a useful tool to diagnose intestinal lymphoma, but cannot be used for the differentiation of histological types.

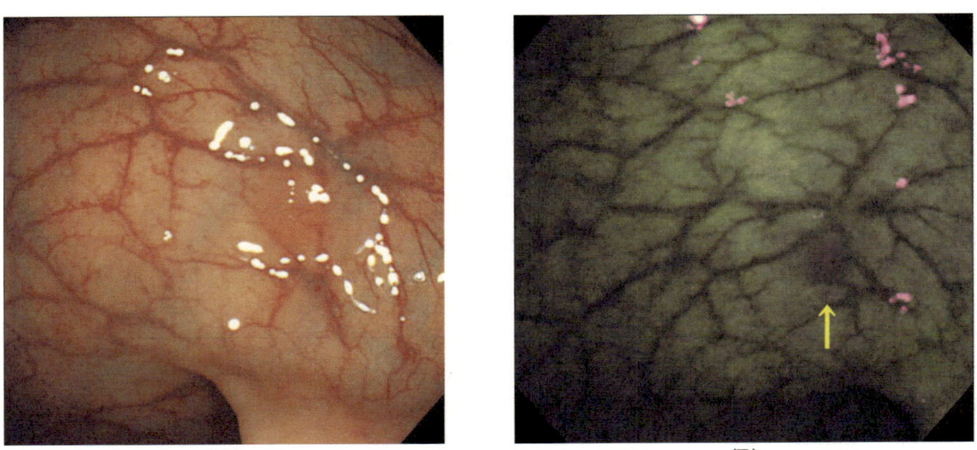

(A) (B)

Fig. 21. HRE reveals a very faint change in the way the light is caught (A). AFI clearly detects a small lesion (arrow) of an intestinal lymphoma as a magenta spot (B) (These pictures are cited from Ueno et al. Endoscopy (in press)).

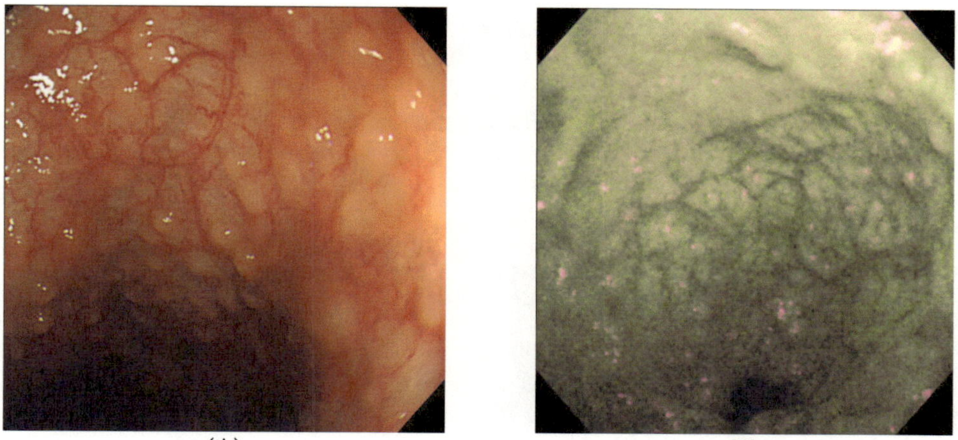

(A) (B)

Fig. 22. HRE reveals multiple polyps in the ileum (A). AFI does not enhance the polyps (B) (This picture is cited from Ueno et al. Endoscopy (in press)).

3.3 Ulcerative colitis

Ulcerative colitis is a chronic refractory colitis whose etiology is still unknown. Various therapeutic strategies for ulcerative colitis are performed according to the type and activity of the disease, thus, the evaluation of the activity is important to choose an appropriate treatment. While clinical symptoms are essential to assess the activity of ulcerative colitis, endoscopic assessment helps to predict the relapse or evaluate the grade of mucosal healing **(Fujiya M, et al. 2002)**.

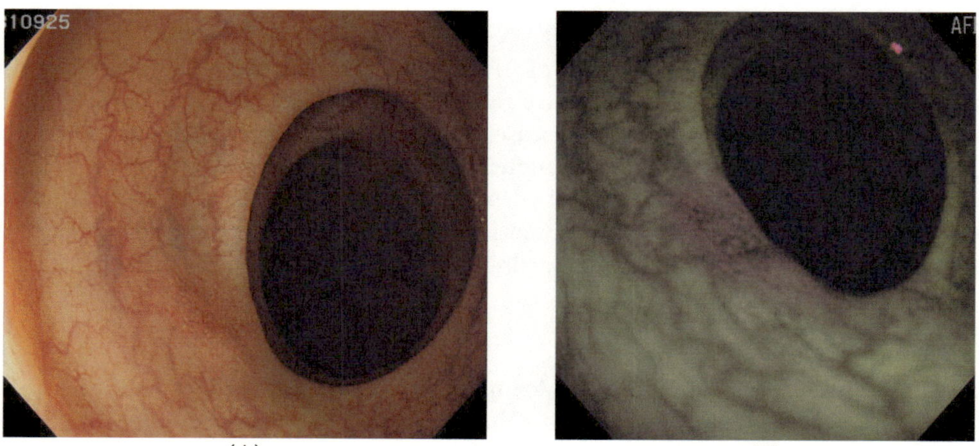

(A) (B)

Fig. 23. HRE reveals a small amount of redness with minute erosions (A). AFI clearly describes the lesion as a magenta area, suggesting the limited active inflammation in the area (B).

Our previous investigation proposed that the intensity of fluorescence captured by AFI was inversely proportional to the histological activity in ulcerative colitis **(Fujiya M, et al. 2007)**. Even a small lesion with slightly active inflammation can be clearly detected by AFI

(Figures 23 and 24). This suggests that when a numerical analysis of the fluorescence intensity is performed, AFI can evaluate the activity of ulcerative colitis with quite a high reproducibility and inter-observer consistency. Furthermore, it has been reported that AFI may be used to detect dysplasia in the inflamed mucosa of ulcerative colitis **(Matsumoto T, et al. 2007)**. The future analysis of the efficacy of AFI to assess the disease activity and detect dysplasia is therefore expected to confirm the significance of AFI in the diagnosis of ulcerative colitis.

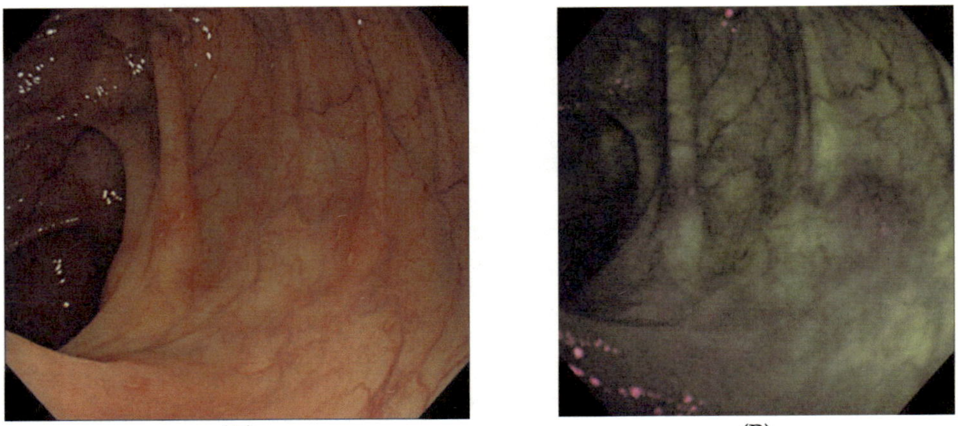

(A) (B)

Fig. 24. HRE reveals several minute erosions (A). AFI detects the erosions with the surrounding inflammation as a magenta area (B)

4. Conclusion

This review describes the typical findings of AFI and the significance of AFI in the diagnosis of intestinal disorders including colon cancer and adenoma, lymphoma, inflammatory bowel diseases, intestinal autoimmune diseases and other conditions. While the efficacy of AFI is still being explored, AFI can definitely be used an efficient tool for objectively assessing intestinal diseases, particularly by less-experienced physicians. In the near future, a numerical analysis of the fluorescence intensity will provide a new diagnostic strategy for intestinal disorders with both high reproducibility and inter-observer consistency.

5. References

Arimura, Y., Kondoh, Y., Kurokawa, S., Azuma, N., Sekiya, M., Nakagawa, N., Endo, T., Satoh, M., & Imai, K. (1998). Chronic ischemic colonic lesion caused by phlebosclerosis with calcification. *Am J Gastroenterol*, Vol.93, No.11, 2290-2, ISSN: 0002-9270

Boparai, K. S., van den Broek, F. J., van Eeden, S., Fockens, P., & Dekker, E. (2009). Hyperplastic polyposis syndrome: a pilot study for the differentiation of polyps by using high-resolution endoscopy, autofluorescence imaging, and narrow-band imaging. *Gastrointest Endosc*, Vol.70, No.5, 947-55, ISSN: 0016-5107

van den Broek, F. J., Fockens, P., Van Eeden, S., Kara, M. A., Hardwick, J. C., Reitsma, J. B., & Dekker, E. (2009). Clinical evaluation of endoscopic trimodal imaging for the detection and differentiation of colonic polyps. *Clin Gastroenterol Hepatol*,Vol.7, No.3, 288-95, ISSN: 1542-3565

van den Broek, F. J., van Soest, E. J., Naber, A. H., van Oijen, A. H., Mallant-Hent, R. Ch., Böhmer, C. J., Scholten, P., Stokkers, P. C., Marsman, W. A., Mathus-Vliegen, E. M., Curvers, W. L., Bergman, J. J., van Eeden, S., Hardwick, J. C., Fockens, P., Reitsma, J. B., & Dekker, E. (2009). Combining autofluorescence imaging and narrow-band imaging for the differentiation of adenomas from non-neoplastic colonic polyps among experienced and non-experienced endoscopists. *Am J Gastroenterol*, Vol.104, No.6, 1498-507, ISSN: 0002-9270

Fearon, E. R., & Vogelstein, B. (1990). A genetic model for colorectal tumorigenesis. *Cell*, Vol.61, No.5, 759–767, ISSN: 0092-8674

Frank, D. Groves., Martha, S. Linet., Lois, B. Travis., & Susan, S. Devesa. (2000). Cancer surveillance series: non-Hodgkin's lymphoma incidence by histologic subtype in the United States from 1978 through 1995. *J Natl Cancer Inst*, Vol.92 No.15, 1240-51, ISSN: 1460-2105

Fujiya, M., Saitoh, Y., Nomura, M., Maemoto, A., Fujiya, K., Watari, J., Ashida, T., Ayabe, T., Obara, T., & Kohgo, Y. (2002). Minute findings by magnifying colonoscopy are useful for the evaluation of ulcerative colitis. *Gastrointest Endosc*, Vol.56, No.4, 535-542, ISSN: 0016-5107

Fujiya, M., Saitoh, Y., Watari, J., Moriichi, K., & Kohgo, Y. (2007). Auto-Fluorescence Imaging is useful to assess the activity of ulcerative colitis. *Digestive Endoscopy*, Vol.19, No. ,145-149, ISSN: 0915-5635

Gurney, K. A., & Cartwright, R. A. (2002). Increasing incidence and descriptive epidemiology of extranodal non-Hodgkin lymphoma in parts of England and Wales. *Hematol J*, Vol.3, No.2, 95-104, ISSN: 0390-6078

International Study Group for Behçet's Disease. (1990). Criteria for diagnosis of Behçet's disease. *Lancet* Vol.335, No.8697, 1078–80, ISSN: 0140-6736

Koppelman, R. N., Stollman, N. H., Baigorri, F., & Rogers, A. I. (2000). Acute small bowel pseudo-obstruction due to amyloidosis: a case report and literature review. *Am J Gastroenterol*, Vol.95, No.1, 294–296, ISSN: 0002-9270

Lengauer, C., Kinzler, K., & Vogelstein, B. (1998). Genetic instabilities in human cancers. *Nature*, Vol.396, No.6712, 643–649, ISSN: 0028-0836

Lindsay, M. Morton., Sophia, S. Wang., Susan, S. Devesa., Patricia, Hartge., Dennis, D. Weisenburger, & Martha, S. Linet. (2006). Lymphoma incidence patterns by WHO subtype in the United States, 1992-2001. *Blood*, Vol.107, No.1, 265-276, ISSN: 0006-4971

Matsuda, T., Saito, Y., Fu, K. I., Uraoka, T., Kobayashi, N., Nakajima, T., Ikehara, H., Mashimo, Y., Shimoda, T., Murakami, Y., Parra-Blanco, A., Fujimori, T., & Saito, D. (2008). Does autofluorescence imaging videoendoscopy system improve the colonoscopic polyp detection rate?—a pilot study. *Am J Gastroenterol*, Vol.103, No.8 , 1926-32, ISSN: 0002-9270

Matsumoto, T., Moriyama, T., Yao, T., Mibu, R., & Iida, M. (2007). Autofluorescence imaging colonoscopy for the diagnosis of dysplasia in ulcerative colitis. *Inflamm Bowel Dis*, Vol.13, No.5, 640-641, ISSN: 1078-0998

Modlin, I.M., Lye, K.D., & Kidd, M. (2003). A 5-decade analysis of 13,715 carcinoid tumors. *Cancer*, Vol.97, No.4, 934–59, ISSN: 0008-543X

Nakashima, A., Miwa, H., Watanabe, H., Kobayashi, O., Ogihara, T., & Sato, N. (2001). A new technique: light-induced fluorescence endoscopy in combination with pharmacoendoscopy. *Gastrointest Endosc*, Vol.53, No. 3, 343-8, ISSN: 0016-5107

Rembacken, B. J., Fujii, T., Cairns, A., Dixon, M. F., Yoshida, S., Chalmers, D. M., & Axon, A. T. (2000). Flat and depressed colonic neoplasms: a prospective study of 1000 colonoscopies in the UK. *Lancet*, Vol.355, No.9211, 1211–1214, ISNN: 0140-6736

van Rijn, J. C., Reitsma, J. B., Stoker, J., Bossuyt, P. M., van Deventer, S. J., & Dekker, E. (2006). Polyp miss rate determined by tandem colonoscopy: a systematic review. *Am J Gastroenterol*, Vol.101, No.2, 343–350, ISSN: 0002-9270

Robertson, D. J., Greenberg, E. R., Beach, M., Sandler, R.S., Ahnen, D., Haile, R. W., Burke, C. A., Snover, D. C., Bresalier, R. S., McKeown-Eyssen, G., Mandel, J. S., Bond, J. H., Van Stolk, R. U., Summers, R. W., Rothstein, R., Church, T. R., Cole, B. F., Byers, T., Mott, L., & Baron, J. A. (2005). Colorectal cancer in patients under close colonoscopic surveillance. *Gastroenterology*, Vol.129, No.1, 34–41, ISSN: 0016-5085

Saitoh, Y., Waxman, I., West, A. B., Popnikolov, N. K., Gatalica, Z., Watari, J., Obara, T., Kohgo, Y., & Pasricha, P. J. (2001). Prevalence and distinctive biologic features of flat colorectal adenomas in a North American population. *Gastroenterology*, Vol.120, No.7, 1657–1665, ISSN: 0016-5085

Sato, R., Fujiya, M., Watari, J., Ueno, N., Moriichi, K., Kashima, S., Maeda, S., Ando, K., Kawabata, H., Sugiyama, R., Nomura, Y., Nata, T., Itabashi, K., Inaba, Y., Okamoto, K., Mizukami, Y., Saitoh, Y., & Kohgo, Y. (in press) The diagnostic accuracy of high-resolution endoscopy, autofluorescence imaging and narrow-band imaging for differentially diagnosing colon adenoma. *Endoscopy,* ISSN: 0013-726X

Winawer, S. J., Zauber, A. G., Ho. M. N., O'Brien, M. J., Gottlieb, L. S., Sternberg, S. S., Waye, J. D., Schapiro, M., Bond, J. H., Panish, J. F., Ackroyd, F., Shike, M., Kurtz, R. C., Hornsby-Lewis, L, Gerdes, H., Stewart, E. T., & The National Polyp Study Workgroup. (1993). Prevention of Colorectal Cancer by Colonoscopic Polypectomy. N Eng J Med Vol.329, No.27, 1977-1981, ISSN: 0028-4793

Ueno, N., Fujiya, M., Moriichi, K., Ikuta, K., Nata, T., Konno, Y., Ishikawa, C., Inaba, Y., Ito, T., Sato, R., Okamoto, K., Tanabe, H., Maemoto, A., Sato, K., Watari, J., Ashida, T., Saitoh, Y., & Kohgo, Y. (in press). Endosopic auto-fluorescence imaging is useful for the differential diagnosis of intestinal lymphomas resembling lymphoid heyperplasia. *J Clin Gastroenterol*, ISSN: 0192-0790

Westermark, P. Aspects on human amyloid forms and their fibril polypeptides. (2005). FEBS J, Vol.272, No.23, 5942–9, ISSN: 1742-464X

15

Intestinal Dynamic Color Doppler Sonographic Tissue Perfusion Measurement

Thomas Scholbach[1], Jörg Hofmann[1] and Jakob Scholbach[2]
[1]*Hospital for Children and Adolescents, Chemnitz Clinincs, 09116 Chemnitz*
[2]*University of Münster, Mathematical Institute, 48149 Münster*
Germany

1. Introduction

The evaluation of intestinal diseases encompasses morphological as well as functional aspects. The proper function of any organ depends on a sufficient blood supply to meet its actual metabolic needs. Blood flow though is a measure of physiological and pathophysiological tasks which are accomplished by the respective organ. Thus, many of these tasks can be described by measuring the amount of blood passing through tissues. Inflammation is an excellent example of such a response to a stimulus which increases tissue perfusion. The measurement of perfusion intensity would be helpful to monitor inflammatory processes. In contrast to the obvious advantages of such an approach only very limited methods exist to quantify perfusion of the bowel today. Contrast media in MRI, CT and angiography can give a vague impression of the quality of bowel perfusion but are not usable to quantify perfusion. Doppler ultrasound is used to record changes of blood flow velocity in the main intestinal arteries to calculate the so called Resistance Index (RI) and the related Pulsatility Index (PI). Both cannot describe the amount of intestinal blood since they lack the information of the width of the intestinal vascular network. Besides the actual flow velocity inside each vessel the vessel width is the other necessary constituent to calculate flow intensity or volume inside a tissue. We developed a novel method to overcome these limitations - the Dynamic Color Doppler Sonographic Tissue Perfusion Measurement (DTPM). The following chapter describes the principle of DTPM and its use in gastroenterology.

DTPM was developed to meet so far unsatisfied daily needs in clinical practice, to quantify tissue perfusion in order to answer pressing clinical questions: is the tissue viable, is it damaged and to which extent, is there an inflammatory hyperperfusion, is the blood supply to an organ sufficient to fulfill its tasks properly.

2. Dynamic Color Doppler Sonographic Tissue Perfusion Measurement (DTPM)

2.1 Idea

The idea behind DTPM is that we all are used to estimate by the naked eye the intensity of blood flow in a tissue by watching the strong or less strong coloration of a tissue during a routine color Doppler ultrasound examination – but unfortunately this feeling that the blood flow is strong or weak cannot be used for a sound decision on treatment. All we see remains a vague impression. To discuss our findings with others or to refer to our own previous observations we need a reliable basis for comparison – we need a measurement of what we see. This is not easily accomplished since the pumping heart causes an ever changing picture of sparkling color dots inside the tissue under investigation. We need to measure these changes from beginning to the end of the heart beat to calculate a mean perfusion value referring to a complete heart beat. Moreover we know that perfusion is blood volume per time running through the vascular bed of a tissue. Volume per time per tissue unit is but perfused area multiplied by perfusion velocity (the area is virtually lifted at a certain height per time thus creating a volume made up of tiny cylinders which stand more or less dispersed between nonperfused (extravascular) parts (the non-colored background of the color Doppler image). The product of perfused area and perfusion velocity needs to be referred to the total area of the tissue section which is actually examined.

2.2 Principle

DTPM is a software assisted method to extract and use color Doppler data from standardized color Doppler videos in order to measure the perfusion of a tissue (Scholbach et al., 2004; Scholbach et al., 2005a, 2006; Scholbach et al., 2005b). The perfusion intensity (Q) is calculated as product of perfusion velocity and perfused area (A) inside a region of interest (A_{ROI})

$$Q = v^*A/\ A_{ROI} \quad \text{with the unit } [cm/s] = [cm/s\ ^*cm^2/cm^2].$$

All colored pixels code a certain number of red blood cells moving with a certain velocity towards the transducer. The color represents the flow direction (red symbolizes flow towards the transducer and blue the opposite direction or vice versa). The shade of both colors from dark to light nuances represents a certain velocity value. Each pixel has a certain area and is the elementary unit of image resolution. Perfused parts of a tissue are depicted in color whereas nonperfused parts remain non-colored (black, gray or white). DTPM comprises the complete information, which is necessary to describe the perfusion intensity i.e. perfused area and velocity values of all pixels, which is extracted and referred to the tissue area under investigation. This way a description of perfusion is achieved which goes far beyond existing techniques of conventional Doppler sonographic perfusion evaluation as RI and PI (Resistance and Pulsatility Index) (Scholbach et al., 2005b). Thus DTPM is applicable for all tissues which can be depicted by means of ultrasound (Rouviere et al., 2004; Scholbach & Scholbach, 2009; Wieczorek et al., 2009).

2.3 Technical requirements

The equipment to perform DTPM is a conventional color Doppler ultrasound machine with transducers that are suitable for a detailed and fast color Doppler imaging. For the investigation of the intestinal tract a linear transducer is mandatory with a B-mode frequency above 5 MHz and a color Doppler frequency of at least 3 MHz. The machine must display the color bar inside the image and must show the maximum values of the depicted flow velocities at the end of the color bar. Moreover the recording of short videos must be possible (at least 2 sec duration) and these files should be recorded and transferred to an external PC via network, USB-stick or other data storage media for the subsequent DTPM with the PixelFlux-software. DICOM file format is preferred over avi-file format since information about image and recording details as well as patient data are included in the header of the DICOM-file but lack in the avi-file. Despite this avi files are suitable too but need more manual processing than DICOM files thus requiring more time and manpower to be processed.

2.4 Standardization

The standardization of image acquisition is crucial for DTPM. A preset of all machine settings must be defined in the beginning of a DTPM study to define in detail the best imaging conditions for the tissue in question. The following parameters must be kept constant in all times to ensure a comparability of the DTPM (others may be also fixed – depending on the parameters offered by the equipment in use): gain, frequency, persistence, color bar, time and spatial resolution, transducer type, ultrasound machine type, wall filter, depth compensation.
If the actual patient requires an other imaging preset then the primary one, it must be confirmed by statistical comparisons, that the measurement results of both presets are not significantly different. If significant differences are found in a preliminary investigation with the same probands or calibrating devices a special reference range must be established to compare those data with the normal range established with the new preset.
In general daily practice this strict confinement to the own standard preset does not interfere with a smooth work-up of the imaging requests. It is a general practice to define presets for special purposes and all manufacturers offer a variety of them as default settings for different organs and transducers. In most cases these presets can be used or need to be adapted only slightly. Such a preset should be named and can be reinstituted then by preselection before starting the imaging.

2.5 Phantom perfusion measurements

DTPM is basically a pixelwise evaluation of perfusion using the color Doppler image data as delivered by the ultrasound machine. To prove if the concept yields reliable results we made interobserver correlation studies as well as phantom flow comparisons of the actually pumped volumes and the perfusion intensities measured by DTPM. In a phantom study with a perfused tube in a water basin we found a highly significant correlation to the actual perfusion as pumped by a precision laboratory pump (Pearson's $r = 0{,}987$; $p < 0{,}001$) (Scholbach et al., 2011). Moreover in a clinical setting the ultrasound of the thyroid revealed a good correlation between two independent researchers measuring the same video sequences (Spearman's $r = 0{,}870$, $p < 0{,}001$) (Scholbach et al., 2011).

2.6 Output

With DTPM the following parameters are calculated from a video sequence recording at least one full heart cycle.

- Perfusion intensity throughout the entire ROI: Perfusion intensity [cm/s] = mean perfused area [cm^2] * mean flow velocity [cm/s] /area of the ROI [cm^2]
- Mean flow velocity throughout the entire region of interest (ROI)
- Mean perfused area in relation to the ROI
- Area of the ROI
- Tissue Pulsatility Index (TPI) of velocity / of area / of perfusion intensity

- TPI = (maximal systolic value – minimal diastolic value) / mean value - "value" may be velocity, area or intensity
- Tissue Resistance Index (TRI) of velocity / of area / of perfusion intensity
- TRI = (maximal systolic value – minimal diastolic value) / maximal systolic value - "value" may be velocity, area or intensity
- Spatial distribution of flow across the tissue
- an overlay of false colors upon the ROI shows local distribution of flow intensity
- Quantitative distribution of perfusion intensity throughout the tissue section
- the whole range of flow intensity (resp. perfused area) over a full video sequence is divided into percentiles. Each interval's fraction of the ROI describes the distribution of perfusion intensity in numerical values.
- Time lines of above explained perfusion parameters of individual patients can be displayed and statistically evaluated

An example of a DTPM is given below (fig 1a-d).

2.7 Performing a DTPM

The first step to perform a DTPM is to record a standardized color Doppler video of the respective tissue. In the case of intestinal diseases the bowel or gastric wall is focused on. Liver, pancreas and lymph nodes are equally useful targets of a DTPM investigation. In the following a typical procedure for examining the bowel in chronic inflammatory bowel diseases (IBD) is outlined.

With a linear Doppler probe the respective bowel segment is imaged. Colon segements are in most cases easily distinguished from small bowel segments by their haustra. Inflamed bowel segments expose themselves by their typical inflammatory changes: they are much thicker, darker and less mobile than normal ones (fig 2).

The bowel segment is then imaged with color Doppler ultrasound. The patient is asked to stop breathing for 3 seconds to prevent movements of the bowel segment. Most inflamed bowel segments are rather immobile so breathing sometimes can be continued. In all cases flushing movement color artifacts, which may veil larger parts of the image behind a curtain of a single color shade (which unmasks them as artifacts easily) have to be avoided. A video of 2 to 3 seconds duration is recorded then and transferred to the PC with the PixelFlux-software. The video file is then opened and calibrated according to the distances and the color hues. This is done by the software in DICOM-files and must be supported in avi-files by the investigator. The calibration is necessary to calculate areas and flow velocities. Flow velocities are calculated by direct comparison of each color pixel with the color bar. Since the software deciphers the velocity values from the color bar, it can assign to each pixel inside the bowel wall an individual velocity value. All pixels are measured and the sum of all colored pixels' area and the mean of all color pixels' velocity values is calculated. This is repeated automatically from the beginning to the end of a heart cycle. The software recognizes automatically complete heart cycles. The mean values of all colored areas (A) from one or more complete heart cycles and of all velocities (v) are calculated and referred to the area of the entire region of interest (A_{ROI}) to calculate the perfusion intensity Q (see above). Besides this most important parameter of perfusion more than 50 others are displayed and may add to the perfusion measurement (for details see www.chameleon-software.de) (Chameleon-Software, 2009). The perfusion intensity is used as the parameter to describe blood flow inside the bowel wall and can be used to grade hyperperfusion in inflammatory disorders. The grade of hyperperfusion is a measure of actual inflammatory processes at the investigation site.

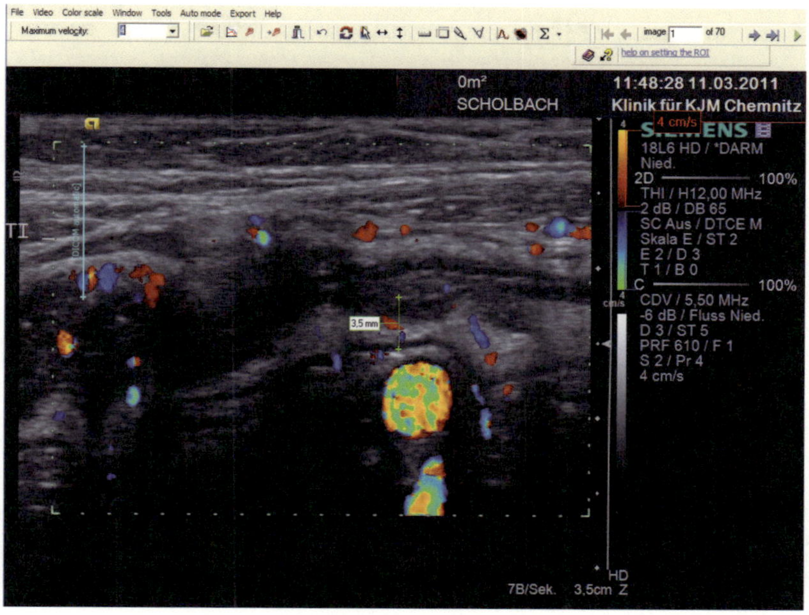

Fig. 1a. Color Doppler sonogram of the terminal ileum in a patient with Crohn disease

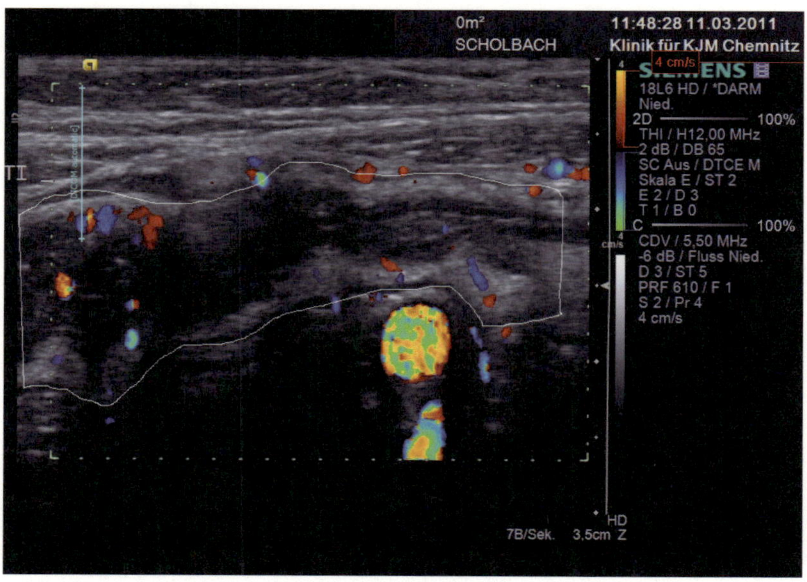

Fig. 1b. Freehand encirclement of the ROI. Posterior and anterior wall are included

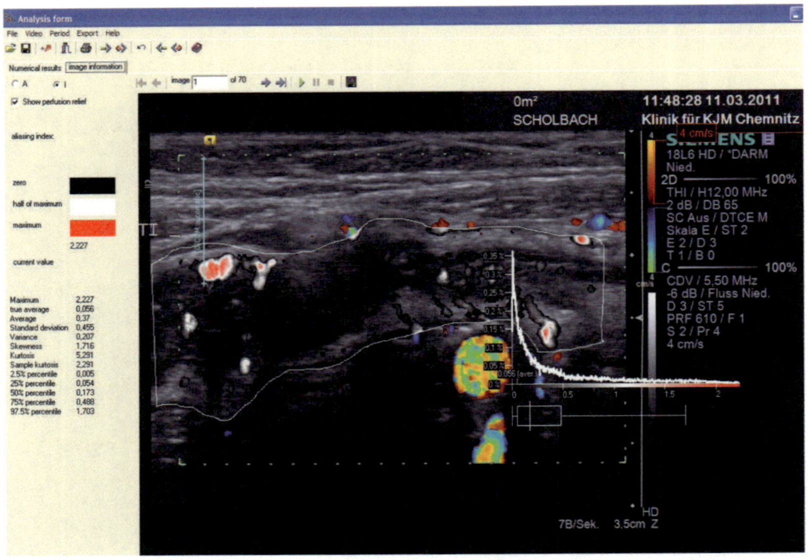

Fig. 1c. False color map of the terminal ileum in a patient with Crohn disease and diagram of the distribution of perfusion intensities with quartile boxplot (inset)

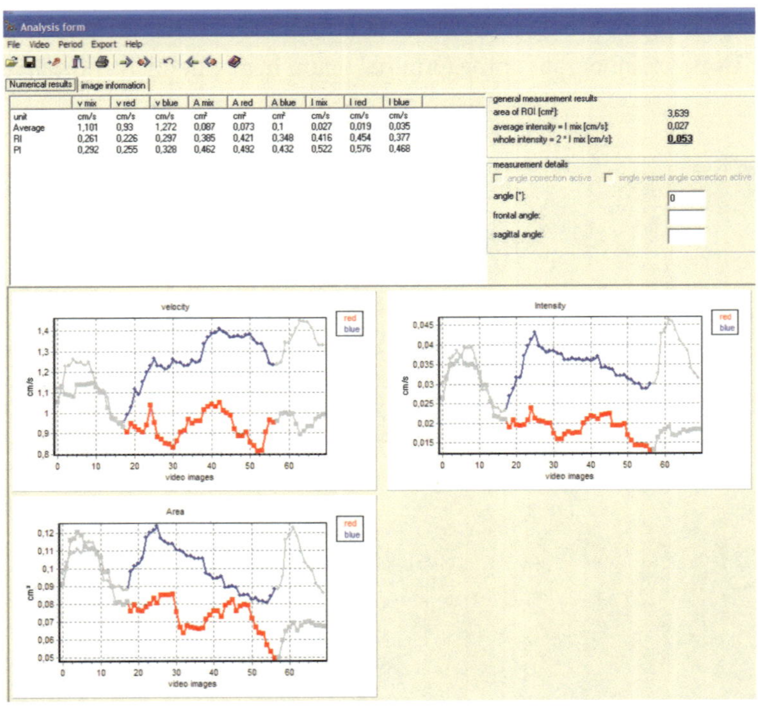

Fig. 1d. PixelFlux-output (abridged) indicating clue parameters as table and diagrams. The diagrams show the time course of flow velocities and perfused areas as well as the calculated perfusion intensities from the first to the last image of the respective video. Colored parts of the curves highlight the automatically recognized heart cycles.

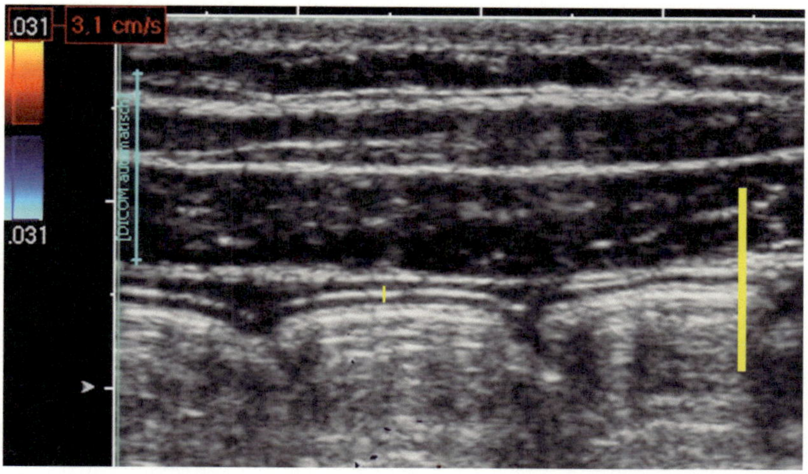

Normal colon wall. (thick bar: 1 cm; thin bar anterior wall with three clearly discernable layers)

Fig. 2a. Color Doppler image of the wall of the ascending colon in a healthy proband

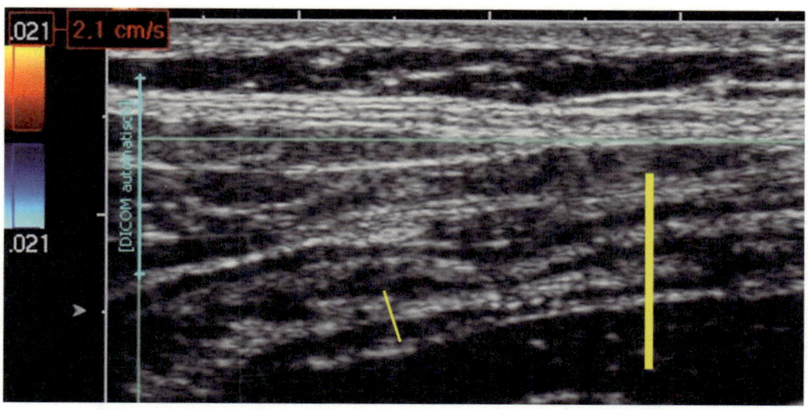

Normal wall of the terminal leum (thick bar: 1 cm; thin bar thickness of the posterior wall with three clearly discernable layers)

Fig. 2b. Color Doppler image of the wall of the erminal ileum in a healthy proband

2.7 Interpretation and normal values

Bowel wall perfusion intensity is low in healthy probands (tab.1, fig. 2a and 2b). Significant differences exist only between perfusion of the terminal ileum and some parts of the large bowel (tab. 2).

Bowel segment	N	Median of perfusion intensity [cm/s]	25. percentile [cm/s]	75. percentile [cm/s]	90. percentile [cm/s]	95. percentile [cm/s]
TI	13	0,008	0,002	0,015		
CA	18	0,007	0,001	0,009		
CT	11	0,004	0,001	0,007		
CD	15	0,003	0,001	0,007		
SI	18	0,003	0,002	0,006		
all	75	0,004	0,002	0,009	0,013	0,034

Table 1. Perfusion intensity in healthy probands

Bowel segment	TI	CA	CT	CD
CA	p=0,230			
CT	p=0,082	p=0,514		
CD	p=0,072	p=0,395	p=0,815	
SI	p=0,036	p=0,319	p=0,770	p=1,000

TI: terminal ileum
CA: ascending colon
CT: transverse colon
CD: descending colon
Table 2. Differences of perfusion intensities of different bowel segments in healthy probands (Mann-Whitney-U-test)

There are no overt differences of the bowel wall perfusion in fasting probands and probands examined without regard to the time interval to the last meal (fig 3).
The thickness of large and small bowel segments (terminal ileum) is significantly different in healthy probands (tab. 3 and 4) (Hormann, 2011):

Bowel segment	N	Median of bowel wall thickness [mm]	Maximum of bowel wall thickness [mm]
TI	13	1,9	2,1
CA	18	1,5	2,0
CT	11	1,5	1,8
CD	15	1,5	2,2
SI	18	1,4	2,1

Table 3. Bowel wall thickness of different segments in healthy adult probands

Bowel segment	TI	CA	CT	CD
CA	p=0,001			
CT	p < 0,001	p=0,412		
CD	p=0,008	p=0,817	p=0,357	
SI	p=0,003	p=0,650	p=0,877	p=0,556

Table 4. p-values of the two-tailed Mann-Whitney-U-test for differences of the bowel wall thickness of different segment in healthy adult probands

There is a weak inverse correlation (Spearman p=0,018, r=-0,535, n=19) of bowel wall perfusion intensity and the body mass index (BMI) (fig. 3)(Hormann, 2011).
In contrast to this no correlation was found between BMI and the bowel wall thickness (fig. 4).
In children similar results as in adults could be found (table 5 and 6) (Hormann, 2011).

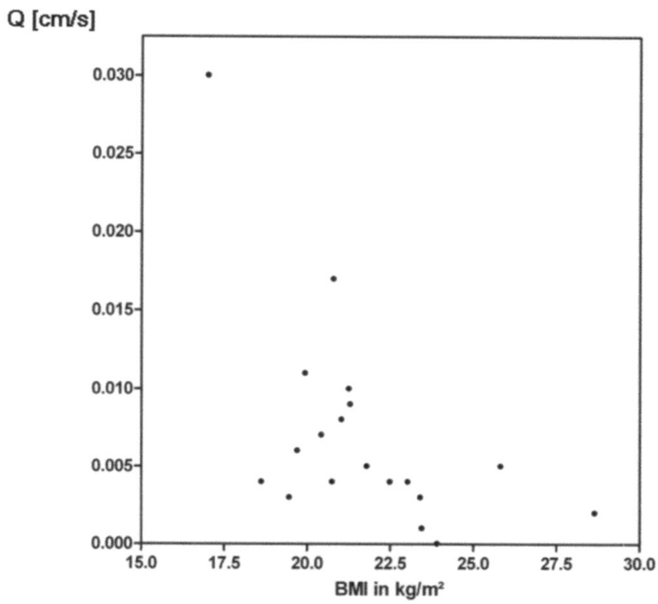

Fig. 3. Correlation between bowel wall perfusion and BMI

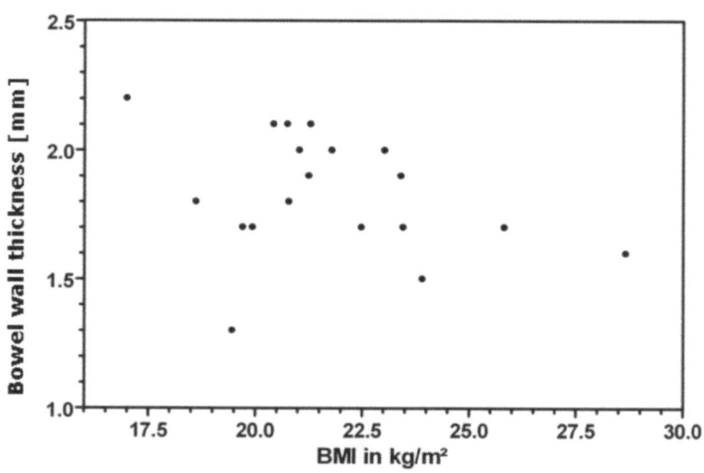

Fig. 4. Correlation of bowel wall thickness and BMI, n=19

Bowel segme nt	N	Median of perfusion intensity [cm/s]	25. percentile [cm/s]	75. percentile [cm/s]	90. percentile [cm/s]	95. percentile [cm/s]
TI	8	0,008	0,002	0,016		
CA	8	0,002	0	0,005		
CT	5	0,007	0	0,015		
CD	7	0,007	0,001	0,014		
SI	6	0,007	0,001	0,059		
all	34	0,007	0,001	0,014	0,028	0,071

Table 5. Median values and percentiles of bowel wall perfusion in healthy children in different bowel segments

Bowel segment	TI	CA	CT	CD
CA	p=0,130			
CT	p=0,524	p=0,621		
CD	p=0,694	p=0,281	p=0,755	
SI	p=0,852	p=0,181	p=0,537	p=0,731

Table 6. p-values of the two-tailed Mann-Whitney-U-test for differences of the bowel wall thickness of different segment in healthy children

Bowel segment	N	Median of bowel wall thickness [mm]	Maximum of bowel wall thickness [mm]
TI	8	1,9	2,6
CA	8	1,5	2,6
CT	5	1,5	2,5
CD	7	1,5	2,6
SI	6	1,4	2,8

Table 7. Bowel wall thickness of different segments in healthy children

Bowel segment	TI	CA	CT	CD
CA	p=0,232			
CT	p=0,524	p=0,755		
CD	p=0,382	p=0,955	p=0,833	
SI	p=0,181	p=0,836	p=0,537	p=0,950

Table 8. Differences of perfusion intensities of different bowel segments in healthy children (Mann-Whitney-U-test)

Between healthy adults and children no significant differences of the bowel wall perfusion could be demonstrated in comparison of all bowel segments (TI, CA, CT, CD, SI) (figure 5) and also no significant differences could be demonstrated in perfusion intensity (fig. 6) (Hormann, 2011).

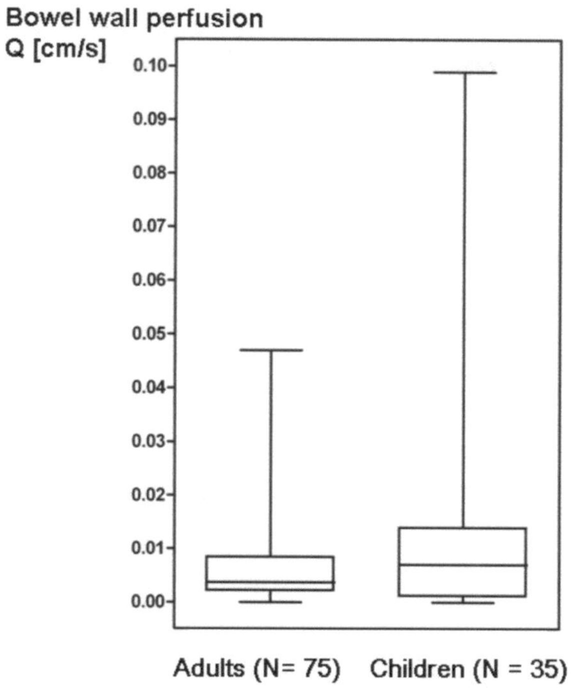

Fig. 5. Comparison of bowel wall perfusion between healthy adults and children - no significant differences (Mann-Whitney-U-test: p=0,783; N: number of bowel segements).

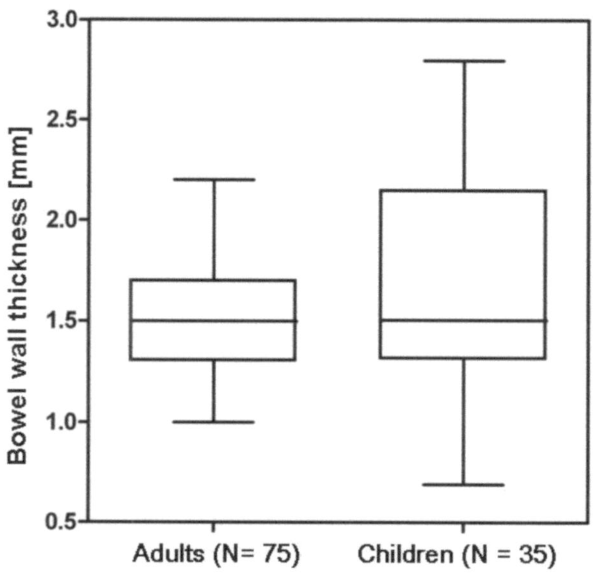

Fig. 6. Comparison of bowel wall thickness between healthy adults and children - no significant differences (Mann-Whitney-U-test: p=0, 680; N: number of bowel segements).

3. DTPM in gastroenterology

3.1 Chronic inflammatory bowel diseases (IBD)

IBD constitute a diagnostic and therapeutic challenge as their symptoms start creepingly and are unspecific. Their course is unpredictable and complicated by spontaneous recovery as well as unexpected outbreaks. The diagnostic gold standard today is the histology and endoscopic description. The threshold for endoscopy is high due to its invasiveness, need for preparation, discomfort and pain for the patient, often requiring general anesthesia, and costs. Non-invasive methods are therefore urgently wanted to make the diagnosis and to describe the natural course of IBD, their intestinal extent and the effects of treatment. Ideally complications should be also evaluated with noninvasive techniques. Imaging modalities hold the promise of being non-invasive (aside from the need of contrast media injection for CT, MRI or angiography or the necessity to infuse or drink enemas). Ultrasound combines the advantages of being noninvasive too while offering a spatial resolution which other techniques cannot achieve. Moreover this is combined with hemodynamic information displayed as color Doppler signals that give functional information and direct insight into the local inflammatory reaction which is from ancient times described as a process characterized by rubor, tumor, calor, dolor and functio laesa. All of them are reflected in color Doppler sonography as increased perfusion causing redness resp. increased coloration, heat resp. increased temperature by activated metabolism fueled by hyperperfusion, pain which can be traced by one finger palpation during the ultrasound investigation directly, swelling to be detected in B-mode ultrasound images and disturbed function which is reflected, among others, by stiffness of the thickened bowel wall and dampened peristalsis.
It is therefore a logical step to use color Doppler ultrasound to describe this inflammation. Unfortunately conventional approaches fall short compared to the inherent potential of the method. Perfusion estimates from changes of the Resistance index (Britton et al., 1998) in the superior mesenteric artery do not take into account the blood volumes passing through the intestines and do not elucidate the specific increase caused by a certain affected bowel segment. More precise insight is possible by direct evaluation of the affected intestinal segment. To quantify inflammatory hyperperfusion inside the bowel wall scores have been proposed which count vessels or perfused area inside a bowel wall segment in still images. DTPM expands these approaches. It does not only count vessels but measures each pixel's velocity value and area but refers these data to the area of the bowel wall and to full heart cycles. This way changes of these parameters which cause relevant spread of measurements in still images can be overcome and the error of measurement reduced which on the other hand is inevitable with the use of still images in describing a dynamic phenomenon as cyclic perfusion basically is.
The following section describe in detail the advantages of DTPM in Crohn disease and ulcerative colitis.

3.1.1 Crohn disease (CrD)

CrD is diagnosed in increasing frequency in the industrialized countries (Munkholm et al., 1993; Pozler et al., 2006; Shoda et al., 1996; Vind et al., 2006). Its main localization is the terminal ileum which is easily accessible with ultrasound. Other intestinal sites may be also affected. Even with small bowel affections others than the TI the diseased site can be retrieved by ultrasound since the inflammation causes prominent swelling and hyperperfusion which are readily found.

CrD is a transmural inflammation which typically causes a disruption of the clear borders between the intestinal layers which in healthy intestines can be clearly distinguished in all parts of the intestines (fig. 2a and 2b). This blurring of the inner wall structure may resolve and a thickened submucosal layer may point to chronic fibrotic changes. In acute stages prominent fat wrapping encapsulating the inflamed loops may be quite impressive. This mesenteric fat may host dilated vessels running in intervals to the inflamed segment to feed shorter pieces of the intestinal tube. Enlarged local lymph nodes accompany the inflammation but may be not differentiated in B-mode alone from resting but still enlarged ones. Here the use of color Doppler ultrasound is quite helpful or even necessary. As in the bowel wall in the surrounding structures perfusion intensity can be measured and thus compared to the bowel perfusion. Thus it is possible to discriminate different degrees of inflammation and to determine its focus. DTPM has proven to give valuable diagnostic and treatment-relevant information in patients with CrD (Scholbach et al., 2005b).
An example of CrD with transition from normal to inflamed bowel segments is given in figures 8a and 8b. B-Mode alone is suspicious for IBD but cannot tell resting from exacerbated disease. Color Doppler, in a standardized fashion of image acquisition, however, can show, that there is actually an inflammation going on. But to which degree this inflammation has already evolved cannot be deduced from such an image. To accomplish this, a semiquantiative method (Heyne et al., 2002; Rogoveanu et al., 2003; Ruess et al., 2000; Spalinger et al., 2000), contrast enhanced sonographic perfusion evaluation (Girlich et al., 2009; Ripolles et al., 2009) or even better, since not requiring invasive and costly procedures, DTPM is necessary. An example of its results is shown in fib. 8b. The red column refers to the perfusion intensity in the thin-walled segment, whereas the green one describes perfusion intensity on the neighboring segment. So it is very easy to compare different parts of the intestinal tract with respect to their actual involvement into an IBD. This holds true for the effects of treatment too. Figure 9 shows the differing impact of treatment onto various bowel segments highlighting where the disease is still active. This may aid the planning of future treatment modalities in selected cases. In this case the ascending colon responded much quicker and stronger than the descendent colon in a patient with CrD.

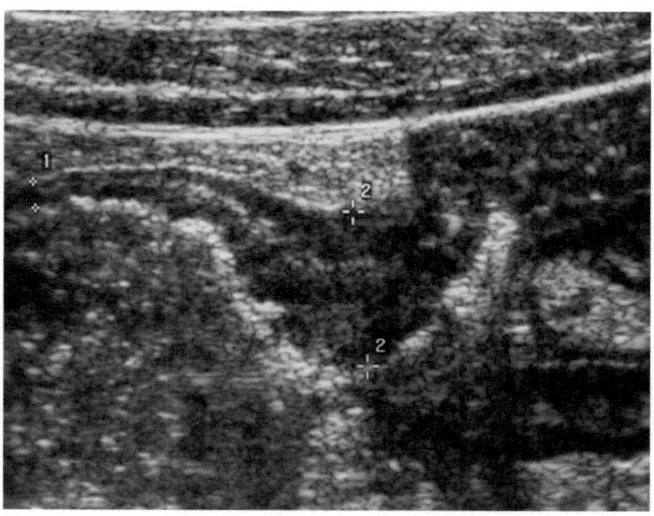

Fig. 8a. B-mode ultrasound image of the transition from normal to inflamed colon in CrD

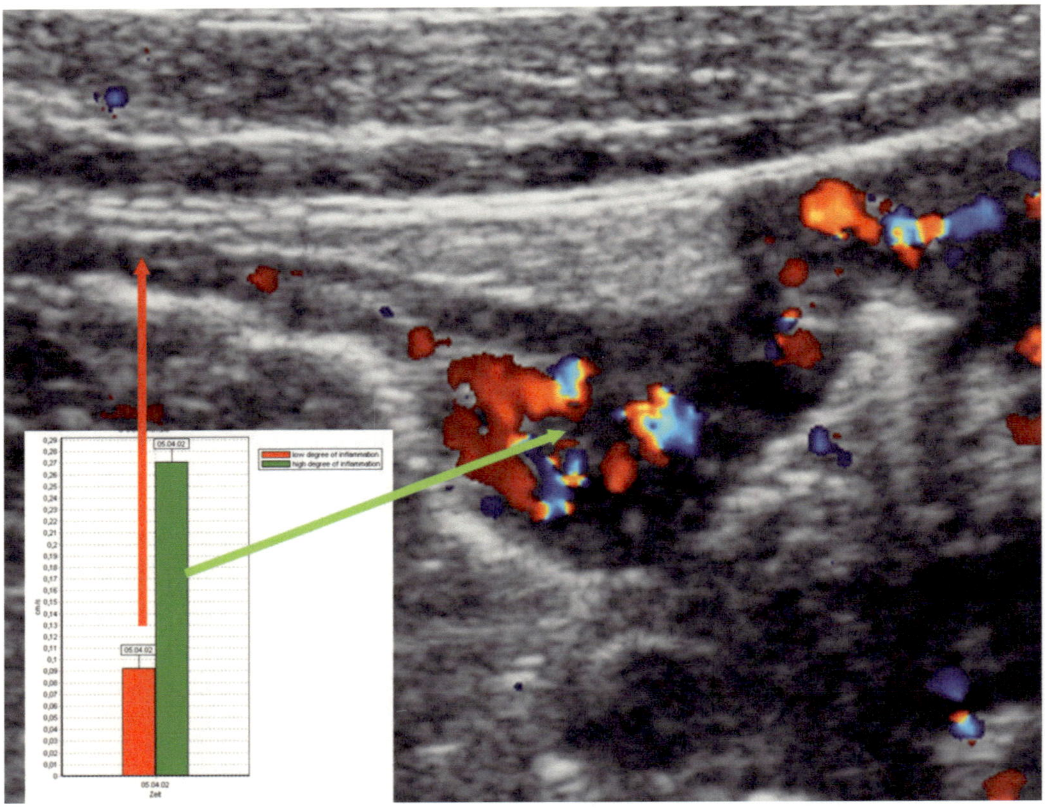

Fig. 8b. Same image as in fig. 8a in color Doppler mode. Inset showing the results of dynamic tissue perfusion measurement in both segments.

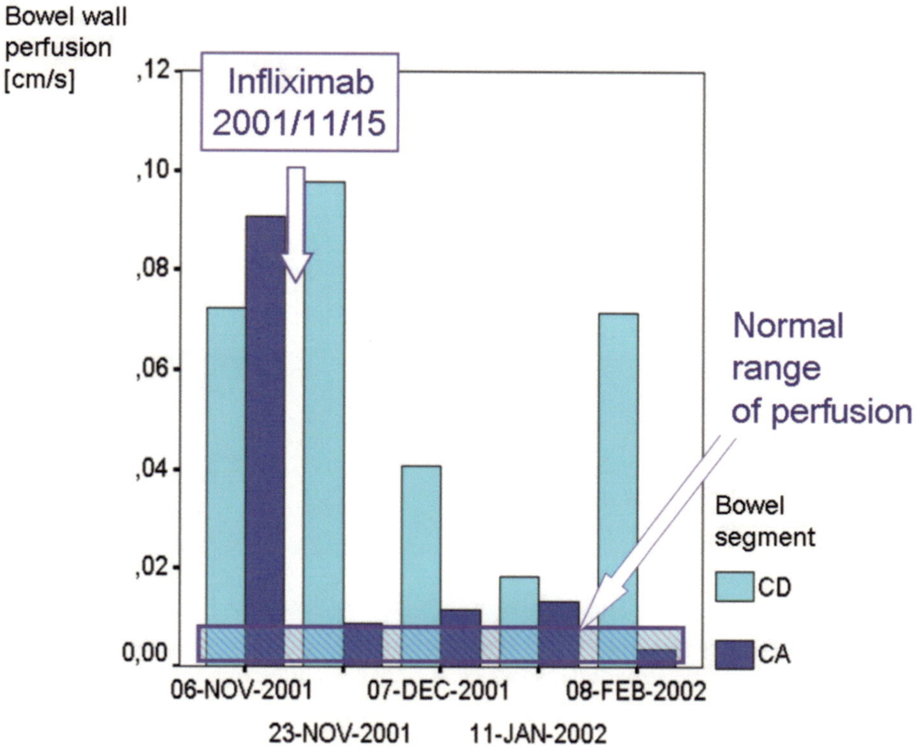

Fig. 9. Differing response of different bowel segments to Infliximab treatment. Descending colon (CD) responding later and less pronounced than ascending colon (CA). Normal range highlighted as semitransparent box.

Complications of CrD as fistulas can be described with great scrutiny. In figure 10a the cutaneous mouth of a fistula in CrD is shown and its closure is documented shortly after treatment with Infliximab. One might assume, that a profound suppression of the inflammation occurred. However, DTPM shows the details of fistula perfusion thus demonstrating, that there is a clear reduction of hyperperfusion but to a remaining value of 61% of the original one. The investigation of the intestinal opening of the fistula gives more information (fig. 10b). Here it becomes quite obvious, that further treatment is necessary to dampen the inflammation in order to prevent a new outbreak of the fistula. Repeated Infliximab infusions eventually led to a normalization of the initial hyperperfusion and resulted clinically in a permanent closure of the fistula. The terminal ileum, away from the fistula bearing colon, showed a different but substantial response too (fig. 10c).
Clinical assessment of disease activity might be difficult, especially in children. Often activity indices are sought to establish a basis to compare activity scores along with treatment and over time. These indices are a composition of clinical, anamnestical and laboratory data. They cannot describe the disease activity at its origin but are used when other tools cannot be applied (repeated endoscopies) or are lacking. DTPM can fill this gap. We found a weak but significant correlation of Children's Crohn Activity Index to bowel wall perfusion intensity measured with DTPM (fig. 11a). An individual example (fig. 11b) demonstrates that there may be a clear discrepancy between the locally measured disease activity and the pediatric CAI. Striking changes of local inflammatory hyperperfusion fail to

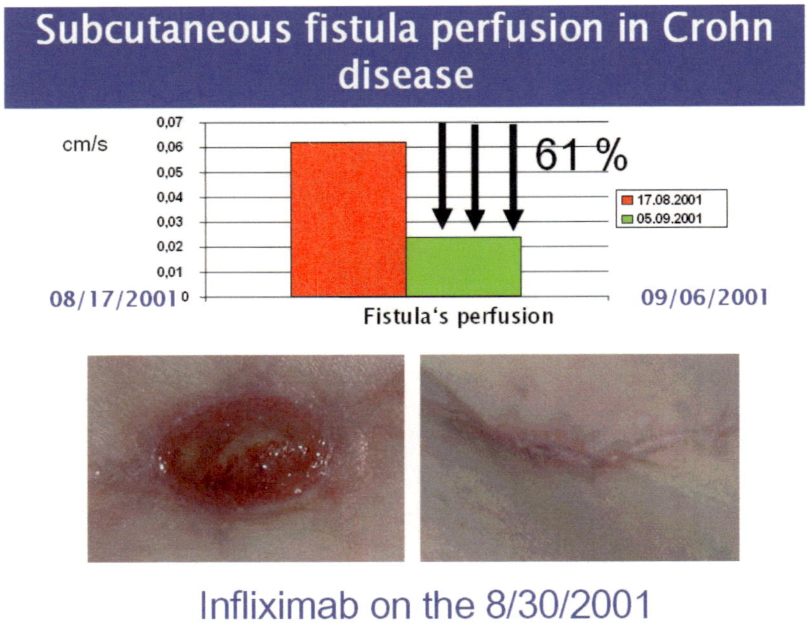

Fig. 10a. Enterocutaneous fistula in CrD evaluated clinically (below) and by means of DTPM (upper part). Infliximab treatment caused a closure of the cutaneous mouth and a reduction of fistula's hyperperfusion to 61%.

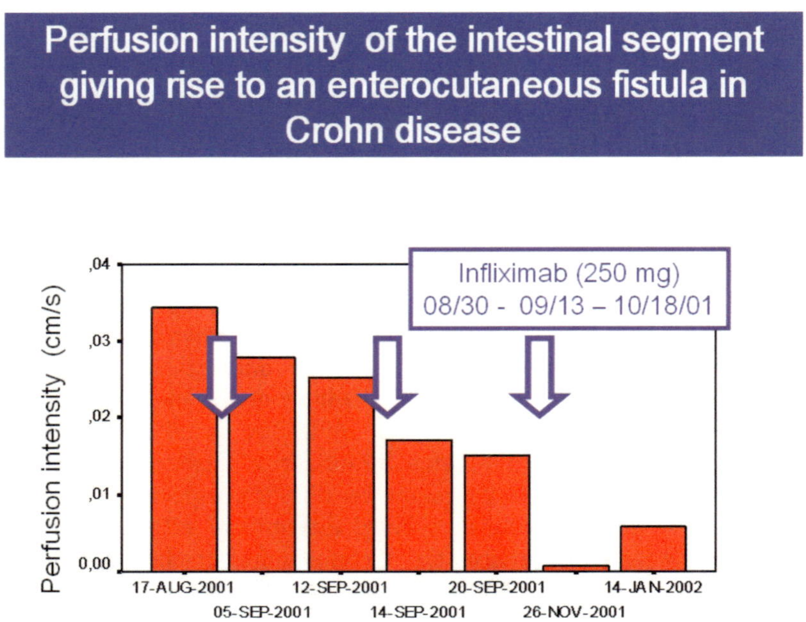

Fig. 10b. Same patient as in fig. 10a. Here DTPM of the colonic segment around the enteric opening of the fistula. In contrast to the proper fistula bowel perfusion drops less readily and signals the need of further treatments, which, after all, led to a normalization of perfusion.

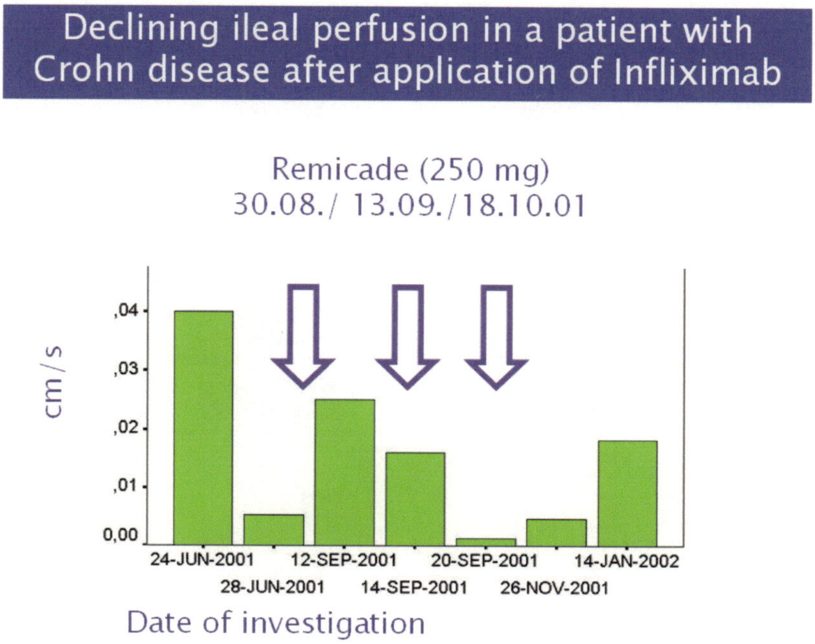

Fig. 10c. Same patient as in 10 a and 10b. The terminal ileum responds differently compared to fistula and colonic fistula origin.

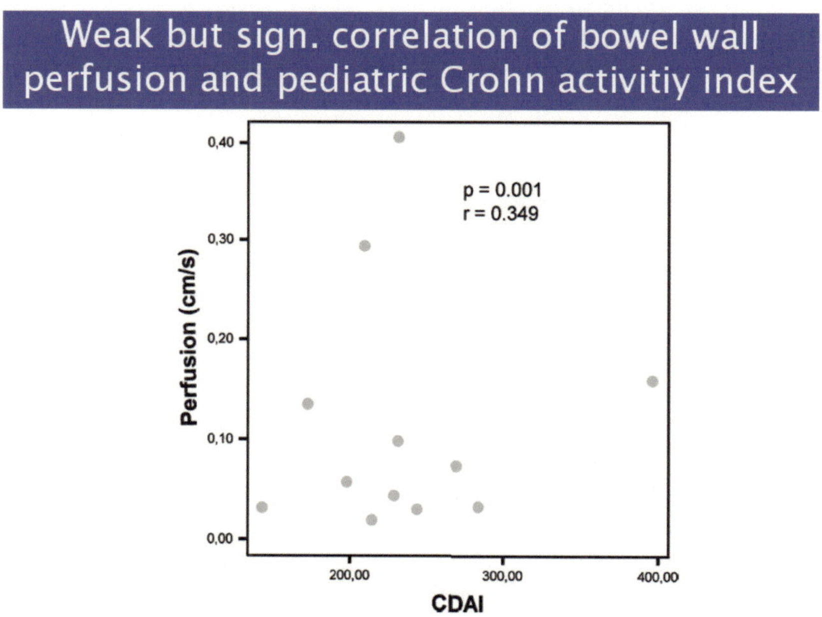

Fig. 11a. Weak but significant correlation of bowel wall perfusion intensity and pediatric Crohn activity index.

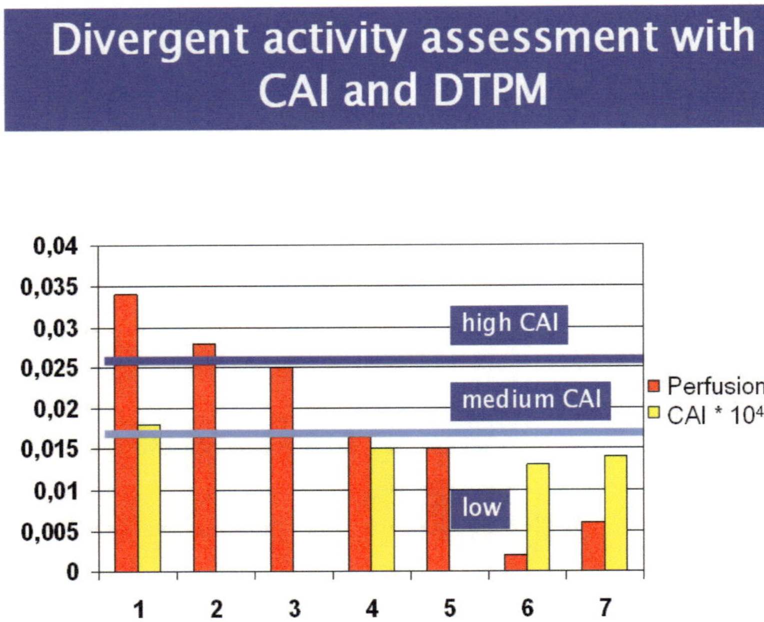

Fig. 11b. Obvious differences of inflammation evaluation in an individual with CrD by means of DTPM and pediatric Crohn activity index (CAI). Red columns: Perfusion intensity; yellow columns: CAI. Perfusion intensity follows the actual inflammation more closely than CAI leading to diverging assessment of disease activity.

be mirrored by an adequate fluctuation of the CAI. However, this is not surprising with regard to the different sources of information in both methods. DTPM measures local perfusion whereas the indices refer to indirect criteria only. Similar results were found by others comparing bowel wall thickening and biochemical indices of inflammation (Mayer et al., 2000)

3.1.2 Ulcerative colitis (UC)

As in CrD UC-incidence is increasing too (Jakobsen et al., 2008) but contradictory reports have been also published (Loftus et al., 2007; Molinie et al., 2004). In less industrialized regions similar incidences as in industrialized countries were found for both CD and UC (Sood et al., 2003). This stresses the need for a fast and reliable, cheap and non-invasive diagnostic tool for these conditions. DTPM, which meets these needs, can affirm the presence of colonic inflammation and describe its activity quite clearly.

We correlated several histological parameters (table 9) of UC with DTPM at the site of the biopsies in 19 patients with UC (Scholbach et al., 2010).

Patients with UC demonstrated a weak but significant correlation of their bowel wall perfusion intensity and wall thickness (fig. 7).

A synopsis of histological, endoscopic and color Doppler images underscores the advantage of a perfusion measurement (figure 12). It is helpful to describe the degree of inflammation numerically in order to substantiate the visual impression of imaging and the verbal description of findings. The columns demonstrate clearly how DTPM can tell severe from medium and low grade inflammation whereas the images themselves are important and impressive but cannot convey such precise information that would make them numerically

Score points	0	1	2	3
Changes of crypt architecture (Bentley et al., 2002)	none	minor	moderate	severe
Depletion of goblet cells(Guindi & Riddell, 2004; Hendrickson et al., 2002; Morson, 1971)	no	minor	moderate	severe
Paneth cells distal of the left colon flexure (Bentley et al., 2002)	none	few	some	many
Lymphocytes (Ajioka et al., 2005; Bentley et al., 2002; Eksteen et al., 2008)	normal concentration	minor increase	relevant increase	severe increase
Plasma cells (Bentley et al., 2002; Morson, 1971)	normal concentration	minor increase	relevant increase	severe increase
Eosinophils (Eksteen et al., 2008; Schmitz-Moormann & Himmelmann, 1988)	normal concentration	minor increase	relevant increase	severe increase
unspecific inflammatory infiltrates (Bentley et al., 2002)	none	minor	moderate	severe
PMNs in Lamina propria and Lamina epithelialis (Glickman et al., 2004; Reaves et al., 2005; Wang et al., 2004)	normal concentration	minor increase	relevant increase	severe increase
Crypt abscesses (Bentley et al., 2002; Glickman et al., 2004; Hendrickson et al., 2002; Morson, 1971)	none	few	some	many
Edema (Hendrickson et al., 2002)	none	minor	moderate	severe

Score points	0	1	2	3
Erosions or ulcerations (Bentley et al., 2002; Hendrickson et al., 2002)	none	erosion	large erosions	ulcera
regenerative epithelium (Lee, 1987; Morson, 1971)	none	scarce	relevant	
Fibrosis (Mitomi et al., 2005; Schmitz-Moormann & Himmelmann, 1988)	none	minor	moderate	severe
Increased cryptal distance to muscularis mucosae (Morson, 1971; Robert et al., 2004; Schmitz-Moormann & Himmelmann, 1988)	none	minor	moderate	severe

Table 9. Histological criteria compared with DTPM from the biopsy site

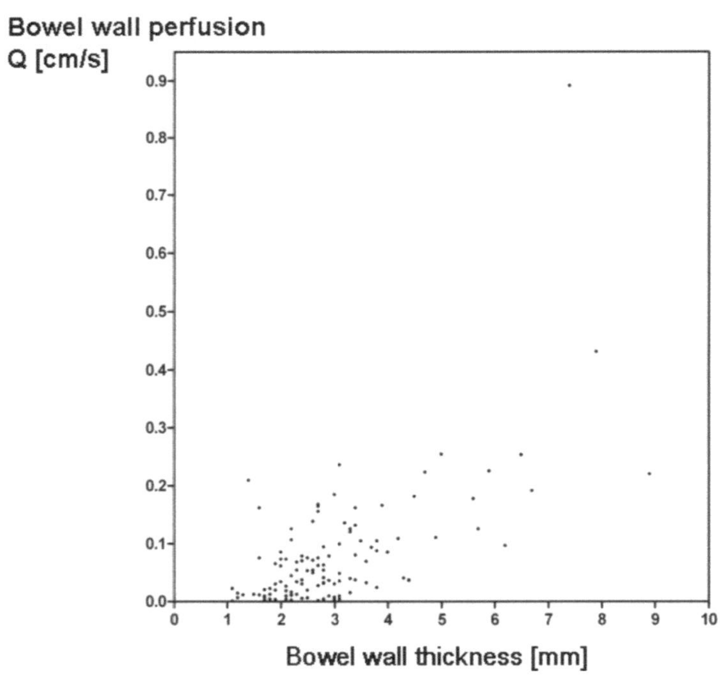

Fig. 7. Correlation of bowel wall perfusion and wall thickness in patients with ulcerative colitis (Spearman p<0,001, r=0,563)

comparable. With respect to the color Doppler images it must be stressed, that the information given by single images may be misleading since the image is taken from an undefined point of the heart cycle. The visual impression changes profoundly from systole to diastole. DTPM, in contrary evaluates all images of an entire heart cycle, thus ruling out this error.

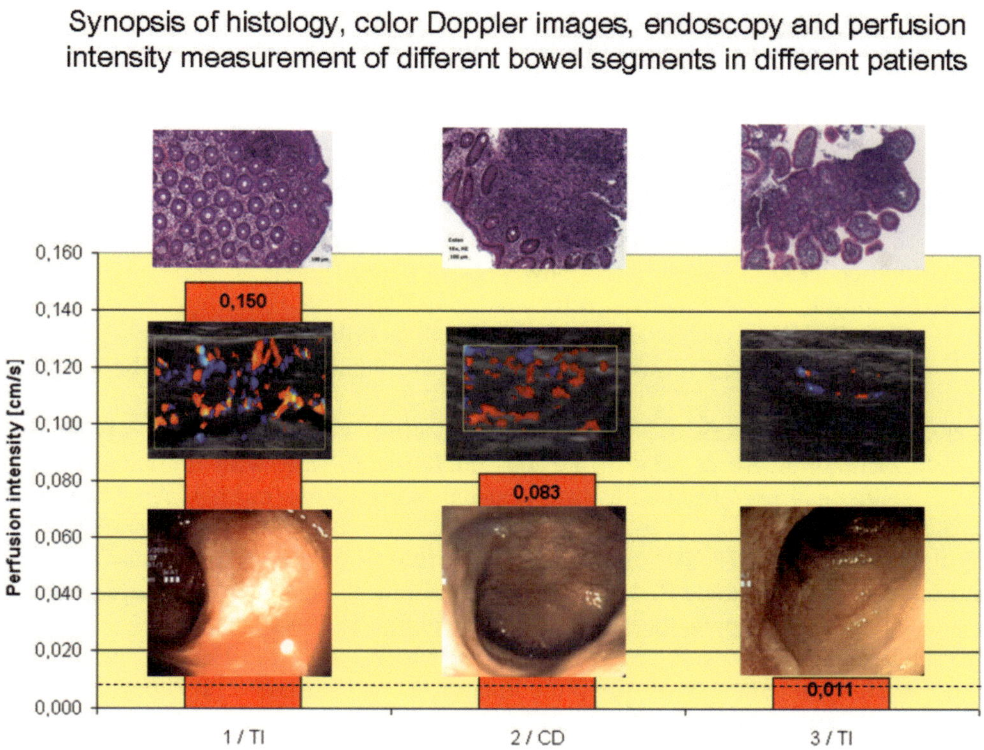

Fig. 12. Synopsis of histology (upper row), color Doppler images (central row), endoscopy (lower row), and perfusion intensity measurement (red columns) of different bowel segments (TI: terminal ileum, CD: descending colon) in different patients (1-3). Normal range limit indicated by dashed line.

4. Summary

In IBD, in CrD as well as in UC, a fast, convenient, inexpensive and reliable assessment of the intestinal inflammation is possible without preparation of the patient. DTPM allows a true comparison of measurement results in the course of the disease by the use of standardized imaging conditions, defined ultrasound presets and an objective software-based calculation of inflammatory hyperperfusion. Significant correlations could be demonstrated with established histological criteria. DTPM is thus an adjunct to colonoscopy quantifying inflammation with minimal effort. In some cases it may even replace a control endoscopy. In all cases it will add to the endoscopic findings what cannot be perceived from the luminal perspective: the reliable, since numerical description of the periintestinal structures and their perfusion as well as a refined description of the changes inside the submucosal layers of the intestinal wall.

5. References

Ajioka, Y., Nishikura K. & Watanabe G. 2005. [Pathomorphology of ulcerative colitis]. Nippon Rinsho 63:763-769.

Bentley, E., Jenkins D., Campbell F. & Warren B. 2002. How could pathologists improve the initial diagnosis of colitis? Evidence from an international workshop. J Clin Pathol 55:955-960.

Britton, I., Maguire C., Adams C., Russell R. I. & Leen E. 1998. Assessment of the role and reliability of sonographic post-prandial flow response in grading Crohn's disease activity. Clin Radiol 53:599-603.

Chameleon-Software. 2009. PixelFlux. www.chameleon-software.de

Eksteen, B., Liaskou E. & Adams D. H. 2008. Lymphocyte homing and its role in the pathogenesis of IBD. Inflamm Bowel Dis 14:1298-1312.

Girlich, C., Jung E. M., Iesalnieks I., Schreyer A. G., Zorger N., Strauch U. & Schacherer D. 2009. Quantitative assessment of bowel wall vascularisation in Crohn's disease with contrast-enhanced ultrasound and perfusion analysis. Clin Hemorheol Microcirc 43:141-148.

Glickman, J. N., Bousvaros A., Farraye F. A., Zholudev A., Friedman S., Wang H. H., Leichtner A. M. & Odze R. D. 2004. Pediatric patients with untreated ulcerative colitis may present initially with unusual morphologic findings. Am J Surg Pathol 28:190-197.

Guindi, M. & Riddell R. H. 2004. Indeterminate colitis. J Clin Pathol 57:1233-1244.

Hendrickson, B. A., Gokhale R. & Cho J. H. 2002. Clinical aspects and pathophysiology of inflammatory bowel disease. Clin Microbiol Rev 15:79-94.

Heyne, R., Rickes S., Bock P., Schreiber S., Wermke W. & Lochs H. 2002. Non-invasive evaluation of activity in inflammatory bowel disease by power Doppler sonography. Z Gastroenterol 40:171-175.

Hormann, J. 2011. Farbduplexsonografische Gewebeperfusionsmessung im Vergleich mit histologischen Untersuchungen der Darmwand bei pädiatrischen Patienten mit Colitis ulcerosa

Jakobsen, C., Wewer V., Urne F., Andersen J., Faerk J., Kramer I., Stagegaard B., Pilgaard B., Weile B. & Paerregaard A. 2008. Incidence of ulcerative colitis and Crohn's disease in Danish children: Still rising or levelling out? J Crohns Colitis 2:152-157.

Lee, R. G. 1987. Villous regeneration in ulcerative colitis. Arch Pathol Lab Med 111:276-278.

Loftus, C. G., Loftus E. V., Jr., Harmsen W. S., Zinsmeister A. R., Tremaine W. J., Melton L. J., 3rd & Sandborn W. J. 2007. Update on the incidence and prevalence of Crohn's disease and ulcerative colitis in Olmsted County, Minnesota, 1940-2000. Inflamm Bowel Dis 13:254-261.

Mayer, D., Reinshagen M., Mason R. A., Muche R., von Tirpitz C., Eckelt D., Adler G., Beckh K. & Kratzer W. 2000. Sonographic measurement of thickened bowel wall segments as a quantitative parameter for activity in inflammatory bowel disease. Z Gastroenterol 38:295-300.

Mitomi, H., Okayasu I., Bronner M. P., Kanazawa H., Nishiyama Y., Otani Y., Sada M., Tanabe S., Igarashi M., Katsumata T. & Saigenji K. 2005. Comparative histologic assessment of proctocolectomy specimens from Japanese and American patients with ulcerative colitis with or without dysplasia. Int J Surg Pathol 13:259-265.

Molinie, F., Gower-Rousseau C., Yzet T., Merle V., Grandbastien B., Marti R., Lerebours E., Dupas J. L., Colombel J. F., Salomez J. L. & Cortot A. 2004. Opposite evolution in incidence of Crohn's disease and ulcerative colitis in Northern France (1988-1999). Gut 53:843-848.

Morson, B. C. 1971. Pathology of ulcerative colitis. Proc R Soc Med 64:976-977.

Munkholm, P., Langholz E., Nielsen O. H., Kreiner S. & Binder V. 1993. [Increased incidence of Crohn disease in the county of Copenhagen]. Ugeskr Laeger 155:3199-3202.

Pozler, O., Maly J., Bonova O., Dedek P., Fruhauf P., Havlickova A., Janatova T., Jimramovsky F., Klimova L., Klusacek D., Kocourkova D., Kolek A., Kotalova R., Marx D., Nevoral J., Petro R., Petru O., Plasilova I., Seidl Z., Sekyrova I., Semendak N., Schreierova I., Stanek J., Sykora J., Sulakova A., Toukalkova L., Travnickova R., Volf V., Zahradnicek L. & Zeniskova I. 2006. Incidence of Crohn disease in the Czech Republic in the years 1990 to 2001 and assessment of pediatric population with inflammatory bowel disease. J Pediatr Gastroenterol Nutr 42:186-189.

Reaves, T. A., Chin A. C. & Parkos C. A. 2005. Neutrophil transepithelial migration: role of toll-like receptors in mucosal inflammation. Mem Inst Oswaldo Cruz 100 Suppl 1:191-198.

Ripolles, T., Martinez M. J., Paredes J. M., Blanc E., Flors L. & Delgado F. 2009. Crohn disease: correlation of findings at contrast-enhanced US with severity at endoscopy. Radiology 253:241-248.

Robert, M. E., Tang L., Hao L. M. & Reyes-Mugica M. 2004. Patterns of inflammation in mucosal biopsies of ulcerative colitis: perceived differences in pediatric populations are limited to children younger than 10 years. Am J Surg Pathol 28:183-189.

Rogoveanu, I., Saftoiu A., Cazacu S. & Ciurea T. 2003. Color Doppler transabdominal ultrasonography for the assessment of the patients with inflammatory bowel disease during treatment. Rom J Gastroenterol 12:277-281.

Rouviere, O., Curiel L., Chapelon J. Y., Bouvier R., Ecochard R., Gelet A. & Lyonnet D. 2004. Can color doppler predict the uniformity of HIFU-induced prostate tissue destruction? Prostate 60:289-297.

Ruess, L., Blask A. R., Bulas D. I., Mohan P., Bader A., Latimer J. S. & Kerzner B. 2000. Inflammatory bowel disease in children and young adults: correlation of sonographic and clinical parameters during treatment. AJR Am J Roentgenol 175:79-84.

Schmitz-Moormann, P. & Himmelmann G. W. 1988. Does quantitative histology of rectal biopsy improve the differential diagnosis of Crohn's disease and ulcerative colitis in adults? Pathol Res Pract 183:481-488.

Scholbach T, Scholbach J. & Stöppler M. 2011. unpublished results.

Scholbach, T., Dimos I. & Scholbach J. 2004. A new method of color Doppler perfusion measurement via dynamic sonographic signal quantification in renal parenchyma. Nephron Physiol 96:p99-104.

Scholbach, T., Girelli E. & Scholbach J. 2005a. Dynamic tissue perfusion measurement: a novel tool in follow-up of renal transplants. Transplantation 79:1711-1716.

Scholbach, T., Scholbach J., Krombach G. A., Gagel B., Maneschi P. & Di Martino E. 2005b. New method of dynamic color doppler signal quantification in metastatic lymph nodes compared to direct polarographic measurements of tissue oxygenation. Int J Cancer 114:957-962.

Scholbach, T., Girelli E. & Scholbach J. 2006. Tissue pulsatility index: a new parameter to evaluate renal transplant perfusion. Transplantation 81:751-755.

Scholbach, T., Hormann J. & J. S. 2010. Dynamic tissue perfusion measurement of the intestinal wall - correlation to histology in ulcerative colitis. . Journal of Medical Ultrasound 18:62-70.

Scholbach, T., Kobrle A. & Bergner N. 2011. unpublished results.

Scholbach, T. & Scholbach J. 2009. Can We Measure Renal Tissue Perfusion by Ultrasound? . Journal of Medical Ultrasound 17:9-16.

Shoda, R., Matsueda K., Yamato S. & Umeda N. 1996. Epidemiologic analysis of Crohn disease in Japan: increased dietary intake of n-6 polyunsaturated fatty acids and animal protein relates to the increased incidence of Crohn disease in Japan. Am J Clin Nutr 63:741-745.

Sood, A., Midha V., Sood N., Bhatia A. S. & Avasthi G. 2003. Incidence and prevalence of ulcerative colitis in Punjab, North India. Gut 52:1587-1590.

Spalinger, J., Patriquin H., Miron M. C., Marx G., Herzog D., Dubois J., Dubinsky M. & Seidman E. G. 2000. Doppler US in patients with crohn disease: vessel density in the diseased bowel reflects disease activity. Radiology 217:787-791.

Vind, I., Riis L., Jess T., Knudsen E., Pedersen N., Elkjaer M., Bak Andersen I., Wewer V., Norregaard P., Moesgaard F., Bendtsen F. & Munkholm P. 2006. Increasing incidences of inflammatory bowel disease and decreasing surgery rates in Copenhagen City and County, 2003-2005: a population-based study from the Danish Crohn colitis database. Am J Gastroenterol 101:1274-1282.

Wang, B., Saha P. K., Udupa J. K., Ferrante M. A., Baumgardner J., Roberts D. A. & Rizi R. R. 2004. 3D airway segmentation via hyperpolarized 3He gas MRI by using scale-based fuzzy connectedness. Comput Med Imaging Graph 28:77-86.

Wieczorek, A. P., Wozniak M. M., Stankiewicz A., Bogusiewicz M., Santoro G. A., Rechberger T. & Scholbach J. 2009. The assessment of normal female urethral vascularity with Color Doppler endovaginal ultrasonography:preliminary report. Pelviperineology 28:59-61

16

Towards Intelligent Systems for Colonoscopy

Jorge Bernal, Fernando Vilariño and Javier Sánchez
Computer Vision Center and Computer Science Department,
Universitat Autònoma de Barcelona
Spain

1. Introduction

Colorectal cancer is one of the leading causes of cancer related deaths. Colorectal cancer's survival rate depends on the stage in which it is detected, decreasing from rates higher than 95% in the first stages to rates lower than 35% in stages IV and V (Tresca, A. (2010)); hence the importance of detecting it on its early stages by using screening techniques, such as colonoscopy (Hassinger, J.P., Holubar, S.D. et al. (2010)), which is still considered the gold standard for the screening of patients for colon cancers and lesions. Classical focal colonoscopy has been proved to be a successful tool for colon screening, although other tools are being also used for this purpose, such as Virtual Colonoscopy, Computed Tomography Colonoscopy, Chromoendoscopy or Wireless Capsule Video Endoscopy, among others.

In this chapter we present tools that can be used to build intelligent systems for colonoscopy. The idea is, by using methods based on computer vision and artificial intelligence, add significant value to the colonoscopy procedure. Intelligent systems are being used to assist in other medical interventions. For instance, we can build systems that can be used to develop the knowledge bases used by expert systems, such as KARDIO (Bratko et al. (1990), which was developed to interpret electrocardiograms. Another example can consist of developing a system that, in the context of anesthesia, provides a robust/reliable control system that could determine the optimal infusion rate of the drugs (muscle relaxant, anesthetic, and analgesic) simultaneously, and titrate each drug in accordance to its effects and interactions. Such a system would be a valuable assistant to the anesthetist in the operating theater. An example of such a system can be found in the work of Nunes et al. (2005). More close to our topic of interest, colonoscopy, we can find many examples of intelligent systems build to assist in cancer detection. Such is the case of breast cancer detection (Wei et al. (2011)) or prostate cancer detection (Viswanath et al. (2011)).

The question that arises now is: how can intelligent systems help in colonoscopy? What kind of applications these systems can be built for? In Figure 1 we depict some of the potential areas related to colonoscopy where an intelligent system can play a key role.

As shown in Figure 1, we foresee four different areas where an intelligent system can be introduced and add significant value to the colonoscopy procedure:

1. The most manifest application of this kind of systems could be the **assistance in the diagnosis procedure** during the intervention or in post-intervention time. This could be very useful in order to reduce the miss rate associated to polyp identification.

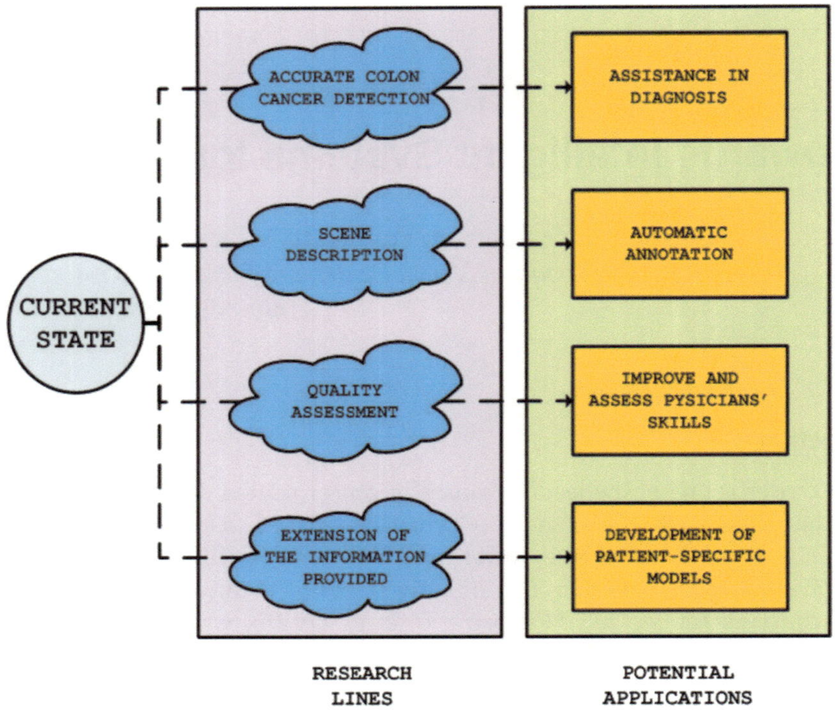

Fig. 1. Research lines and potential applications in the scope of intelligent systems for colonoscopy.

2. We can make use of the scene description provided by an automatic system -including the presence of salient traits, such as informative frames, anatomical structures, insertion or withdrawal phases, etc.- in order to **automatically annotate colonoscopy videos**. This would potentially provide a very efficient way of case annotation, with multiple uses in different applications.

3. In addition, an intelligent system may offer a quality assessment of the colonoscopy intervention, which could provide a non-subjective way of assessment. This could also be used as a way to train physicians in a way such they can **assess and improve their skills** without the cost associated to a real interventions, and it would allow to compare different performance metrics objectively.

4. We can also build intelligent systems that extend and provide additional information from colonoscopy data. Belonging to this area we can think of applications such as the **development of patient-specific models**, that can be re-used later, when a new study arrives, to check for coincidences that can help in the diagnosis and enrich in this way a final case report.

From the examples mentioned above, we can see that intelligent systems can indeed play a role in the future of colonoscopy. The objective of this chapter is to give an insight into this future, to expose what tools could be used to build an intelligent system for colonoscopy. In the next section we present the object of analysis in colonoscopy video by introducing the endoluminal scene. In Section 3 we deploy the different methods proposed to extract information from the endoluminal scene by explaining the techniques for image processing, the methods for scene description, the current proposals for polyp detection, the approaches pointed for quality assessment, and an insight into the potentiality of developing patient specific models. Next, we address the problem of the construction of databases of colonoscopy video and the acquisition of the ground truth. Finally, in Section 4 we fully develop our contribution with one example of a polyp segmentation algorithm.

2. Endoluminal scene

Before starting with the explanation of the several methods that can be used in building intelligent systems for colonoscopy, it is necessary to identify what is present on the endoluminal scene. This is compulsory because by knowing what we may find in images, we can develop methods that are devoted or attracted to the individual parts or objects of interest in the image.

As presented in Figure 2, the colonoscopy endoluminal scene shows the intestinal lumen, i.e., the inner region of the colon. The colon presents a tubular shape defined by the intestinal walls. Throughout a colonoscopy screening, the appearance of the intestinal walls varies in color and texture not only among different subjects but also among some of the different regions of the colon (ascending, transverse, descending and also sigmoid colon). Regardless of this intrinsic variability, the endoluminal scene consistently shows the lumen (1), the folds and wrinkles of the intestinal walls (2), the blood vessels (3), and eventually, diverticulosis

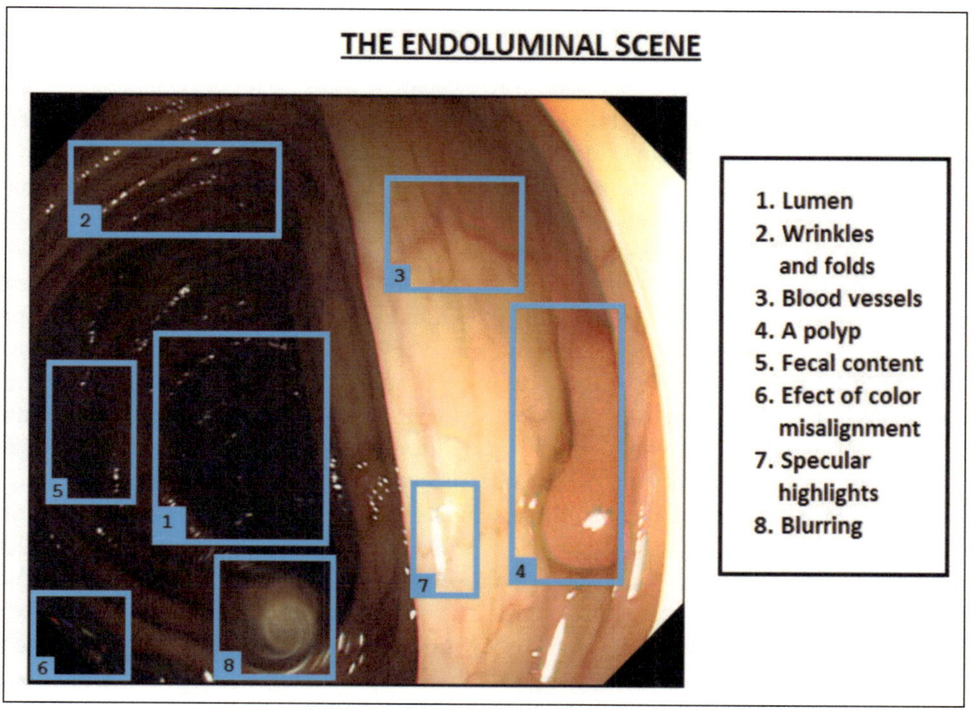

Fig. 2. Complete endoluminal scene: 1) Lumen, 2) wrinkles and folds, 3) blood vessels, 4) a polyp, 5) fecal content, 6) effect of the color misalignment, 7) specular highlights, and 8) blurring.

and lesions, such as ulcer, localized bleeding or polyps (4). Due to the flexible and extendible nature of the colon, and in part owed to the impact of the probe insertion or withdrawal in its deformation, it is difficult to find a perfect tubular appearance in the colon lumen because intestinal walls can be bent and folded. In addition, the wrinkles associated to the colon physiological structure appear in the scene as radial protuberances which modify the flat surface of the intestinal walls. On the intestinal walls, blood vessels are observed with their characteristic tree ramifications, presenting a certain variability associated to their width. Diverticulosis are shown as cavities or holes in the intestinal wall. The lesions related with bleeding are generally identified by its characteristic color. Polyps present a large variety in shapes, and seldom show a discriminative change in texture and/or color in comparison to the surrounding area. Despite a preparation is required for most of the colonoscopy interventions -with the aim of eliminating all fecal matter so that the physician conducting the colonoscopy can have a clear view- in many cases intestinal content is still present after the preparation procedure, and this intestinal content will hinder the right visualization of the intestinal walls. The procedure of elimination of the remaining fecal matter (5), consisting of the direct injection of water through the colonoscope in order to dilute the intestinal contents, turns out into the blurring of the video sequence and the appearance of bubbles. Finally, during the time of intervention, some tools used by the physician for different tasks -i.e., biopsy, cauterization, etc-. can be part of the visual scene.

In addition to the difficulties associated to the characterization of the colonoscopy scene due to its high variability and complexity, there are many visual artifacts the impact of which should be taken into account in order to tackle a robust system for the automatic analysis of colonoscopy video. The nature of these artifacts is twofold: 1) On the one hand, image acquisition systems are usually based on a tree-channel RGB image sensor which acquires each color component at a different time. In the event of motion, this delay on the acquisition time can yield to color phantoms (6) (Dahyot et al. (2008)). In addition to the former, and in order to optimize the dimensions of the image sensor and minimize its price, the video sequence is usually a composition of two interlaced fields (odd and even), corresponding to a compound of the RGB channels at different times. The result is an interlacing effect which is perceptually filtered by the observer during the video screening, but which is present at a frame level, carrying out the characteristic textured pattern of interlaced video. Finally, a different artifact, technically designated as specular highlights (7), is produced when the camera is frontally focusing a reflecting surface, the outcome of which is a white saturation in the image frame. 2) On the other hand, due to the limited bandwidth and frame rate of the video capture device, fast movements of the colonoscope can give away blurred images with diffused visual features (8). All these artifacts can have a potential impact into the automatic systems, and for this reason these artifacts should be addressed efficiently in order to guarantee an optimal performance.

Diverse endoscopy techniques, such as capsule endoscopy (both for small bowel and colon), bronchoscopy, gastroendoscopy, etc. show different endoluminal scenes, each of them with particular features. Besides, there is a variety of imaging methods to be used to enhance particular physiological targets, which is the case for narrow band imaging or chromoendoscopy, just to mention a few. This situation sets up a heterogeneous scenario from the perspective of automatic analysis using computer vision, and makes it not feasible to tackle the endoscopic image problem as a whole. However, it is possible to take some of the methods used in a given technique and adapt them to the specific particularities of colonoscopy video. For example, the automatic detection of intestinal content is a topic addressed in the bibliography of capsule endoscopy (as it can be seen in Vilariño (2006)) by means of the analysis of color distribution and texture, and its equivalent to the detection of intestinal content in colonoscopy would require relatively minor modifications. The identification of elliptical shapes in the image in order to detect potential polyps is a recurrent subject in virtual colonoscopy, and evolved versions of some of these techniques can be tried to colonoscopy video by adapting the search context, as we propose in Section 4.

3. Building up an intelligent system for colonoscopy

Once we know what can appear in the endoluminal scene, which is where we will extract all the information from, we present in this section several tools that can provide information from the image frames. Since the number of works that apply computer vision and artificial intelligence is large, we have grouped them into the four potential areas suggested in Section 1. As an introduction, we first analyze which are the preliminary steps that should be performed in colonoscopy video.

3.1 Image preprocessing

Image preprocessing is needed in order to eliminate or minimize the impact of image artifacts associated to colonoscopy video, which fundamentally consist of the color phantoms and the presence of specular highlights.

The problem of color phantoms associated to the temporal misalignment of the color channels has been addressed in the work of Dahyot et al. (2008). This happens because most colonoscopy devices use monochromes cameras, in which the RGB components are taken at different times. This causes a worsening in the quality of the images, as it can be seen in Figure 3 a,b), which may difficult posterior image analysis tasks. The method proposed involves both color channels equalization and the estimation and compensation of the camera motion. The experimental results that can be found in Dahyot et al. (2008) show a global improvement in the quality of the images, failing only in cases when the quality of the original image is very low, although the evaluation is done qualitatively.

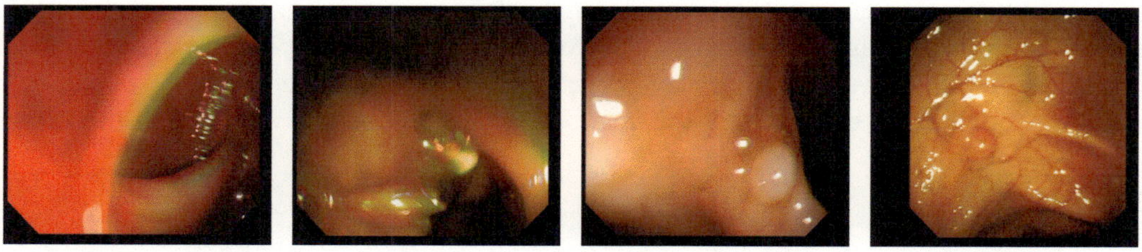

(a) (b) (c) (d)

Fig. 3. Examples of: (a-b) color channel misalignment (c-d) specular highlights.

Adding a solution to a different problem, the work of Arnold et al. (2011) presents a method to improve the quality of colonoscopy videos. More precisely, the authors offer a solution for two problems, the already mentioned color channel misalignment and the apparition of specular highlights. Specular highlights appear on the intestinal surface as an effect of frontal illumination, as can be seen in Figure 3 c,d). The issue of specular highlights is addressed using two methods: 1) segmentation based on nonlinear filtering and a posterior color image thresholding and 2) fast inpainting method. We have also faced the problem of correction of specular highlights, as it can be seen in Bernal, J. and Sánchez, J. and Vilariño, F. (2011). In our case our objective was to provide a fast method that replaces the specular highlights with an interpolative approximation of what could really be under them, based on the information that surrounds the specular highlights.

3.2 Scene description for automatic video annotation

The majority of the existing literature devoted to scene description in colonoscopy video can be grouped according to three different topics, namely: 1) segmentation of the lumen; 2) definition of non-informative frames, and 3) polyp detection. Taking into account the importance of the latter we will analyze the first two topics, and later on we will deploy the different approaches to polyp detection in a full subsection.

3.2.1 Lumen segmentation

The detection of the lumen and its position can be crucial, for example, in post-intervention video processing. Frames where the proportion of lumen out of all the image is large can be related to the progression of the colonoscope through the patient (Figure 4 a-b)). On the other hand, frames where the amount of lumen presence is low (Figure 4 c-d)) may potentially indicate areas of the image where the physician has paid more attention. In addition to that, an efficient lumen segmentation may lead to remove great part of the image for a further computational analysis.

Several works are centered on lumen detection, such as the work of Gunduz-Demir et al. (2010), which aims at decomposing the tissue image (where lumen may be present) into a set of primitive objects and segment glands making use of the organizational properties of these objects. In this approach, an image is first decomposed into its tissue components that, as they are difficult to locate, are approximately represented transforming the image into a set of circular objects (nucleus and lumen objects). Following a similar line of research, the work of Tian et al. (2001) presents an automatic segmentation algorithm for lumen region and boundary extraction from endoscopy images which uses an adaptative Iris filter applied to the Region of Interest (segmented by an adaptative progressive thresholding method).

The work of Zhang et al. (2010) presents an approach for lumen segmentation which uses the information that contrast agents provide. Following this trend, the work of Bevilacqua et al. (2009) addresses lumen segmentation by first estimating the centerline, which can be achieved by first removing the background and then extracting air regions with a threshold filter.

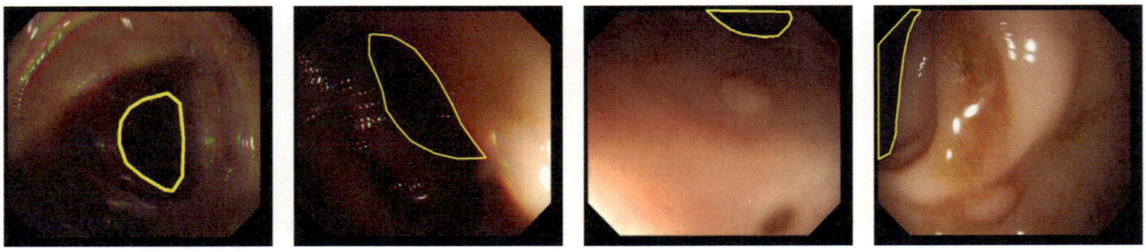

(a) (b) (c) (d)

Fig. 4. Examples of lumen (surrounded by a yellow boundary): a) and b) full view, c) and d) partial view.

Although used in CT and virtual colonoscopy respectively, the extension of these methods to focal colonoscopy may lead to more efficient lumen segmentation techniques due to their bidimensional nature.

3.2.2 Definition of non-informative frames

The content of the image itself can lead to the definition of informative and non-informative frames. In this domain of application, non-informative frames are those that, either their quality is so damaged (by the artifacts, hindering intestinal content, etc.) that it is difficult to extract information from them, or they are clinically uninteresting for a given task. For instance, frames where the instrumental take up great part of the image may not be relevant for polyp detection tasks. An accurate detection of the non-informative frames could also lead to a great reduction in the processing time of a stored colonoscopy intervention. Fundamentally, this information may be used for automatic video annotation and efficient video indexing and retrieval.

There are a few works that are centered on the **identification of non-informative frames**. The work of Arnold et al. (2009) addresses the identification of clinically uninteresting frames by analyzing the energy of the detail coefficients of the wavelet decomposition of a given image, which is used as the input to the classification system. In this case non-informative frames are those which do not carry any useful clinical information, such as those that occur when the camera is covered with liquids or when it is very close (even touching) the mucosa. These cases do occur frequently in colonoscopy procedures leading to extremely blurry images. This method is based on the 2D discrete wavelet transform which results in a set of approximation and detail coefficients. The approximation coefficients represent the low frequency content of the image while the detail coefficients hold the complementary high frequency information. The authors use detail coefficients to distinguish between informative and non-informative frames holding on the fact that the norm of the detail coefficients will be lower for low contrast images, making them more likely to be classified as non-informative.

The work of Cao et al. (2007) presents a method that extract those frames which correspond to a diagnostic or therapeutic operation, following work done in other domains (i.e., detecting important semantic units such as scenes and shots). This work takes profit of several characteristics that colonoscopy videos present, such as the presence of many blurred frames due to the frequent shifts of the camera position while it is moving along the colon. The identification of the operation shots is based on the detection of diagnostic or therapeutic instruments. In this case the authors map the problem of detecting instruments to the problem of detecting the cables of these instruments as they are present in the operation, regardless of their type. The architecture scheme shown in Figure 5 consists of five different steps which involve: 1) image preprocessing, to remove the effects of the specular highlights; 2) identification of the insertion direction of an instrument; 3) region filtering, where regions that are not part of the cable are removed; 4) region merging, which combines regions where parts of the instrument appears and 5) region matching, which matches the candidate regions in the image with the cable and without the cable.

Apart from the two methods presented related to the identification of non-informative frames, other approaches have been carried out such as the work of Oh et al. (2003) where a measure called the *isolated pixel ratio* (IPR) is used to classify the frames into informative, ambiguous and non-informative. The IPR measure is calculated from the edges of the image: an edge pixel that is not connected to any other edge pixel is defined as an isolated pixel. Those

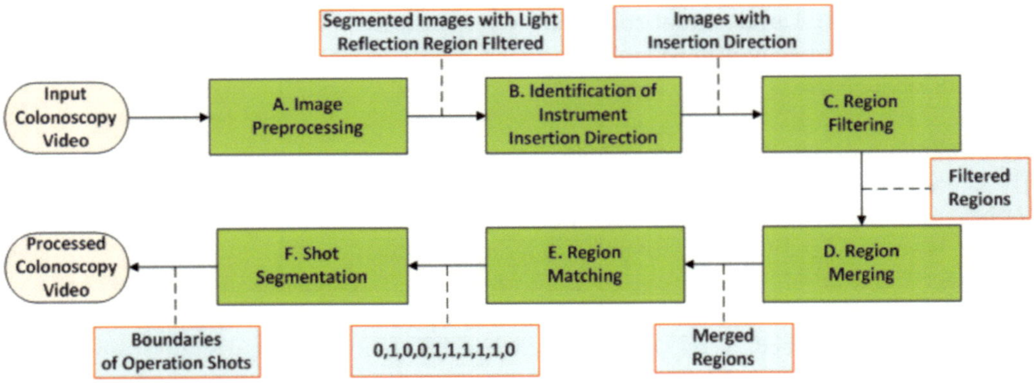

Fig. 5. A system architecture for operation shot detection as described in Cao et al. (2007).

isolated pixels are counted for each frame and are put in relation with the total number of edge pixels to obtain the IPR ratio.

Finally, an example of an endoscopic full multimedia information system for video annotation implementing many of these approaches is described in the work of Liu et al. (2007).

3.3 Automatic polyp detection

The main objective of the colonoscopy procedures is to check the status of the colon and to find possible lesions and cancer polyps on it. The general appearance of the polyps has been covered widely by medical bibliographic sources. However, there is a great variability in polyp appearance in colonoscopy videos, since there are some challenges that hinder polyp detection, namely: 1) the non-uniform appearance of polyps (see Figure 6 a-b); 2) their shape, flat or peduncular (Figure 6 c-d); 3) the effects of image acquisition, such as changes in pose, blurring, occlusions, specular highlights (Figure 6 e-g), and 4) the high similarity between the tissues inside and outside the polyp, which disables the possibility of relying only on texture or color cues (Figure 6 f), just to mention a few. The direct application of the methods presented in this section can be the potential assistance in the diagnosis, both during and in post-intervention time.

In the case of polyp detection, the great majority of the approaches is based on the analysis of features detected in the image. In the context of image processing, features can be defined as singular visual traits, associated to the visual primitives that constitute an object, such as edges, corners or lines, among others. The usual procedure is to use *feature detection* methods to locate the potential ROIs of the image and then describe them using one or many *feature descriptors*. After doing an extensive research on the different types of feature descriptors (Bernal, J. and Vilariño, F. and Sánchez, J. (2010)), we have divided them into four groups: shape, texture, color and motion.

Shape-based approaches

These approaches observe the structure of polyps as they appear in images and find the shapes which polyps commonly have. In general, polyps present two different shapes: flat or peduncular, as can be seen in Figure 6 a-b). What makes polyp detection by shape features difficult is that, in many times, we do not have a perfect shot of the polyp but an image where its pose, size and appearance can vary largely. Thus, many of the approaches presented try to

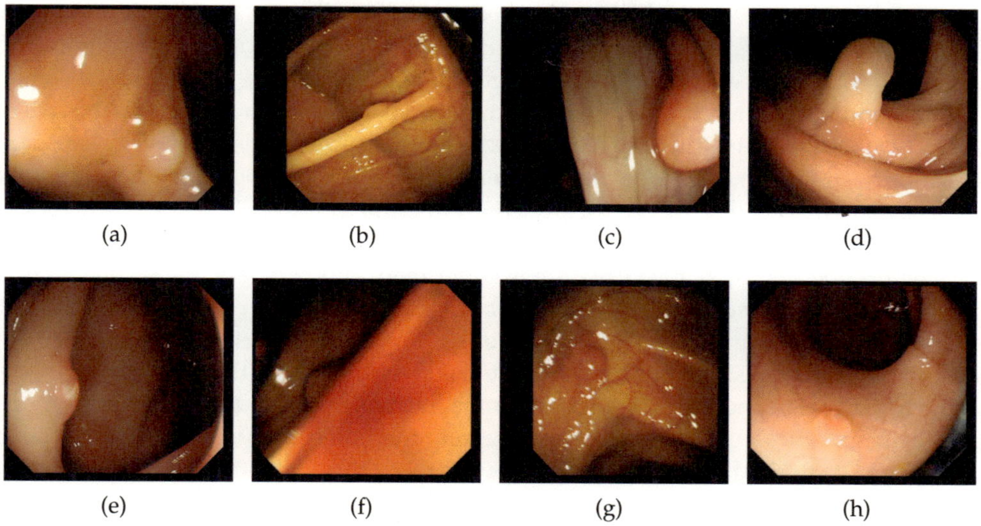

Fig. 6. Challenges in polyp detection: (a-d) non uniform appearance, e) partial (lateral) views, f) blurred images, g) specular highlights, and h) uniform texture and color inside and outside the polyp.

detect polyps not by detecting its whole shape but by detecting parts of the image that may indicate polyp presence.

For instance, flat polyps are meant to have elliptical shapes so one way to detect polyps is trying to find which structures in the image are surrounded by boundaries that constitute ellipses. The difficulty in this case is that in many occasions we do not have complete boundaries or the point of view makes it difficult to fit elliptical shapes (such is the case of lateral views). The works presented in this subsection could also be classified into two categories, namely: 1) detection by curvature analysis and 2) detection by ellipse fitting.

As it has been mentioned, **curvature analysis** is used to perform polyp detection. We can use curvature in different ways. For instance, we can check the curvature profile of the boundaries that appear in the image, that may have been detected by means of an edge detector. An example of the former can be consulted in the work of Krishnan et al. (1998), where the authors present an approach to polyp detection by means the extraction of contours. These contours are smoothed afterwards to make them suitable for curvature computation.

The work of Zhu et al. (2010) elaborates on the use of curvature-based shape measures (such as the shape index, curvedness or mean curvature) to analyze the local shapes in the colon wall. The problem in this case can appear in spurious calculations indicating high curvature, which is observed when the kernel contains two surfaces. Another problem that can appear is the discontinuities in curvature, which is shown when the gradient magnitude necessary to calculate the curvature vanishes. One possible solution to this is the redefinition of curvature as the magnitude of the change of the surface normal.

A different approach can be found in the work of van Wijk et al. (2010). The authors present a method that enables automated detection and segmentation of colorectal polyps, proposing a method that measures the amount of protrudedness of a candidate object in a scale adaptative fashion. The work uses the second principal curvature flow as a way to remove protruding elements from a curve in 2-D. We can suppose that the the points on the convex region of the polyp (the polyp head) are iteratively moved inwards, flattening the object. The convex region expands during the process and will ultimately include the polyp neck. After a certain amount of deformation, the surface flattening is such that the protrusion is completely removed, as if the object was never there. The idea here is to observe the second order differential properties of the implicit surface embedded. If we consider the colon as a long elongated structured tube, for a perfect perfect cylinder shape the principal curvatures are smaller than or equal to zero everywhere. However, the colon contains many folds, i.e., structures which are bended only in one direction: the first principal curvature is larger than zero, whereas, the second principal curvature is close to zero. Protruding objects, such as polyps, have positive values for the first and second principal curvature. Therefore, an operator is designed to affect only on points with a positive second principal curvature and in such a way that the second principal curvature decreases. The distinction between the head and neck is made by the sign of the second principal curvature. On the line connecting the inflection points, which in this case separate head to neck, the curvature is 0. It is clear that this method works well for images where we have clearly identified what is tissue and what is not so, in this case, the use of curvature measures can lead to good results in polyp detection.

The other category that collects many works is polyp detection by **ellipse fitting**. The general idea is, once we have a set of boundaries in the image, try to fit elliptical shapes in them. Belonging to this group we can observe in the work of Kang, J. and Doraiswami, R. (2003), which performs an edge detection in each of the R, G and B channels after applying a contrast enhancement algorithm. In order to classify the several regions (connected by closed edges) this method uses area, color and elliptical shape.

An approach that combines both curvature and ellipse fitting can be found in the work of Hwang, S. and Oh, J.H. and Tavanapong, W. et al. (2007). The method presented consists of fitting ellipses into the frontiers obtained after a first segmentation, and then classifying candidate regions by considering curvature, distance to edges and intensity value. Without entering into many details, in order to detect the ellipses an edge image is needed, where desirable edges should be grouped. Taking into account the challenges that colonoscopy images present, only some parts of the polyp boundary will have strong edge information so, based on this, the method uses the marker-controlled watershed (Vincent, L. , Soille, P. (1991)) algorithm for polyp segmentation because it can handle the gap between broken edges properly. Then, using the edges in each segmented region, the method generates an ellipse using an ellipse fitting method. Finally the number of final ellipses is reduced by removing those which do not represent actual polyps filtering by curve direction and curvature, by edge distance and by intensity value.

There are some works that cannot be assigned to an specific category because they use methods that appear in both curvature and ellipse-fitting categories. For instance, the work of Dhandra et al. (2006) also starts with a watershed segmentation but it performs its detection scheme by using color information. As it will be presented later for the case of texture descriptors, in the work of Coimbra & Cunha (2006), MPEG-7 descriptors are used in polyp detection tasks. In the field of shape descriptors, *region-based shape descriptor* is presented. RBS descriptor belongs to the broad class of shape-analysis techniques based on moments. A set of separable angular radial transformation (ART) basis functions is defined that classifies shape along various angular and radial directions. The RBS descriptor obtains 35 coefficients from the ART transform.

Finally, the work of Krishnan, S.M. and Goh, P.M.Y. (1997) is devoted to describe polyp appearance. Several parameters are evaluated, such as the response in the red channel of the image (which may indicate the presence of malignant tumors), the perimeter, the enclosed boundary area or the the *form factor*, which can give indication of possible presence of abnormalities in the colon (the more irregular the shape of the lumen, the smaller the value of the *form factor*).
Our work (Bernal, J. and Sánchez, J. and Vilariño, F. (2011)) cannot be easily assigned to a single group too, because it also starts with a basic segmentation but in this case it is based on the definition of a model of polyp appearance. This model defines a polyp as a region enclosed by intensity valleys. While we will explain it in more depth in Section 4, our results show that our model is a valid starting point that can be used in polyp detection, applicable for most types of polyp appearance.
Texture-based approaches
The use of texture descriptors on polyp detection has been gaining interest during last years. There is a number of works that are based on the use of **wavelet descriptors**. In this case the wavelet transform is calculated for each frame and the attention is put on the detail and approximation coefficients.
The work of Li et al. (2005) takes into account that, when detecting abnormalities in colonoscopic images, the location, shape and size of the abnormal regions in the image are unknown and vary across images therefore it is difficult to determine the appropriate patch-size to use for searching. In this case the solution is to use multi-size patches and ensemble them in order to achieve good performance. The features extracted from these patches are taken from both approximating and detail coefficients from wavelet decomposition of the image patches in the three channels of the CIE-Lab color space.
Also in the context of texture-based approaches we can observe the works of Karkanis et al. (2003). In these works the first operation that is done to the image is wavelet transformation, which is combined with other texture descriptors, such as co-ocurrence matrices or local binary patterns. The same group of researchers developed of a tool to detect colorectal lesions in endoscopic frame, which was named CoLD (colorectal lesions detector, Maroulis et al. (2003)). This tool provides a graphical user interface so both novice and experts user can take advantage of its use. In this case wavelets' information is used to discriminate amongst regions of normal and abnormal tissue.
There are some other texture descriptors that have been used to develop polyp detection method, such as the already mentioned local binary patterns or co-ocurrence matrices. The work of Ameling et al. (2009) combine both of them, with the novel use of local binary patters in opponent color space. As the authors state, texture can be seen as a local property and therefore, each image is divided into small image patches and four different methods were implemented, which combine co-ocurrence matrices (using different statistical measures such as energy, homogeneity or entropy) and local binary patterns. The analysis of the performance results points out that the inclusion of color characteristics (in this case, in local binary patterns) gives better results so color should be considered as an important feature for polyp detection.
As in the case of shape-based approaches, MPEG-7 also offers texture descriptors that can be used to build polyp detection methods. In the work of Coimbra & Cunha (2006), although applied to a different type of endoscopic process, several texture and color descriptors are presented. In the sub-field of color descriptors, methods such as *dominant color*, *scalable color*

or *color structure* are presented (see Bernal, J. and Vilariño, F. and Sánchez, J. (2010) for a further explanation of them). Related to texture descriptors, *homogeneous texture* and *local edge histogram* are introduced. These methods are evaluated in a big database and, in order to quantify the performance of each descriptor, several measures were used such as descriptor's redundancy or the variation of the descriptors' value. The experimental results show the superiority of *scalable color* over other color descriptors due to its higher resolution. On the other hand we have the apparently strong *local edge histogram* that performs worse than other simpler approaches, such as *homogeneous texture*, since it pays too much attention to the small texture variations in the image.

Not all the texture-based methods are built on the use of a certain descriptor. The work of Tjoa et al. (Tjoa et al. (2002) and Tjoa & Krishnan (2003)) introduces the concept of texture unit (TU) and texture unit number (NTU). Texture units characterize the local texture information for a given pixel and its neighborhood, and the statistics of all the texture units over the whole image reveal the global texture aspects. Without entering into details, each pixel value is compared with the value of the pixels in its neighborhood and then the value for this pixel in the TU matrix is assigned according to the comparison. The texture information is presented in the texture spectrum histogram, which is obtained as the frequency distribution of all the texture units. Six statistical measures are used to extract new features from each texture spectrum, which include energy, mean, standard deviation, skew, kurtosis and entropy.

3.4 Quality assessment

Currently, there are several metrics for the assessment of the quality of the colonoscopy intervention, such as the insertion time and withdrawal time. For instance, current ASGE (American Society for Gastrointestinal Endoscopy) and ACG (American College of Gastroenterology) guidelines suggest that, on average, withdrawal time should last a minimum of 6 minutes. Other works propose the use of additional metrics that include the quality of preparation, among others (Morán et al. (2009)). In the case of Europe, a very good work on quality assessment in colonoscopic interventions can be found in the work of Segnan et al. (2011), which defines from how to prepare conveniently the patient to an intervention to a classification of the polyps that can be found. These metrics can be potentially used into training programs for physicians, in order to assess their skills.

3.4.1 Obtention of metrics from colonoscopy videos

Unfortunately, there is not a lot of information about what metrics could be extracted from a colonoscopy video in terms of computer vision analysis. One interesting approach can be found in the work of Hwang et al. (2005), which was extended in Oh et al. (2009). These works presents a method to measure automatically the quality metrics for colonoscopy videos, based on analysis of a digitized video file created during colonoscopy and produces information regarding insertion time or withdrawal time. The process to calculate these metrics involve some results that have been already presented in previous subsections, such as: 1) detection of non-informative frames; 2) estimation of the camera motions, performed to find a boundary between insertion and withdrawal phases; 3) segmentation of the colonoscopy video based on camera motions (proximal and distal direction), with the objective of finding the end of insertion phase (cecum); 4) lumen identification, performed to decided if an informative frame contains the colon lumen or not and 5) computation of seven metrics: insertion time, withdrawal time, clear withdrawal time and ratio, number and ratio of camera motion changes and clear operation-free withdrawal time. The authors have considered a combination of the metrics in a single quality score but the idea has been abandoned due the fact that several components affect the final quality of a colonoscopy, some patient-related (such as the preparation of the colon), some equipment-related (quality, color or contrast of the image) and some endoscopist-related.

3.4.2 Applications for training

Intelligent systems can be used to provide information oriented to build up training systems for the physicians to improve and test their skills. The work ofVilariño et al. (2009) proposes the evaluation of the skills of the trainees, and their evolution during learning processes, by using eye-tracking methodologies as a tool for the assessment of abilities such as active visual search and reaction time to the presence of polyps, among others. This study presents a novel method which compares visual search patterns between the skilled specialists and the trainees. This is done by tracking the eye position of two groups of physicians (experts and novices) while they are shown a set of colonoscopy videos. Several measures were computed by analyzing the eye-tracker results, such as eye movement speed or number of fixations. The obtained results show that colonoscopy experts and novices show a different behavior in their visual search patterns, and therefore the proposed eye-tracking based procedure can provide automatic and objective measures for their evaluation. A method similar to the one presented in Vilariño et al. (2009) can be potentially used both for assessment of the skills of the trainees during their learning process or to assess the quality of the whole procedure in intervention time. In addition, the inclusion of the models of appearance and the item categorization from the tools for scene description can provide an objective ground-truth against which to check the abilities of the trainee. This can potentially be implemented by analyzing the extent to which the trainee identifies the regions of interest.

The link between the attention models that guide the physicians visual search and the visual descriptors which discriminate between the regions of interest is an open and most paramount line of work, that can help in a twofold way: On the one hand, by providing essential information for the deepening in the understanding of the processes associated to the target abilities in colonoscopy (such as the active search of polyps or the accurate navigation throughout the colon), and on the other hand, by allowing the simulation of these processes in computer models that can be potentially used for assessment.

3.5 Development of patient-specific models

Approaches identified in the previous sections deploy the state-of-art about a novel conception regarding the role that computer-assisted technologies may potentially play in the discipline of colonoscopy. These contributions aim at increasing the quality of the intervention by adding in complementary information which is not currently at the reach of the hand of the physician. Since the described methods allow the detection, segmentation and characterization of anatomical structures, lesions and physiological behavior, there is a manifest potential to use these strategies in order to endow current techniques with architectures ready to work with patient-specific models. The patient-specific approach has been one of the main trends in clinical research lately and it has been one of the pillars of the research funding schemes for Information and Communication Technologies related to health care in Europe during the last Framework Programs (ICT Programme Commitee (2011)). The patient-specific orientation focuses on the adaptation of existing methodologies so that they can take profit of the particular information, traits, clinical details or characteristics associated to each patient. Thus, the patient-specific viewpoint aims at the focalization of the (general) outcomes provided by each technique onto the (particular) specificities of each case. The extent to which this perspective can be exploited by using intelligent systems in colonoscopy is an open field of work. Here, we expose only as a matter of example a tentative list of a few prospective ideas:

- On the one hand, the use of feature detection in colonoscopy video could provide a way to the characterization of the inner walls of the colon, based on the identification of unique traits. This could be used for the tagging or annotation of physiological features as markers, and apply this information in a further step for the identification of the exact place of the situation of region close to a polyp.
- A system storing the visual traits of the colon from a given patient could make use this information in order to find those very specific locations when a new colonoscopy intervention is performed on that patient. This could provide a method for a precise spatial localization of regions of interest. The straightforward application of this potential implementation would be oriented to the registration and study of evolution of lesions in time (or whatever other item of interest) in the sequential routine interventions carried out on a particular patient, by automatically providing the specialist with a measure of certainty about the location of those lesions.
- The generalization of this methodology could be addressed towards the definition of a patient-specific atlas of the colon, in a way in which the specialist could have track of landmark positions in intervention time. This perspective presents a scenario in which the specialist is endowed with a road map for the navigation in intervention time, allowing the specialist to address specific targets with high reliance, reduced time and a potential shrinking of the miss rates.

Finally, and since the former ideas can be intrinsically implemented at the intra- and inter-patient levels, one of the major challenges for a patient-specific approach consists of the efficient definition of the video database, together with a solid ground truth against which obtaining qualitative and quantitative performance assessments of the different methods. The next section deals with the headlines related to the building-up of such databases.

3.6 Ground-truth and database building

In order to carry out an objective assessment of a given method or system, a ground-truth must exist. The ground truth consists of set of samples from a given number of case studies, with the corresponding annotations provided by an expert or group of experts. In our context, a video annotation can be of different natures, among which we can highlight, only to mention a few: 1) a whole frame, indicating that it is that frame which contains a particular event -e.g., the first image in a sequence showing a polyp-; 2) a given region of interest (ROI) -e.g., indicating the bounding box surrounding the polyp itself-; 3) any textual information -e.g., a qualitative assessment of the clinical relevance of a polyp-, etc. These annotations are used to check the performance of a new expert or a new method against the results provided by the annotator, who is considered the reference. In the ideal case, the annotation procedure should be repeated by each expert, in order to get a intra-observer variability measure, and by different experts, in order to get a inter-observer variability measure. A good database with

a solid ground-truth is an invaluable resource and a key point for the objective assessment of different methods under a common context of evaluation.
Unfortunately, databases of annotated colonoscopy videos are scarce, and even the access to small databases is very restricted (few examples can be found at National Cancer Institute (2011)). The reason of this (without taking into account the natural motivations related to ethical and administrative issues) has to do with the generalized fact that colonoscopy video interventions are not routinely saved, since no a-posteriori analysis is needed after the intervention. In many cases, the only image saved consist of a single picture of the ileo-cecal valve, which serves as a prove of the its achievement during the phase of introduction and indicates the start of the withdrawal phase (Malik (2010)). In the computer vision bibliography, some authors proposed pilot approaches that were validated in a few frames, with no significant inference for the case of a large video. In other cases, when the number of cases was higher, the database used for the results was not available. We provide our own test set of annotated videos with polyp sequences, which is accessible to the interested researchers by direct email petition to the authors. This dataset will be described in Section 4.

3.6.1 Building up of a database

The building-up of a colonoscopy database consists of two different parts, namely: 1) The video acquisition system, and 2) the video annotation procedure. The video acquisition system must be able to grab HD frames from the colonoscopy source and store them to hard disk, with no lose of frame rate or frame quality. Although the posterior analysis of the frames must not need HD size, by storing the HD version of the video we assure the maximum image quality provided by the device. In order to capture the HD frames, a HD frame grabber must be installed into a PC which will play the role of data repository. Finally, in order to keep the frame rate and video quality, the frames must be compressed with a fast lossless compression codec, and stored with a high speed RAID 1 configuration (parallel disc write). Figure 7 a) shows a graphical representation of the set-up.

3.6.2 Annotation of colonoscopy video

The video annotation procedure can be performed in different ways. In the case of frame annotation, a keyboard interaction can be potentially enough to select the desired frames. A navigation system must be implemented if the the expert is allowed to go forward and backwards in the video sequence. If the annotation task consist of the definition of ROIs, a mouse, a digital pen, or a tactile device can be used. More sophisticated techniques, such as the use of eye-tracking (Vilariño et al. (2007)), can be implemented in case that the video is to be annotated by using attention/perception models -see Figure 7 b) for a general scheme.

4. Polyp detection by means of a model of polyp appearance

Our current work, as it has been stated in Section 3, can be enclosed into polyp detection by means of shape descriptors. The difference between our work and the works by other authors is that in order to develop our approach we started by defining a model of polyp appearance. This model is based on how polyps are shown in colonoscopy videos, and the aim of our work is to build up our polyp detection system by taking into account as many types of polyp appearances as possible. Hence, we rely on methods that are based on the detection of the elliptical shape of flat polyps but we also consider the detection of peduncular polyps.

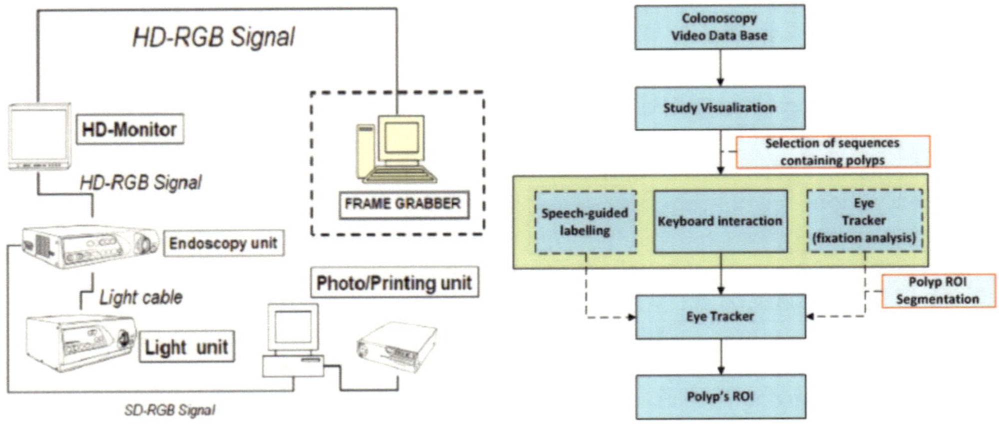

(a) (b)

Fig. 7. a) Schematics of the HD colonoscopy data acquisition system. b) Data annotation scheme.

Our processing scheme consists of three stages (see Bernal, J., Sánchez, J., Vilariño, F. (2011)), namely: *region segmentation*, *region description* and *region classification*. The segmentation stage is stated as follows: Given an input image showing a polyp, our objective is to divide the image into meaningful separate regions, provided that one and only one of these regions will contain the whole polyp. The resulting regions from the segmentation stage will be then analyzed for region description. In the *region description* stage, our plan is to find the descriptor that best characterizes the region in terms of likelihood for polyp presence. The descriptions of the segmented regions will be introduced into the *region classification* stage whose aim is to decide, considering the data that receives and previous knowledge, if a region contains a polyp or not. This section focuses exclusively on the region segmentation stage, since its good performance is crucial for the consecutive phases of the method.

4.1 Region segmentation by means of a model of polyp appearance

As mentioned above, our model of polyp appearance is based on how polyps are shown in colonoscopy videos. More precisely, the analysis of different frames from our database leads to the conclusion that the lighting of the probe gives us hints about how the polyps appear. As light falls perpendicularly to the colon walls, it creates shadows around the surfaces, and when the light falls into a prominent surface it creates a bright spot surrounded by darker areas. Finally, the surrounding shadows define boundaries, and boundaries are identified as edges and intensity valleys in the processed images. We can see in Figure 8 a graphical example of our method and how it can be valid for both lateral and overhead views.

Although this model of prominent surface appearance under the lighting conditions of the colonoscope appears to be valid, there are some challenges to be overcome which are those previously exemplified in Figure 6, namely: non-uniform appearance of polyps, different point of view, specular highlights, image blurring and color channel misalignment, among others. Taking all this into consideration, we base our segmentation method on a model of polyp appearance where we define a polyp as *a prominent shape enclosed in a region with presence of edges and valleys around its frontiers.*

A complete example of how our *region segmentation* method works can be seen in Figure 9. Recall that the objective of this stage was: given an input image, divide it into a minimum number of informative regions. In our case, the term *informative regions* is used here for regions candidate to contain polyps, which will be classified in a later stage into polyp- vs. non-polyp. Finally, one and only one of the informative regions will contain the whole polyp. Conversely, *non-informative regions* are those assumed not to contain a polyp inside, and therefore there will be no need of further processing for polyp detection (Bernal, J., Sánchez, J., Vilariño, F. (2010))). The proposed region segmentation scheme consists of 3 different stages:

1. **Image Preprocessing:** Before applying any segmentation algorithm there are some operations that should be done: 1) converting the image into gray-scale (Figure 9 b)), 2) de-interleaving (since our images come from a high definition interleaved video source), 3) correction of the specular highlights (Figure 9 c)), and 4) inverting the grey-scale image (Figure 9 d)).
2. **Image Segmentation:** Following some of the approaches presented in Section 3, we apply watersheds as a first segmentation method. The improvement of our contribution is that instead of using the original image we use gradient information, which makes the boundaries between the regions obtained this way closer to the boundaries that separate the different structures (see Bernal, J., Sánchez, J., Vilariño, F. (2010)).
3. **Region Merging:** Since it is difficult to obtain perfect segmentation results from a basic segmentation process, the output of the previous stage will be a high number of regions

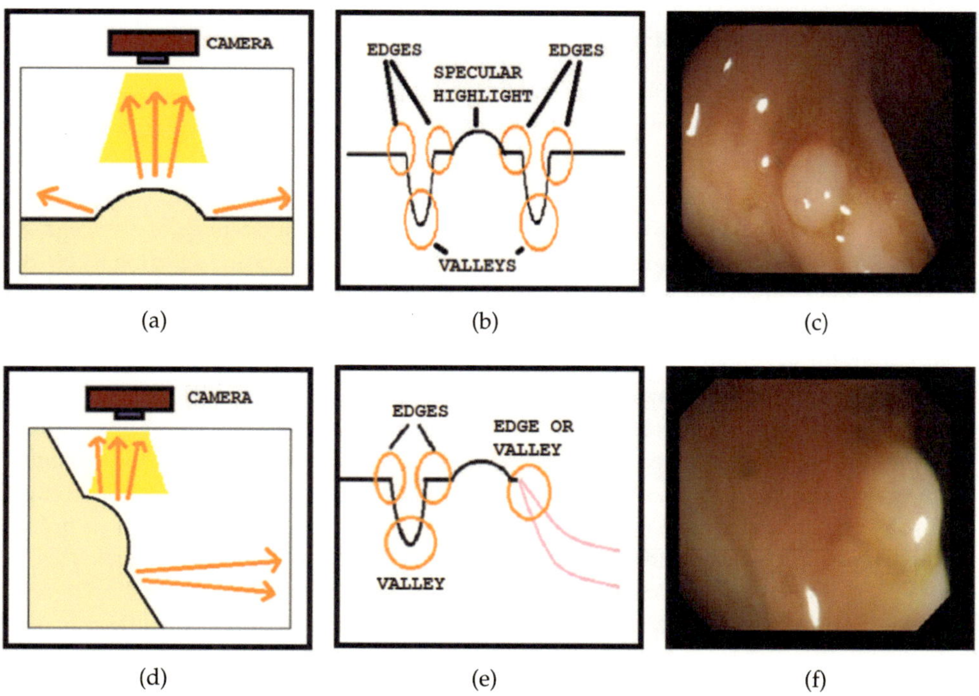

Fig. 8. a) and d): Simulation of an illuminated prominent surface. b) and e): Grey-scale profile. c) and f): Example images.

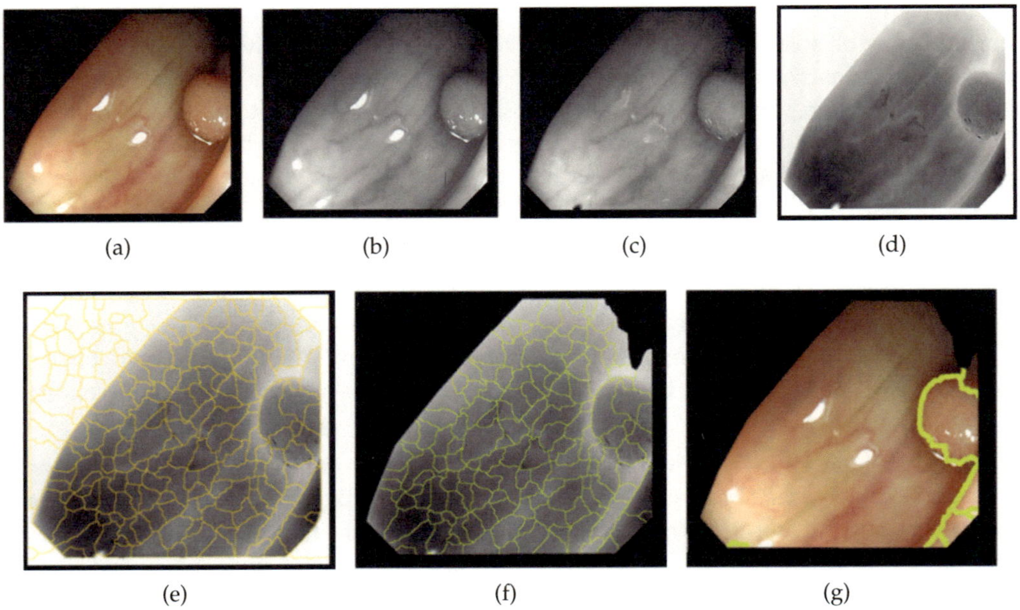

Fig. 9. Complete example of segmentation: a) Original image, b) grey-scale image, c) correction of reflections, d) complemented image, input to watershed segmentation, e) first watershed segmentation, f) segmentation results after region information-based region merging, and g) final segmentation

that should be reduced. In this case our region merging method takes into account the previously-defined model of polyp appearance to combine neighbor regions into larger ones. We apply a joint strategy: 1) Region information-based region merging, and 2) Depth of valleys-based region merging.

a) *Region information-based*: We first calculate the neighborhood map of the segmented image (Figure 9 e)) and identify the frontiers between each pair of regions. Next, we categorize the regions and frontiers in terms of the amount of information that they contain (Bernal, J., Sánchez, J., Vilariño, F. (2010)). For instance, a low information region will have a very high (or very low) mean grey level, and also a very low standard deviation of grey level. We will only merge regions: 1) with the same kind of information, and 2) separated by weak frontiers. In this case, in order to consider a frontier as weak we propose a frontier weakness measure as defined in Equation 1. This measure combines the information of the mean gradient of the frontier pixels (weighted by the coefficient α) and the strength of the frontiers (weighted by the coefficient β). The latter is measured as the percentage of frontier pixels remaining after applying two median filters of increasing order -this helps removing spurious regions created by blood vessels-. We merge and categorize regions until their number is stabilized or there are no weak frontiers left (Figure 9 f)).

$$FrontierWeakness = \alpha * gradient + \beta * strength \quad (1)$$

b) *Depth of valleys-based*: We define a *depth of valleys* measure that combines the output of a ridges and valleys detector (see López, A.M., Lumbreras, F. et al. (1999) for details) with the

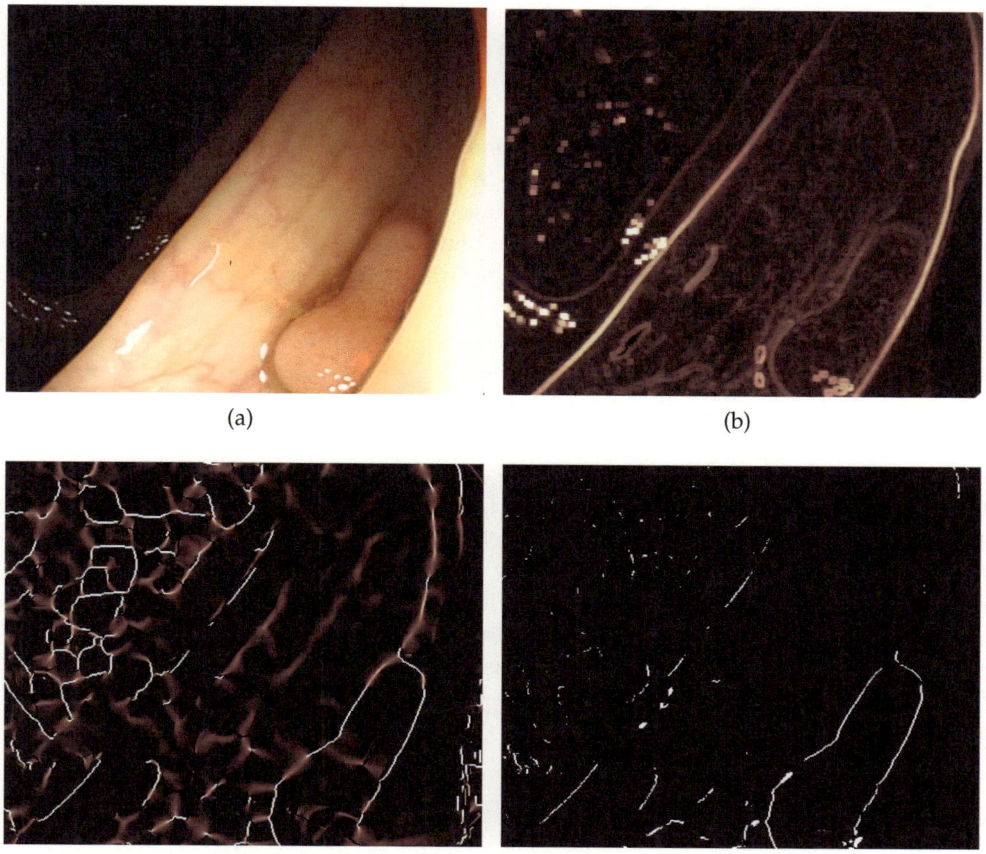

(a) (b) (c) (d)

Fig. 10. Creation of the depth of valleys image: a) Original image. b) morphological gradient image, c) valleys image, and (d) depth of valleys image.

output of the morphological gradient. This gives information about the depth of the pixels in the valley image. The pixels that constitute the frontier of the region will have high values for both the valley and gradient magnitudes (both measures will be smaller for the inner pixels, as can be seen in Figure 10). Using this information we can continue merging regions, keeping only those whose frontiers are strong in terms of *depth of valleys*. We merge regions until there are no weak frontiers according to the depth of valleys threshold or when the number of regions is stabilized (Figure 9 g)).

In order to assess the quality of our *region segmentation* method, we have created a database with different studies of polyp appearance. We were provided 15 random cases, in which the experts (physicians) annotated all the sequences showing polyps, and a random sample of 20 frames per sequence was obtained. The experts guaranteed that all these 20 frames showed a significantly different point of view within the scene by rejecting similar frames. This allows us to maximize the variability of the images used, while not jeopardizing any bias at all.
We will evaluate the performance of our method by using two different measures: Annotated Area Covered (AAC) and Dice Similarity Coefficient (DICE). Both measures are

complementary as the former calculates the amount of annotated polyp area while the latter complements it with the amount of non-polyp information that is kept in the region. We will compare our final segmentation results with the ones obtained using one state-of-the-art method such as *normalized cuts*.

We also have to consider that colonoscopy images have black borders around them. Our region segmentation method consider their presence and use the results of non-informative region identification (which borders of the image are part of) to avoid further processing of this areas. In order to test the effect that these borders have in the segmentation results, we have also created a database that eliminates the borders of the images, although it may lead to a loss of information.

In Table 1 we show results for polyp region detection, comparing the performance of our method with the performance achieved by normalized cuts, using the same number of final regions. We get better results than normalized cuts in terms of AAC and DICE. This means that our method outperforms normalized cuts by providing regions that do not separate the polyp, and the polyp is always present in only one region.

The elimination of the borders in the image, in terms of AAC, has almost no effect for our method but it has more incidence for normalized cuts. DICE results improve for both methods by using the image without borders (better as the threshold value increases), although normalized cuts results are better. But, as it can be seen in Figure 11, normalized cuts non-polyp regions tend to be larger than our non-polyp regions (in our case we know that the larger region corresponds always to the background).

With Borders						
Measure / Method	Ours	NCuts	Ours	NCuts	Ours	NCuts
Threshold Value	0.6		0.7		0.8	
AAC	61.91%	63.66%	70.29%	69.06%	75.79%	70.86%
DICE	55.33%	44.97%	44.6%	37.75%	36.44%	34.01%
Without Borders						
Measure / Method	Ours	NCuts	Ours	NCuts	Ours	NCuts
Threshold Value	0.6		0.7		0.8	
AAC	60.71%	60.2%	70.29%	63.98%	74.32%	64.24%
DICE	55.68%	63.15%	48.01%	61.84%	45.01%	56.73%

Table 1. Comparison between the results obtained by our method and normalized cuts with respect to the value of the depth of valleys.

In Figure 11 (a-d) we can see examples of the output of each method. It can be seen that the final regions that our method provides (c) are closer the polyp mask -the ground-truth segmented by experts-.

4.2 Analysis of results

As it has been shown in the previous subsection, we have developed a region segmentation method which takes into account the model of polyp appearance. The preliminary results obtained indicate that our model can be valid for polyp segmentation, although there are some problems that need to be overcome. Although the numerical results are satisfactory in terms of accuracy, DICE results must be improved. The number of final regions should be

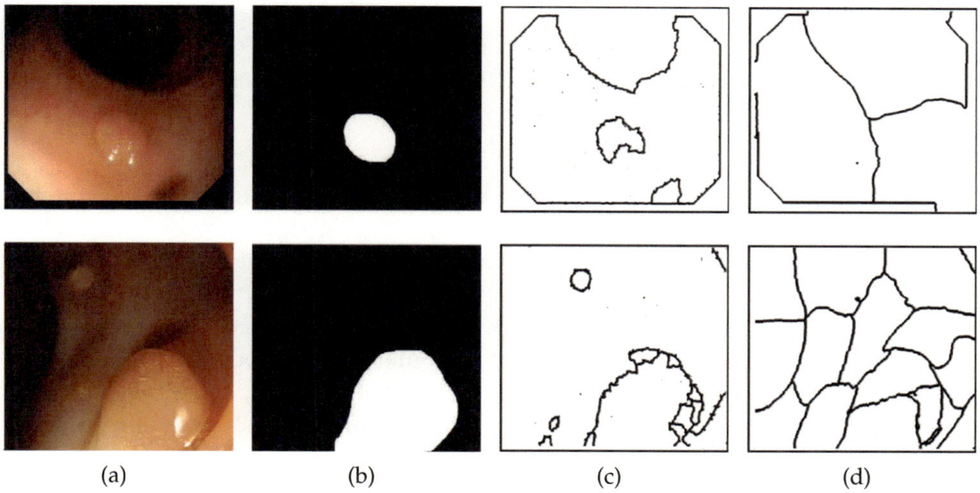

Fig. 11. Comparison of segmentation results: a) Original images, b) polyp masks, c) output of our method, and d) output of normalized cuts.

reduced to the minimum possible if we do not want to hurt, in terms of computation time, the following stages in the pipeline. One possible solution will be to start discarding regions that will not be passed to posterior stages. We have already used the term of non-informative regions (as we proposed in Bernal, J., Sánchez, J., Vilariño, F. (2010)) but we can also take profit of some of the works presented in this chapter: for instance, we can use some results for lumen segmentation in order to help our description of what is on the scene. Segmentation results could be potentially improved by applying a size threshold to discard some of the smallest regions. It would not have an impact in terms of polyp detection if the hypothesis of a minimum size for detection of polyps is considered. The DICE results could be also potentially improved by merging some small regions that appear inside the polyp region.

Our efforts now are focused on developing more the approach of depth of valleys. Our idea is that polyps appear in the image surrounded by intensity valleys and contours where the light falls perpendicularly on them. We complement the information that a valley detector provides with the morphological gradient in order to achieve a method that enhances both valley and contour information, because in certain type of views (in general, in lateral views) we do not have a whole valley surrounding the polyp. However, non-connected edges are available in these cases, and once we have this information, that can be complete or incomplete, our next steps will be focused on finding out the points which are inside or outside the polyp. To achieve this goal, we will use the depth of valleys image as the seed for an object identification algorithm. This algorithm is based on the fact that if a point is interior to an object, it will be surrounded by boundaries (in this case, high values in the depth of valleys image) in many directions. Conversely, if a point is exterior to an object, it will be surrounded only in a few directions. This concept can be better understood by following the representation shown in Figure 12.

Finally, this method needs an accurate and robust boundary detector, although these contours can be partially incomplete. This method could also be adapted to the idea of ellipse-fitting (Hwang, S. and Oh, J.H. and Tavanapong, W. et al. (2007)) in order to fit points interior to objects to those which would be interior to an ellipse. The development of a method that identifies accurately which points are interior and which are exterior to objects may lead to an efficient pruning of the regions obtained from the region segmentation stage.

5. Conclusions and prospective

As mentioned in our introduction, we believe that there is a great potential to use intelligent systems in colonoscopy. Throughout this chapter we have shown several methods that, starting from a description of what is on the scene, can be used to add in valuable information to the output of the colonoscopy intervention.

We have shown how the quality of colonoscopy videos can be improved, by eliminating some of the artifacts that can alter the performance of computer vision-based systems, such specular highlights or color channel misalignment. We have also shown that, by a general analysis of the image and the motion of the camera, it is possible to automatically annotate the different parts of the intervention for video indexation and retrieval.

There is a vast majority of methods in the literature devoted to lesions and cancer detection. Several approaches have been carried out, which involve from the direct analysis of the shapes of the objects that appear on the image to an analysis of the texture of the tissues. We argued that these methods (included ours) should be tested on a benchmark database with a solid common ground truth, which is not available yet, in order to have solid inference about their actual performance. Despite this, the contributions presented show that the particular results could be potentially used to aid the diagnosis of the physician, both during and post-intervention.

We have proposed methods that could be used to assess the physician skills in training programs. By analyzing training results we can improve our systems or, as one method presented show, we can use the physicians' reaction of what they see in colonoscopy videos to learn about what can be relevant in each colonoscopy frame. This provides a baseline to understand how the attention models are working in intervention time, and which and why the regions of interest call the physician's attention.

In the near future, we can think of colonoscopy interventions where intelligent systems add key information in real-time and allow objective metrics for the assessment of the quality

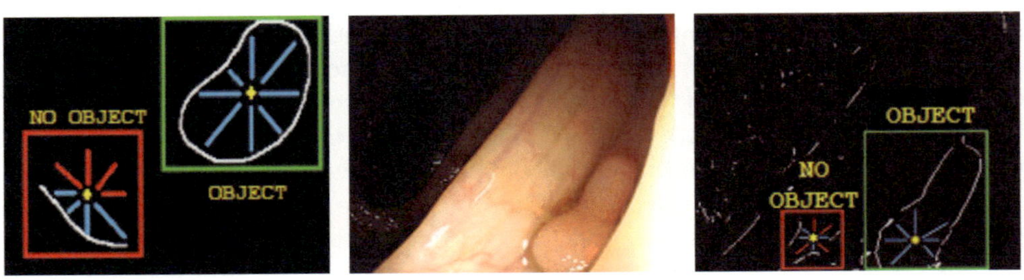

(a) (b) (c)

Fig. 12. a) Graphical example for the definition of points exterior and interior to objects. Blue lines indicate directions where the point is surrounded by a strong boundary and red lines indicate the direction where the point is not surrounded by a strong boundary. b) Original image, and c) intuitive approximation for the performance of the method in the previous image.

of the intervention. Whether it is an alert to the physician by highlighting some part of the image where the intelligent system observes some evidence of lesion or cancer presence, or by automatically storing a patient-specific report of the patient's colon, intelligent systems are called to be a relevant tool in the future of colonoscopy.

6. Acknowledgements

This work was supported in part by a research grant from Universitat Autonòma de Barcelona 471-01-3/08, by the Spanish Government through the founded project "COLON-QA" (TIN2009-10435) and by research programme Consolider Ingenio 2010: MIPRCV (CSD2007-00018).

7. References

Ameling, S., Wirth, S., Paulus, D., Lacey, G. & Vilariño, F. (2009). Texture-based polyp detection in colonoscopy, *Bildverarbeitung für die Medizin 2009* pp. 346–350.

Arnold, M., Ameling, S., Ghosh, A. & Lacey, G. (2011). Quality Improvement of Endoscopy Videos, *Proceedings of the 8th IASTED International Conference on Biomedical Engineering*, Insbruck, Austria.

Arnold, M., Ghosh, A., Lacey, G., Patchett, S. & Mulcahy, H. (2009). Indistinct frame detection in colonoscopy videos, *2009 13th International Machine Vision and Image Processing Conference*, pp. 47–52.

Bernal, J. and Vilariño, F. and Sánchez, J. (2010). Feature detectors and feature descriptors: Where we are now, *Technical Report 154*, Computer Vision Center & Computer Science Department Universitat Autònoma de Barcelona.

Bernal, J. and Sánchez, J. and Vilariño, F. (2011). A region segmentation method for colonoscopy images using a model of polyp appearance, *Lecture Notes in Computer Science. Pattern Recognition and Image Analysis. Proceedings of the 5th Iberian Conference, IbPRIA 2011*, pp. 134–142.

Bernal, J., Sánchez, J., Vilariño, F. (2010). Reduction of Pattern Search Area in Colonoscopy Images by Merging Non-Informative Regions, *Proceedings of the XXVIII Congreso Anual de la Sociedad Española de Ingeniería Biomédica*, Madrid, Spain.

Bernal, J., Sánchez, J., Vilariño, F. (2011). Current challenges on polyp detection in colonoscopy videos: From region segmentation to region classification. a pattern recognition-based approach, *Proceedings of the 2nd International Workshop on Medical Image Analysis and Description for Diagnosis Systems - MIAD 2011*, Rome, Italy.

Bevilacqua, V., Cortellino, M., Piccinni, M., Scarpa, A., Taurino, D., Mastronardi, G., Moschetta, M. & Angelelli, G. (2009). Image processing framework for virtual colonoscopy, *Emerging Intelligent Computing Technology and Applications* pp. 965–974.

Bratko, I., Mozetič, I. & Lavrač, N. (1990). KARDIO: A study in deep and qualitative knowledge for expert systems.

Cao, Y., Liu, D., Tavanapong, W., Wong, J., Oh, J. & de Groen, P. (2007). Computer-aided detection of diagnostic and therapeutic operations in colonoscopy videos, *Biomedical Engineering, IEEE Transactions on* 54(7): 1268–1279.

Coimbra, M. & Cunha, J. (2006). MPEG-7 visual descriptorsï£¡contributions for automated feature extraction in capsule endoscopy, *Circuits and Systems for Video Technology, IEEE Transactions on* 16(5): 628–637.

Dahyot, R., Vilariño, F. & Lacey, G. (2008). Improving the quality of color colonoscopy videos, *Journal on Image and Video Processing* 2008: 1–7.

Dhandra, B., Hegadi, R., Hangarge, M. & Malemath, V. (2006). Analysis of abnormality in endoscopic images using combined hsi color space and watershed segmentation, *Pattern Recognition, 2006. ICPR 2006. 18th International Conference on*, Vol. 4, pp. 695–698.

Gunduz-Demir, C., Kandemir, M., Tosun, A. & Sokmensuer, C. (2010). Automatic segmentation of colon glands using object-graphs, *Medical image analysis* 14(1): 1–12.

Hassinger, J.P., Holubar, S.D. et al. (2010). Effectiveness of a Multimedia-Based Educational Intervention for Improving Colon Cancer Literacy in Screening Colonoscopy Patients, *Diseases of the Colon & Rectum* 53(9): 1301.

Hwang, S. and Oh, J.H. and Tavanapong, W. et al. (2007). Polyp detection in colonoscopy video using elliptical shape feature, *Image Processing, 2007. ICIP 2007. IEEE International Conference on*, Vol. 2.

Hwang, S., Oh, J., Lee, J., Cao, Y., Tavanapong, W., Liu, D., Wong, J. & de Groen, P. (2005). Automatic measurement of quality metrics for colonoscopy videos, *Proceedings of the 13th annual ACM international conference on Multimedia*, pp. 912–921.

ICT Programme Commitee (2011). Fp7. ict - information and communication technologies. work programme 2011-12, Community Research and Development Information Service.

Kang, J. and Doraiswami, R. (2003). Real-time image processing system for endoscopic applications, *IEEE Canadian Conference on Electrical and Computer Engineering*, Vol. 3, pp. 1469 – 1472 vol.3.

Karkanis, S., Iakovidis, D., Maroulis, D., Karras, D. & Tzivras, M. (2003). Computer-aided tumor detection in endoscopic video using color wavelet features, *Information Technology in Biomedicine, IEEE Transactions on* 7(3): 141–152.

Krishnan, S., Yang, X., Chan, K., Kumar, S. & Goh, P. (1998). Intestinal abnormality detection from endoscopic images, *Engineering in Medicine and Biology Society, 1998. Proceedings of the 20th Annual International Conference of the IEEE*, Vol. 2, pp. 895–898.

Krishnan, S.M. and Goh, P.M.Y. (1997). Quantitative parametrization of colonoscopic images by applying fuzzy technique, *Engineering in Medicine and Biology Society, 1997. Proceedings of the 19th Annual International Conference of the IEEE*, Vol. 3, pp. 1121 –1123 vol.3.

Li, P., Chan, K. & Krishnan, S. (2005). Learning a multi-size patch-based hybrid kernel machine ensemble for abnormal region detection in colonoscopic images.

Liu, D., Cao, Y., Kim, K., Stanek, S., Doungratanaex-Chai, B., Lin, K., Tavanapong, W., Wong, J., Oh, J. & de Groen, P. (2007). Arthemis: Annotation software in an integrated capturing and analysis system for colonoscopy, *Computer methods and programs in biomedicine* 88(2): 152–163.

López, A.M., Lumbreras, F. et al. (1999). Evaluation of methods for ridge and valley detection, *IEEE Transactions on Pattern Analysis and Machine Intelligence* 21(4): 327–335.

Malik, A. (2010). *End of insertion detection in colonoscopy videos*, PhD thesis, University of North Texas.

Maroulis, D., Iakovidis, D., Karkanis, S. & Karras, D. (2003). CoLD: a versatile detection system for colorectal lesions in endoscopy video-frames, *Computer Methods and Programs in Biomedicine* 70(2): 151–166.

Morán, S., Torrella, E., Esteban, D., Baños, M., García, A., Ono, A., Pérez, C., Parra, P., Cruzado, Q., Pérez, R. et al. (2009). Colonoscopy quality assessment., *Revista española de enfermedades digestivas: Órgano oficial de la Sociedad Española de Patología Digestiva* 101(2): 107.

National Cancer Institute (2011). Image Archive Resources. URL: *http://tinyurl.com/63n4qo4*

Nunes, C., Mendonça, T., Amorim, P., Ferreira, D. & Antunes, L. (2005). Comparison of Neural Networks, Fuzzy and Stochastic Prediction Models for return of consciousness after general anesthesia, *Decision and Control, 2005 and 2005 European Control Conference. CDC-ECC'05. 44th IEEE Conference on*, pp. 4827–4832.

Oh, J., Hwang, S., Cao, Y., Tavanapong, W., Liu, D., Wong, J. & de Groen, P. (2009). Measuring objective quality of colonoscopy, *Biomedical Engineering, IEEE Transactions on* 56(9): 2190–2196.

Oh, J., Hwang, S., Tavanapong, W., de Groen, P. & Wong, J. (2003). Blurry-frame detection and shot segmentation in colonoscopy videos, *Proceedings of SPIE*, Vol. 5307, p. 531.

Segnan, N., Patnick, J. & von Karsa, L. (2011). *European guidelines for quality assurance in colorectal cancer screening and diagnosis*, Luxembourg: Publications Office of the European Union.

Tian, H., Srikanthan, T. & Vijayan Asari, K. (2001). Automatic segmentation algorithm for the extraction of lumen region and boundary from endoscopic images, *Medical and Biological Engineering and Computing* 39(1): 8–14.

Tjoa, M. & Krishnan, S. (2003). Feature extraction for the analysis of colon status from the endoscopic images, *BioMedical Engineering OnLine* 2(9): 1–17.

Tjoa, M., Krishnan, S. & Doraiswami, R. (2002). Automated diagnosis for segmentation of colonoscopic images using chromatic features, *Electrical and Computer Engineering, 2002. IEEE CCECE 2002. Canadian Conference on*, Vol. 2, pp. 1177–1180.

Tresca, A. (2010). The Stages of Colon and Rectal Cancer, *New York Times (About.com)* p. 1. URL: *http://tinyurl.com/3y4acut*

van Wijk, C., van Ravesteijn, V., Vos, F. & van Vliet, L. (2010). Detection and segmentation of colonic polyps on implicit isosurfaces by second principal curvature flow, *Medical Imaging, IEEE Transactions on* 29(3): 688–698.

Vilariño, F. (2006). *A Machine Learning Approach for Intestinal Motility Assessment with Capsule Endoscopy*, PhD thesis, Universitat Autònoma de Barcelona and Computer Vision Center.

Vilariño, F., Ameling, S., Lacey, G., Ghosh, A., Patchett, S. & Mulcahy, H. (2009). Eye tracking search patterns in expert and trainee colonoscopoist: A novel method of assessing endoscopic competency?, *Book of abstracts from the Digestive Disease Week*, Chicago, America.

Vilariño, F., Lacey, G., Zhou, J., Mulcahy, H. & Patchett, S. (2007). Automatic labeling of colonoscopy video for cancer detection, *Pattern Recognition and Image Analysis* pp. 290–297.

Vincent, L. , Soille, P. (1991). Watersheds in digital spaces: an efficient algorithm based on immersion simulations, *IEEE transactions on pattern analysis and machine intelligence* 13(6): 583–598.

Viswanath, S., Palumbo, D., Chappelow, J., Patel, P., Bloch, B., Rofsky, N., Lenkinski, R., Genega, E. & Madabhushi, A. (2011). Empirical evaluation of bias field correction algorithms for computer-aided detection of prostate cancer on T2w MRI (Proceedings Paper).

Wei, J., Chan, H., Zhou, C., Wu, Y., Sahiner, B., Hadjiiski, L., Roubidoux, M. & Helvie, M. (2011). Computer-aided detection of breast masses: Four-view strategy for screening mammography, *Medical Physics* 38: 1867.

Zhang, D., Zhao, J., Lu, L., Li, L. & Wang, Z. (2010). Virtual eversion and rotation of colon based on outer surface centerline, *Medical physics* 37: 5518.

Zhu, H., Fan, Y. & Liang, Z. (2010). Improved Curvature Estimation for Shape Analysis in Computer-Aided Detection of Colonic Polyps, *Beijing, China* p. 19.

17

Virtual Colonoscopy - Technical Aspects

Andrzej Skalski[1], Mirosław Socha[1], Tomasz Zieliński[2] and Mariusz Duplaga[3]
[1]AGH University of Science and Technology, Krakow
Department of Measurement and Instrumentation
[2]AGH University of Science and Technology, Krakow, Department of Telecommunications
[3]Jagiellonian University Medical College, Krakow
Poland

1. Introduction

Virtual colonoscopy (VC) is a diagnostic method enabling the generation of two-dimensional and three-dimensional images of the colon and rectum from the data obtained with relevant imaging modality, usually spiral computed tomography (CT). If CT is used, the method is also called CT colonoscopy, CT colonography, or CT pneumocolon. The main advantages of the VC which support its broader application in medical practice include: limited invasiveness, improved compliance of patients and value for screening for colorectal cancer.

The introduction of virtual endoscopy technique originates from the extended processing options of the data sets obtained with available imaging modalities. The Visible Human Project and related activities (Hong et al., 1996; Hong, 1997) were of key importance for development of the VC.

The quality of first VC images limited the potential of the clinical use of this technique. But with next generations of the imaging equipment and advanced processing algorithms, their applicability in medical practice was established. VC may be performed with all imaging techniques which result in cross-sections of the abdominal cavity. It can be generated both from CT and magnetic resonance imaging (MRI) cross-sections. However, the CT remains the first choice imaging modality for the VC. It is required that spiral acquisition mode with overlapping reconstructions is applied. The quality of the images generated within VC techniques depends strongly on the spatial resolution obtained with imaging modality. Nowadays, multidetector computed tomography (MDCT) is commonly available and this adds to overall quality of assessment of the colon and rectum resulting from VC.

The patient undergoing helical computed tomography with the intent of obtaining VC should undergo complete bowel preparation as for other procedures within abdomen, e.g. endoscopic colonoscopy. The priority is assigned to evacuation of the contents of the colon before CT. For this purpose, many agents are used including ethylene glycol electrolyte solution, magnesium citrate or oral sodium phospate. Netherless, the quality of bowel preparation for VC varies considerably between different centres (Van Uitert et al., 2008).

The trend for the optimisation of the diagnostic procedures and limitation of the burden to the patient resulted also in a strategy focusing on the performing of the optical colonoscopy just after VC, if it is positive for pathological lesions in the colon, in order to avoid repetition of the bowel preparation procedure. A strategy enabling identification of the artefacts resulting from fecal contents in the bowel in the process of generation of VC images was also proposed. This is achieved by labelling it with some type of contrast agent, e.g. barium or meglumine diatrizoate taken orally before the CT (Iannaccone et al., 2004).

The use of MRI imaging for generating of VC is another attempt to avoid bowel preparation and exposure to the radiation related to the CT imaging (Florie et al., 2007). Finally, the techniques enabling "electronic" colon cleansing before generating VC images were developed to allow for less intensive colon preparation procedures (Lakare et al., 2002). VC without laborious bowel cleansing preparation preceding is related to higher acceptance and compliance from patients. This in turn may be a key condition for successful screening strategy in the society.

Growing use of the VC is supported by its lower invasiveness in the comparison to other diagnostic procedures and potential for higher compliance from patients. These features increase the value of the techniques as a screening test for disorders of the colon. The main indications for VC include screening for colonic polyps or cancer and failure or inadequate results of optical colonoscopy due to anatomical conditions or pathological lesions, e.g. obstruction of the colon lumen. Furthermore, the VC enables also for examination of extracolonic structures not accessible during standard colonoscopy. This may be particularly important for these patients in whom pathological lesions were detected inside the colon lumen.

The first studies focusing on the assessment of the sensitivity of the VC reported usually its lower performance in comparison to optical colonoscopy. The sensitivity of the VC depends considerably on the size of the polyps present in the colon and is lower in less advanced lesions. Introduction of MDCT had significant impact on improving the VC efficiency. Most recent studies indicate that VC sensitivity in detecting polyps of size at least 10 mm is comparable with optical colonoscopy and exceeds 90% (Regge et al., 2009; Graser et al., 2009).

The Guidelines issued in 2008 by American Cancer Society, American College of Radiology and US Multi-Society Task Force on Colorectal Cancer included VC within recommended screening tests for colorectal cancer, which should be performed at 5 years intervals in population of at least 50 years or older (Levin et al., 2008). According to the Guidelines, VC should be performed after complete bowel preparation. The detection of a polyp of size >6 mm in VC necessitates the performance of optical colonoscopy, preferably the same day or second complete bowel preparation is needed.

During classical (optical or video-) endoscopy, the endoscope is inserted into the internal space of a tube-like organ. Colonoscopy is performed with flexible endoscope equipped with a camera. A physician performing examination can bend the tip of the endoscope in two orthogonal directions using small wheels which are placed on the head of the instrument in order to navigate and move it through the colon. Colonoscopy may be associated with different level of discomfort in specific patients and depend on the medication used during preparation and the procedure itself. The VC may be an alternative approach to classical endoscopy. In this chapter, technical aspects of the generation of the VC images are explored. Authors describe all steps which are required to create a 3D computer model of the colon from the CT data. A procedure which allows one to compute the VC is presented in figure 1. It includes CT examination of abdomen, electronic colon cleansing, generation of 3D computer model of the colon with appropriate segmentation techniques. Then a navigation path for virtual camera may be calculated in order to simulate the progression of a real endoscope. Finally, views from colon reconstructed from the CT data are calculated based on visualisation methods.

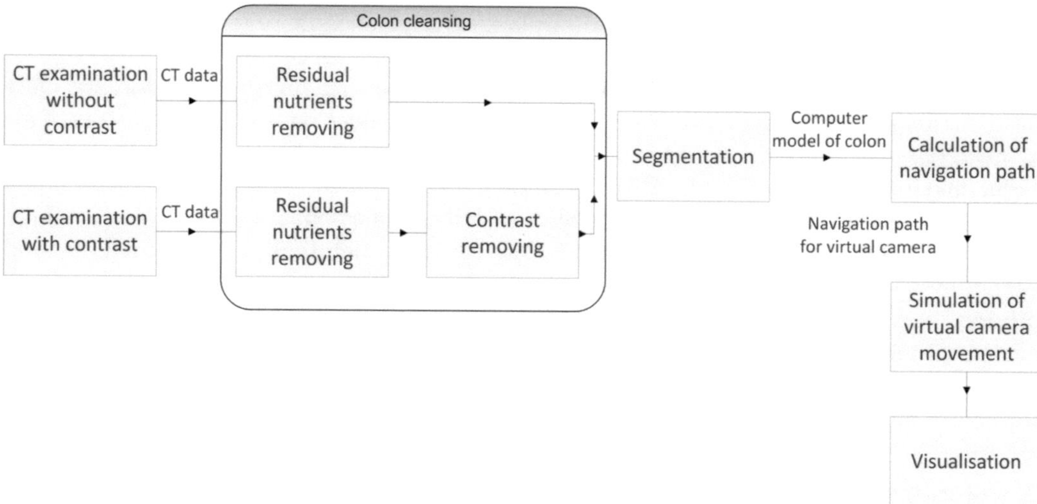

Fig. 1. Block diagram of the Virtual Colonoscopy procedure

2. Computed tomography data

The imaging modality of computed tomography (CT) was developed in the results of the chain of discoveries starting from the year 1895 when Wilhelm Röntgen invented a new type of electromagnetic radiation, called by him as X-rays. The mathematical principles of CT were first investigated by Johann Radon in 1917 and then extended by Kirillov in 1961. The first CT scanner was presented in 1972 by Allan Cormack and Godfrey Hounsfield, who were awarded the Nobel Prize in medicine in 1979. The detailed description of CT was provided in 1988 (Kak & Slaney, 1988). Nowadays, CT imaging is commonly used throughout medical specialities for diagnostic purposes and support of interventional procedures.

Because of easier hardware realization, the fan-beam projection is used in medical CT scanners. In the third-generation CT scanners, the X-ray source and the detector array are rotated around the patient. In helical or spiral cone beam CT scanners, the patient is lying during the procedure on a moving bed and the X-ray source and the detector arrays are rotating around him.

The helical scan method enables for quicker scanning and reduction of the radiation dose (necessary for given resolution) to which the patient is exposed during the procedure. Additionally, the number of rows of detectors in helical CT scanners was increasing from several years. Nowadays, the 64 or 128 multi-slice scanners are frequently encountered in clinical applications. Currently, 256-slice cardiac CT scanners enables for scanning of the heart in less than one second. On the other hand, minimizing the radiation risk to the patient, while maintaining satisfactory CT image quality, becomes urgent especially for colon screening with CT (Wang et al., 2008). Dose reduction for CT imaging can be achieved by scanning patient whit low-mAs protocols (less than 100mAs). Unfortunately, these protocols may result in noisy and streak artefacts in the reconstructed images. This effect can be compensated by the optimisation of data acquisition and the application of iterative image reconstruction algorithm (Wang et al., 2008).

The dataset acquired with the CT scanner can by described by number of slices, the number of pixels per slice and the voxel distances. The number of pixels in one slice is also referred to as image matrix. It is usually set of 512 x 512 pixels. The distances between the voxels are differentiated into the slice distance (out-of-plane) and pixel distance (in-plane). In general, the medical data are anisotropic (pixel and slice distances are not equal).
The data resolution influences the noise level. The data having higher resolution are more noisy for the same radiation dose. The computed intensity values represent the densities of the scanned objects that are normalized into Hounsfield units (HUs). This normalization maps the 12-bit data into two bytes (16 bits). Water is mapped to zero and air is mapped to -1000 value.
Medical images are physically stored together with the data essential for their interpretation. This information is highly standardized. The DICOM standard (Digital Imaging and Communications in Medicine) enables the integration of scanners, servers, workstations, printers, and network hardware from multiple manufacturers into a picture archiving and communication system (PACS). It includes a file format definition and a network communications protocol. The DICOM files can be read by many programs and are supported by numerous libraries (VTK, DCMTK, GDCM).

3. Colon cleansing

The first step of the CT data processing is the electronic cleansing (EC) of the colon, especially if other means were not undertaken to remove fecal contents from the colon. The term EC was first introduced by Wax and Liang (Wax et al., 1998). This is a key operation for ensuring correct segmentation being the next step. In figure 2, we can see fluid (contrast) in the colon. Classical threshold operation does not remove voxels lying on the border between air and fluid (see Fig. 2b). The idea of thresholding operation relies on voxels division into 2 groups making use of a predefined threshold value T:

$$M(x,y,z)=\begin{cases}1 & for\ I(x,y,z)\geq T\\ 0 & for\ I(x,y,z)<T\end{cases} \tag{1}$$

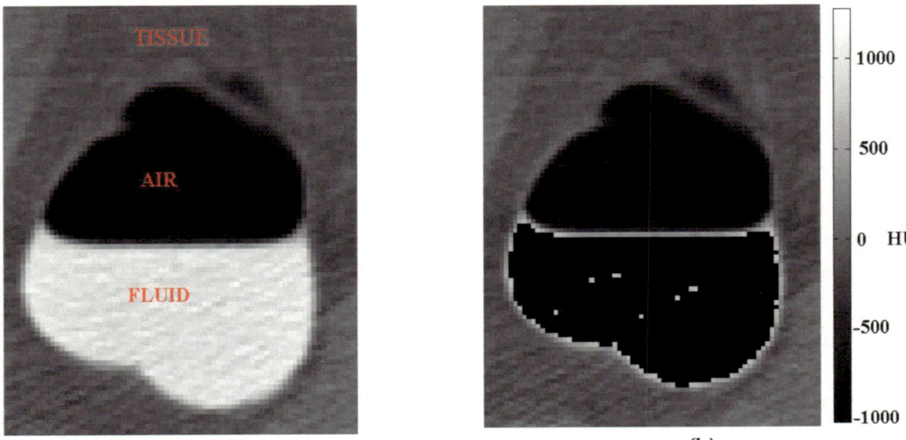

(a) (b)

Fig. 2. 2D slices of: a) 3D CT data; b) 3D CT data after classical thresholding operation

where: $M(x,y,z)$ is a binary mask (1 - indicates object, in this case it should be the colon, 0 - background), and $I(x,y,z)$ denotes a CT data.
The threshold value is usually designated on the basis of the histogram of the CT data or general knowledge about values attributed to anatomical structures. A border between contrast and tissues (see fig. 2b), unwanted but usually being obtained after thresholding operation, is a result of limited resolution of detectors and soft property of reconstruction kernel.

3.1 State of the art

In order to remove voxels representing contrast and residual nutrients, many different computer algorithms were proposed for the electronic colon cleansing (ECC). They differ with the image pre-processing steps, local image features (mainly statistical ones, e.g. 23 features in (Lakare et al., 2003) and 35 in (Cai et al., 2011)), the method of reduction of features dimensionality (vector quantization, principal component analysis), applied modelling (of multi-material objects and their edges/gradients), the use of the segmentation techniques (watershed, active contours, level-set) and classification methods (Markov random fields, expectation maximization, support vector machine). Recent publications in this area (Cai et al., 2011), (Serlie at al., 2010) provide the state-of-the-art and historical perspective of the research focused in the EC.
First works on ECC were based on the application of the statistical image features, vector quantization (for dimensionality reduction), image gradient information and Markov random field classification (Chen at al., 2000). Later methods paid special attention to the application of edge modelling during image segmentation, aiming at efficient delineation of tagged regions. The segmentation ray technique (Lakare et al., 2002) is the most important one in this group. In this method the rays were designed to analyse the intensity profile and to detect the intersection between the air and the residual fluid and between the residual fluid and the soft-tissues. The segmentation rays can accurately detect partial volume regions and remove them if necessary. The same authors (Lakare et al., 2003) proposed a method based on vector quantization but it does not assure correct exclusion of the voxels lying near colon wall. In turn, in another method (Zalis et al., 2004) the image gradient is approximated by Sobel mask filtering followed by a morphological dilation. Recently, Wang (Wang et al., 2006) proposed application of statistical features and an expectation-maximization algorithm for distinguishing voxels belonging to multiple materials while (Serlie at al., 2010) built a scale-invariant three-material transition model between air, soft-tissue and tagged material/fluid and used it for classification of each voxel. The most sophisticated and effective algorithm has been proposed recently in (Cai et al. 2011) that consists of several very carefully designed steps making use of many image features (descriptors), two segmentation procedures (watershed transform, level-set method) and very precise SVM classification/cleansing method (sensitivity 97.1%, specificity 85.3%, accuracy 94.6%).
In order to present problems solved with electronic colon cleansing methods and to demonstrate typical existing solutions, the ECC algorithm developed by the authors of this chapter is briefly described below.

3.2 Electronic colon cleansing using non-linear transfer function and morphological operations

The ECC method proposed by us is based on non-linear value transformation combined with morphological voxels processing (Skalski et al., 2007a).

First, if the CT data has HU values without offset, the voxels values are increased by 1024 and unsigned 16-bit fixed-point integer data format is obtained what results in significant reduction of the calculation time. In order to remove voxels representing contrast one has to find them in the CT data. To reach this aim, we compute two binary masks: a fluid mask and a residual mask. The fluid mask is created by thresholding operation described in section 3: voxels having values greater than 1600 are given value 1. In case of the residual mask we are looking for values greater than 1350 and equal or smaller than 1600 since voxels representing stool and fluid remain within this range. Both masks are dilated using regular hexahedron of size 3. Voxels for which the masks are equal 1 are then processed by two transfer functions, shown in fig. 3, representing Gaussian intensity transformation:

$$I_{new}(x,y,z) = 1000 \cdot \exp\left(-\frac{(I(x,y,z)-1000)^2}{2 \cdot \sigma^2} \right) \quad (2)$$

with $\sigma = 450$ for the fluid mask and 100 for the residual one. This operation is desirable due to necessity to keep smooth changes of intensity on the border between colon and soft tissues.

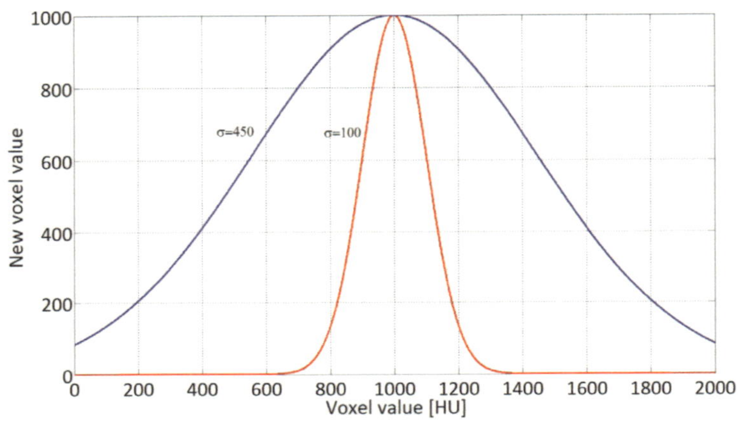

Fig. 3. Gaussian transfer functions; blue line - for fluid mask σ=450 in (2), red line - for residual mask σ=100

In the next step a binary data (M_{Bin}) are created having 0s for the air (v < 300) and 1s for the remaining parts. Then, a sequence of two morphological operations is performed: 1) a 3D erosion operation is applied to each volume by means of a three-cubic matrix, 2) a dilation operation is done on the data resulted from the erosion process. This way, a new volume (M_{Del}) is obtained. After subtraction of M_{Del} from M_{Bin} one receives a binary matrix in which 1s denote voxels that probably lie on the border between air and fluid (stool). Finally, we must check also whether voxels received from the subtraction belong to the border. Since, during the CT scanning the patient lies on his back or abdomen, the border is always parallel to the body surface.
The whole operation can be summarized by the following formula:

$$\begin{aligned} M_{Bin} &= \begin{cases} 1 & for\ I(x,y,z) \geq 300 \\ 0 & for\ I(x,y,z) < 300 \end{cases} \\ M_{Del} &= dilation\left(erode\left(M_{Bin}\right)\right) \\ M_{Pr\_Border} &= M_{Del} - M_{Bin} \end{aligned} \quad (3)$$

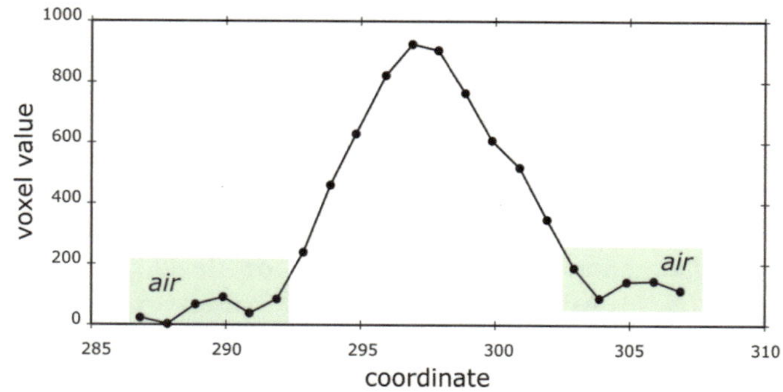

(a)

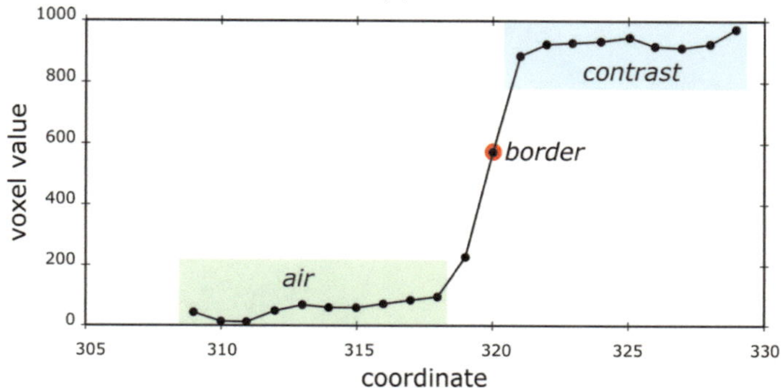

(b)

Fig. 4. The intensity profiles for a voxel which cannot be removed (a) and must be removed (b)

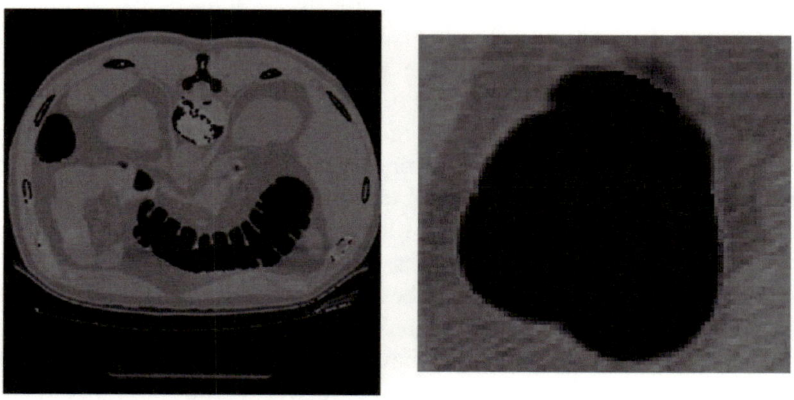

Fig. 5. Exemplary results of usage of the proposed algorithm for colon cleansing

After subtraction we check intensity profile along normal direction to the body surface (fig. 4) for each voxel equal 1 in the M_{Pr_Border} volume: if the profile contains voxels belonging to stool or contrast, this voxel is removed. In figure 4 we can see that the voxel belonging to the border has different characteristic profile than the voxel belonging to the colon wall what allows to distinguish them and remove the border voxel.
Exemplary results from application of the proposed algorithm for electronic colon cleansing are shown in figure 5.

4. Segmentation

Data visualization methods like surface or volume rendering can be used for showing inner structure of the colon. However, inspection of the visualized data requires manual virtual camera movement which make smooth observation difficult. Segmented data may be used for creation of the automatic navigation path for the virtual camera. If we display only segmented structure, we can reduce the time required for visualization. Combined visualization and segmentation algorithms allows for development of 3D models of anatomical structures (fig. 6). Additionally, structures that are external to the colon can be viewed, which improves the assessment of the pathological lesions.

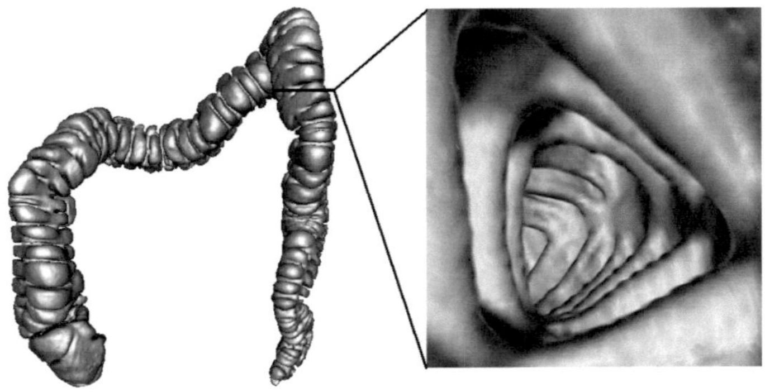

Fig. 6. Colon after segmentation process (Skalski et al., 2007a)

The human abdomen consists mainly of three regions: air, soft tissues and high density materials (bones) and this is reflected by voxels values. Thresholding represents the simplest approach to abdomen segmentation but has many disadvantages, e.g. it does not remove partial volume voxels. For example, voxels near the edge of objects are incorrectly classified when thresholding is used. Therefore, in the VC, segmentation is usually based on region growing (Vilanova et al., 1999; Xie et al., 2003, Sadleir & Whelan, 2005) or active contour methods (Jiang et al., 2005). The idea of the region growing technique is linking thresholding procedure with neighbourhood checking. In first iteration, the algorithm checks membership condition for all voxels of the neighbourhood of voxel being classified. If the voxels pass the membership condition test which can be the same as in classical thersholding procedure, the voxels are added to the object. In next iterations, this process is repeated for all voxels added in the previous iteration until no new voxel can be added. It allows for local operation in contrast to thresholding. Even if in the dataset there are voxels which can pass membership condition, they will not be classified as the object if they have no connection with voxels added before.

Different strategy is applied in the method of active contours, called also "snakes", proposed by Kass et al. (Kass et al., 1988). The active contours method is a segmentation technique in which the problem of object finding in the analyzed data is formulated as energy minimisation. It is usually calculated in iterative routine where contour evaluation is guided by external constraint forces and influenced by image forces that pull the contour towards lines and edges present in the data. The total energy consists of the internal and the external energies which are responsible, respectively, for contour behaviour and image influence. The active contours method is a parametric technique which is susceptible to parameter tuning and this is a one of its main disadvantages. But even then classification of voxels lying near the colon wall is a source of problems.

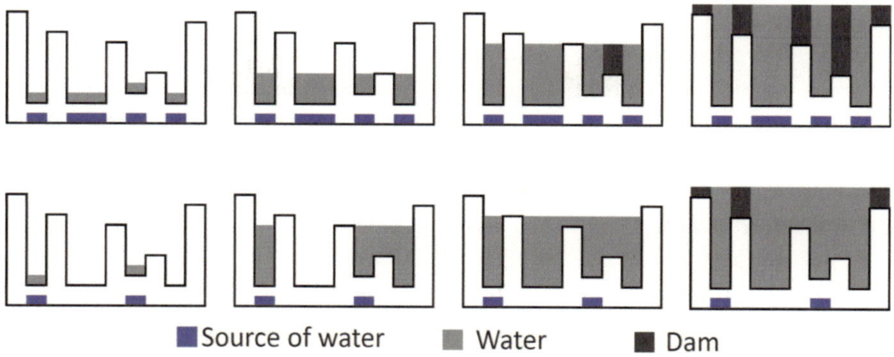

Fig. 7. Idea of the watershed algorithm; First row: classic watershed; Second row: marker-based watershed; description in the text

The 3D segmentation algorithm based on immersion-based watershed method of Vincent and Soille (Vincent & Soille, 1991) can be also applied. The watershed method exploits topographic and hydrology concepts for the development of region segmentation methods. The image may be seen as a topographic relief, in which the value of a pixel (for 2D images) is interpreted as its altitude in the relief. In case of 2D, the principle of watershed algorithm can be illustrated by an idea of immersing the image from water sources. When the neighbouring catchment basins eventually meet, a dam is created to avoid the water spilling from one basin into the other (Vincent & Soille, 1991). When the water reaches the maximum value, the edges of the union of all dams form the watershed segmentation results (fig. 7). In case of 3D, usage of the algorithm leads to receiving 3D objects separated by the dam. If we use local minima of the image as water sources, oversegmentation problem will appear. In consequence, we receive a huge number of objects in the resultant matrix which do not correspond to data.

One of the solutions is a modified strategy of source selection. We used marker-based Watershed transform, where the immersion processes are started from markers computed from the image.

In order to improve results, the absolute value of gradient of the filtered data (fig. 8) is computed using the 3D Sobel's mask and then the data are immersed by the watershed algorithm.

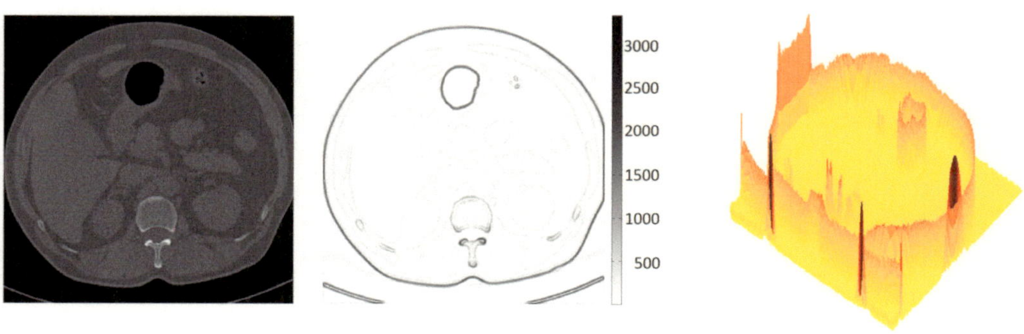

Fig. 8. From left to right: slice of a CT data; Absolute value of the gradient; Gradient visualisation as a topography map

Neubauer et al. (Neubauer et al., 2002) proposed manual placing of markers inside the data. On the contrary, we use automatic methods for markers computation: object markers are obtained from voxels after thresholding operation. We know that voxels having intensity below 300 units represent air, and background markers are voxels which have intensity value corresponding to tissues. This approach eliminates the oversegmentation problem.
The 3D watershed segmentation algorithm computes border between the colon and the soft tissue using the gradient map (fig. 8) calculated as:

$$G_{MOD}(x,y,z) = \sqrt{I_x^2 + I_y^2 + I_z^2} \tag{4}$$

where I_x, I_y and I_z are image gradients in x, y and z directions, respectively.
Thanks to these operations, the colon model, which is traced, reflects details very precisely what we can observe in figure 6.

5. Calculation of navigation path

Fast and accurate navigation path generation is essential for efficient diagnosis using the VC since it allows for simulation of the virtual camera movement inside the segmented structure and the whole colon can be screened by the physician in a short time. The virtual camera can be stopped if a suspicious image is discovered for more careful assessment.
Computation of the colon centerline is not a trivial process. The algorithm should require only minimum operator intervention. Additionally, a centreline approximation of the centre navigation path of the colon must be obtained in reasonable time with acceptable accuracy. Time constraint is a very important factor to evaluate the algorithm especially in a clinical practice.

5.1 State of the art

Centreline calculation methods can be subdivided into three categories since they are mainly based on:

- manual extraction,
- topological thinning (e.g. Xie et al., 2003; Sadleir & Whelan, 2005),
- distance transform (e.g Vilanova et al., 1999).

Manual extraction requires manual identification of the centre of colon slices. It does not guarantee that marked points lie in the centres of slices and that they are directly connected. Furthermore, the allocation is difficult because the colon centreline is oriented in different directions.
Methods based on topological thinning and distance transform are automatic usually. The idea of topological thinning is based on peeling off the colon surface points using morphological operations repeatedly until the centreline is obtained. Though the results of this standard algorithm are well-defined they do not always lie in a proper place. Additionally, the algorithm is extremely inefficient computationally. Therefore, other methods were developed that use 3D topological thinning and graph search algorithm (Ge et al. 1999), optimized 3D topological thinning using Look-up Table (Sadleir & Whelan, 2005), distance transform (Zhou & Toga 1999, Van Uitert and Bitter 2007), minimum energy path (Deschamps and Cohen 2001) or Dijkstra's shortest path algorithm (Bitter et al. 2000).

Some approaches rely on the use of the distance transform. In these methods, the centreline is calculated as a maximum of binary mask representing colon after the distance transformation.
Below an exemplary algorithm of the VC navigation path calculation is presented.

5.2 Exemplary algorithm based on distance transform

In this section we present the colon centreline calculation algorithm based on the distance transform (Skalski et al., 2007b). As an input to the algorithm, the matrix with labelled voxels (label L represents the colon) resulting from the segmentation process is used. The author's algorithm of the colon centreline calculation consists of the steps presented in table 1.

- compute complement IL of the binary mask L (1 – colon, 0 – others)
- choose N, number of points that you want to generate inside the colon
- *iter*=0 (number of iteration)
- **while** (*iter* < N+1) **do**:
  - *iter++*
  - compute distance transform on IL
  - find maximal value *maxD* of the distance transform
  - save location of *maxD*, path $(x_{iter}, y_{iter}, z_{iter})$
  - set sphere to IL (value=1; centre=$(x_{iter}, y_{iter}, z_{iter})$; radius=*maxD*)
- **end**

  as a result we receive points saved in the matrix path (3x*Ndim*)
- sort the path:
  - find a point which has a minimal value of z coordinate or mark a starting point; replace the first point of the path with the starting point; mark this point
  - **for** (i=1 to N-2) **do**:
    - compute the distance between the last marked point path(i) and each other not marked point:
    - find minimal distance d_j based on equation 4 and save its coordinates (x_j, y_j, z_j)
    - replace path($i+1$) and path(j)
    - mark path($i+1$)
  - end
- compute interpolating cubic spline

Table 1. Navigation path calculation algorithm

Firstly, complement of the binary mask resulting from the segmentation process is done. It is a preparation step for the distance transform calculation. The distance transform returns as a result distance to the nearest voxel which belongs to the colon. In order to calculate the distance, the Euclidian metric is usually used:

$$d_{ij} = \sqrt{\left(x_i - x_j\right)^2 + \left(y_i - y_j\right)^2 + \left(z_i - z_j\right)^2} \ . \qquad (5)$$

Maximum value *maxD* is taken from the resultant matrix. It is a point inside the colon in the widest place. Then, spherical neighbourhood of this point is removed. It prevents algorithms from finding next points very close to points found before. This process is repeated in iterative manner. The points received in the previous step become knots of the navigation path. Subsequently, points received from the algorithm are sorted. Finally, points between knots are generated using b-spline cubic interpolation. Exemplary navigation path is presented in figure 9.

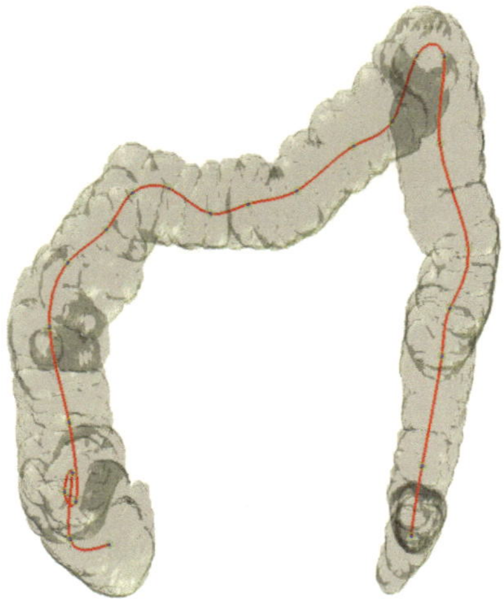

Fig. 9. The colon after the segmentation process with a centreline, number of points $N = 24$

6. Visualisation

The final step in the Virtual Colonoscopy is the data visualization. There are two main methods of 3D medical data visualization: indirect (surface rendering) and direct (volume rendering) (Preim & Bartz, 2007). Both techniques can use fully programmable graphical pipeline.

Surface rendering is one of the indirect methods. This technique produces surfaces in the domain of the scalar quantity. Scalar values, contained in 3D medical data, represents tissue properties, like radiodensity in Hounsfield scale or label mask that contains segmentation results. Surface represents a specific scalar value, the so-called isosurface value. In fact, one iso-surface describes only one scalar value. The interior of the object is not described – surface is the boundary of the volume objects. Surface rendering method includes two stages: generation of the 3D surface from 3D data and proper visualisation relying on the image generation by graphics accelerator. There are numerous methods for implementing the surfaces from a discrete set of 3D data (Preim & Bartz, 2007). One of the most useful is the Marching Cubes algorithm (Lorensen & Cline, 1987). This algorithm has many implementations that solve the problem of ambiguities in first cell triangulation method (holes in surface). Possibly the widely used implementation of the Marching Cubes algorithm comes from The Visualization Toolkit (Schroeder et al., 2004). In the algorithm a polygonal mesh of the isosurface is generated from the 3D scalar field. The polygonal mesh is a collection of vertices (points in 3D) connected to triangles. For high resolution data sets the number of generated graphical primitives can be extremely high. To reduce the number of triangles, the mesh can be decimated or smoothed (Schroeder et al., 1992 and 2004).

Surface can be coloured according to the isosurface value or to another scalar field using a texture mapping technique. To increase the perception of the surface shape in the VC visualization, the virtual lighting is used. The standard model in the OpenGL Application Programming Interface is Phong illumination model (Phong, 1975). This is an empirical model of local illumination. It describes the way a surface reflects the light as a combination of the diffuse reflection of rough surfaces with the specular reflection of shiny surfaces. Phong shading includes a model for the reflection of light from surfaces and a compatible method of estimating pixel colours by interpolating surface normals across rasterized polygons. In fact, at each point of the screen full Phong model calculations are performed (per-pixel lighting). Since the interpolation of surface normals is computationally expensive, the Phong shading is slow. In Gouraud shading algorithm the calculating lighting is performed only in vertex. Next, the screen pixel colour on the triangle are bilinearly interpolated from the vertex colour. This method is fast, but the specular highlight will not be rendered correctly if a highlight lies in the middle of a polygon. This limitation can be solved by increasing a number of triangles by mesh tessellation or by increasing of spatial data resolution. The polygonal data can be efficiently processed in modern graphics card. All shading calculations are done in hardware.

Volume rendering is the process of creating a 2D image directly from 3D volumetric data that operates on the actual data sample without creation of intermediate surfaces consisting of triangles (Preim & Bartz, 2007). The purpose of volume rendering is to effectively convey information present within the volumetric data. It is especially important in case of medical data. All direct volume rendering algorithms can be classified into two main groups: object-space and image-space methods. However, many advanced algorithms cannot by easily classified as one or the other, but fuse aspects from both groups into one hybrid algorithm.

Object-space volume rendering techniques use forward mapping scheme where the data is mapped onto the image plane. One of such approach is the Splatting algorithm that projects the data voxels onto image-plane (Westover, 1989). Texture-mapping algorithms are the other widely used object-oriented algorithms. They are supported by computer graphics hardware. In image-order (image-space) algorithms, a backward mapping scheme is used where rays are cast from each pixel in the image plane through the volume data to determine the final pixel colour. The classic direct volume rendering method is the image-space oriented ray casting algorithm. Moreover, some algorithms use domain-base techniques – the spatial volume data is first transformed into an alternative domain, such as frequency or wavelet, and then a projection is generated directly from this domain (Malzbender, 1993).

Modern graphics cards are characterized by immense ability of 3D data processing. They are developed and optimized for processing triangle meshes, which are used for surface rendering. Furthermore, a fully programmable graphics processing unit (GPU) offer new opportunities to use graphics cards for general purpose computing, especially for volume rendering. Ray-casting volume rendering using CPUs is computationally expensive since it requires the interpolation and shading calculations for every sample point along the ray in the data. Interactive volume ray casting was previously restricted to high-end workstations. GPU implementations of ray-casting rendering approaches have received great attention since they enable interactive visualization of volumetric data (Lee et al., 2009).

The most important in virtual colonoscopy visualization is trustworthy surface presentation. In figure 10, examples of applying different rendering methods are shown. The fastest method in interactive visualization is the surface rendering. Unfortunately, the triangle structure of reconstructed surface has an influence on image quality. The colour interpolation (diamond artefact) are visible. Surface in image generated by the direct volume visualization has better quality (fig. 10 b-d). The shape of wrinkles is kept. However, the computational cost is considerably larger. The texture-mapping technique, supported by the GPU acceleration, can be used in interactive visualization. Unfortunately, this method generates images which contain staircase artefacts caused by interpolation and insufficient depth sampling (fig. 10.d).

To extend the field of view in virtual colonoscopy the multi-cameras are used, especially for visual inspection of the colon wall (Serlie I. et al. 2001). The six cameras are located in the same place, but the view directions are different. They are rotated around, to cover 360 degree of view. Each camera has the 90 degree field of view. Images of this cameras can be mapped into the unrolled-box surface. The sample of this technique is shown in the figure 11. Additionally, the light source moves along with the camera and the position of light source is the same as camera position. The light is configured as positional (headlight), and the cone angle corresponds to camera cone angle. To prevent overexposing nearest surfaces, the irregular light intensity along the cone angle was used. Light fading attenuation was used for distance simulation.

Comparison between real colonoscopic image and virtual one is presented in figure 12.

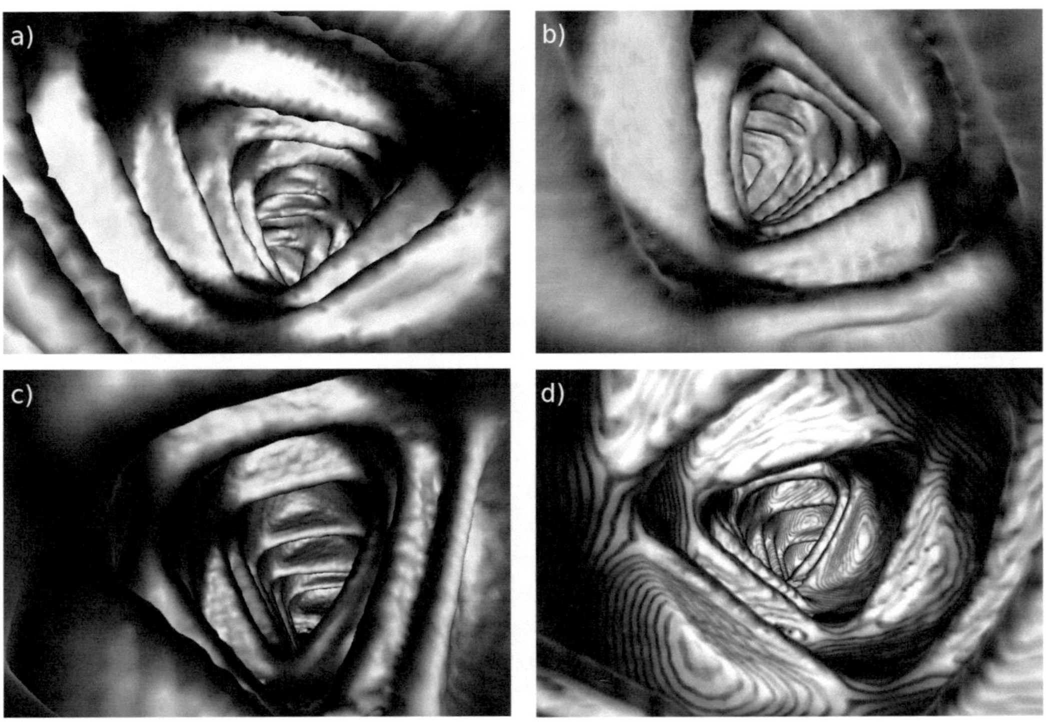

Fig. 10. Exemplary virtual colonography images: a) surface rendering, b) volume rendering by ray-casting, c) isosurface in volume rendering (ray-casting) and d) texture-mapping volume rendering

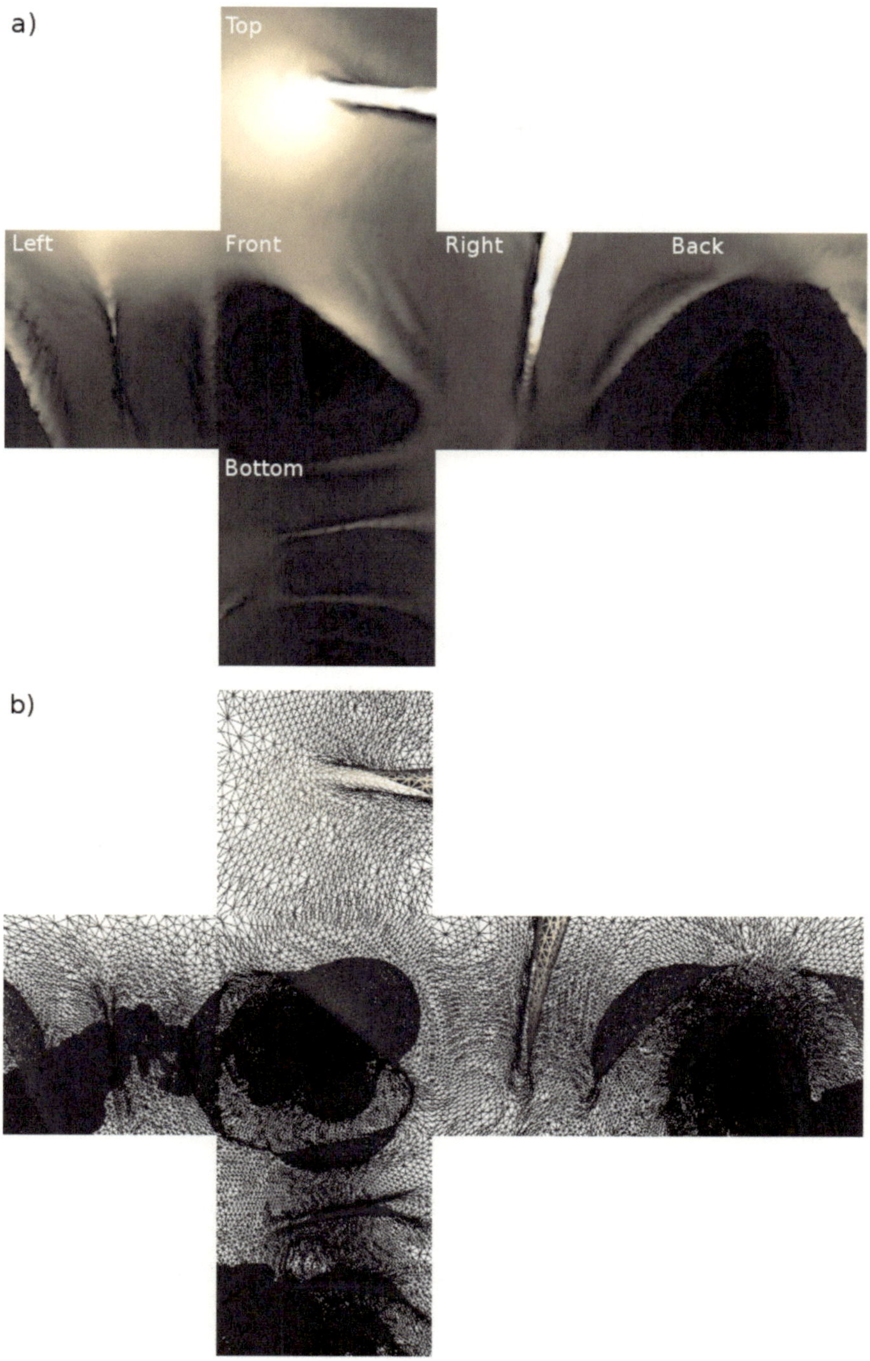

Fig. 11. Extended field of view in virtual colonoscopy by using six cameras: a) surface rendering and b) surface mesh visualization

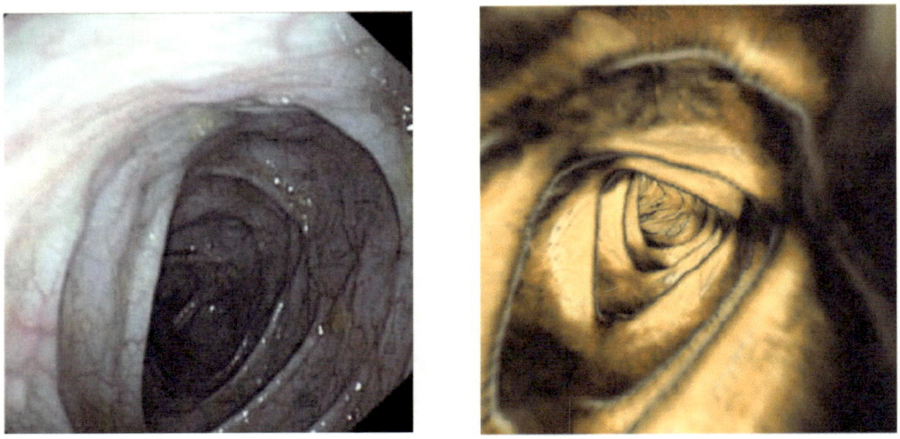

(a) (b)

Fig. 12. a) real endoscopic image, b) virtual colonoscopy image (Bulat et al., 2007).

7. Conclusion

In this chapter virtual colonoscopy has been presented from the point of view of computational sciences. Problems present in the VC software realization have been pointed out and their existing solutions have been cited. For clearity of presentation, to help a reader to understand merits of technical issues associated with the VC, simple examples of computer algorithms have been given, mainly developed by the authors of the chapter. Special attention has been paid to the following technical aspects: electronic colon cleansing, colon lumen segmentation, navigation path calculation and modern 3D visualisation.

8. References

Bitter I., et al. (2000). CEASAR: a smooth, accurate and robust centerline extraction algorithm, *Proceedings of IEEE Visualization 2000,* ISBN 0-7803-6478-3, Salt Lake City, UT, USA, October 2000.

Bulat J., et al. (2007). Data Processing Tasks in Wireless GI Endoscopy: Image-Based Capsule Localization & Navigation and Video Compression. *29th Annual International Conference of the IEEE Engineering in Medicine and Biology Society, 2007. EMBS 2007.* ISBN 978-1-4244-0787-3, pp. 2815 - 2818, Lyon, France, August 2007.

Cai W., et al. (2010). Mosaic decomposition: An Electronic cleansing method for inhomogeneously tagged regions in noncathartic CT colonography. *IEEE Transaction on Medical Imaging,* Vol. 30, No. 3, (March 2011), pp. 559-574, ISSN 0278-0062.

Chen D., et al. (2000). A novel approach to extract colon lumen from CT images for virtual colonoscopy. *IEEE Transaction on Medical Imaging,* Vol. 19, No. 12, (December 2000), pp. 1220-1226, ISSN 0278-0062.

DCMTK - DICOM Toolkit,

http://dicom.offis.de/dcmtk.php.en, accessed on April 2, 2011

Deschamps T. & Cohen L. D. (2001). Fast extraction of minimal paths in 3-D images and applications to virtual endoscopy *Medical Image Analysis,* Vol. 5, No. 4, (December 2001) pp. 281 - 289, ISSN 1361-8415.

DICOM - Digital Imaging and Communications in Medicine, *http://medical.nema.org/*, accessed on April 1, 2011

Florie J., et al. (2007). MR colonography with limited bowel preparation compared with optical colonoscopy in patients at increased risk for colorectal cancer. *Radiology.* Vol. 243, No. 1, (December 2007), pp. 122-131, ISSN 1527-1315.

Frentz S.M. & Summers R.M. (2006). Current Status of CT Colonography. *Academic Radiology,* Vol. 13, No. 12, (December 2006), pp. 1517-1531, ISSN: 1076-6332.

GDCM - Grassroots DICOM library, *http://sourceforge.net/apps/mediawiki/gdcm,* accessed on March 25, 2011.

Ge Y., et al. (1999). Computing the centerline of a colon: a robust and efficient method based on 3D skeletons, *Journal of Computer Assisted Tomography.* Vol. 23, No. 5, (September- October 1999) pp. 786–794, ISSN 0363-8715

Graser A., et al. (2009). Comparison of CT colonography, colonoscopy, sigmoidoscopy and fecal occult blood tests for the detection of advanced adenomas in an average risk population. *Gut,* Vol. 58, No. 2, (October 2008), pp. 241-248, ISSN 1468-3288.

Hong L. et al. (1996). Visible Human Virtual Colonoscopy. *Conference of National Library of Medicine Visible Human Project,* pp. 29-30, October 1996.

Hong L. et al. (1997). Virtual Voyage: Interactive Navigation in the Human Colon. *Proceedings of the 24th annual conference on Computer graphics and interactive techniques, ACM SIGGRAPH'97,* ISBN:0-89791-896-7, pp. 27-34, August 1997.

Iannaccone R., et al. (2004). Computed tomography colonography without cathartic preparation for the detection of colorectal polyps. *Gastroenterology,* Vol. 127, No. 5, (November 2004), pp. 1300-1311, ISSN 0016-5085.

Jiang R.; Berliner L. & Meng J (2005). Computer graphics enhancements in CT Colography for improved diagnosis and navigation. *International Congress Series: CARS 2005: Computer Assisted Radiology and Surgery,* Vol. 1281, ISSN 0531-5131, pp. 109-114. May 2005.

Kak A. C. & Slaney M. (1988). Principles of Computerized Tomographic Imaging. *IEEE Press,* ISBN 0-87942-198-3, New York, NY, USA, also available from http://www.slaney.org/pct/pct-toc.html.

Kass M., Witkin A &, Terzopoulos D. (1988). Snakes: Active contour models. *International Journal on Computer Vision,* Vol. 1, No. 4, (January 1988), pp. 321-331, ISSN 1573-1405.

Lakare S., et al. (2002). Electronic Colon Cleansing using Segmentation Rays for Virtual Colonoscopy. *Proceedings of SPIE Medical Imaging - Physiology and Function from Multidimensional Images.* Vol. 4683, ISBN 9-78081944-428-8, pp. 412-418, April 2002.

Lakare S., et al. (2003). Robust colon residue detection using vector quantization based classification for virtual colonoscopy. *Proceedings of SPIE, Medical Imaging 2003: Physiology and Function: Methods, Systems, and Applications,* Vol. 5031, ISBN 9-78081944-832-3 ,pp. 515-520, May 2003.

Levin B., et al. (2008). Screening and surveillance for the early detection of colorectal cancer and adenomatous polypos, 2008: a joint guideline from the American Cancer Society, the US Multi-Society Task Force on Colorectal Cancer, and the American College of Radiology. *Gastroenterology* Vol. 134, No. 5, (May 2008), pp. 1570-1595, ISSN 1528-0012.

Lee T.-H., et al. (2009) Fast perspective volume ray casting method using GPU-based acceleration techniques for translucency rendering in 3D endoluminal CT colonography, *Computers in Biology and Medicine*, Vol. 39, No. 8, (August 2009), pp. 657-666, ISSN 1879-0534.

Lorensen W.E. & Cline H.E. (1987). Marching Cubes: A high resolution 3D surface construction algorithm. *ACM SIGGRAPH Computer Graphics*, Vol. 21, No. 4, (July 1987), pp. 163-169, ISSN:0097-8930.

Malzbender T. (1993). Fourier volume rendering. *ACM Transactions on Graphics* Vol. 12, No. 3, (July 1993), pp. 233–250, ISSN:0730-0301.

Neubauer A., et al. (2002). Fast and Flexible Iso-Surfacing for Virtual Endoscopy. *Proceedings of the sixth Central European Seminar on Computer Graphics CESCG*. Budmerice, Slovakia, April 22-24, 2002, http://old.vrvis.at/TR/2002/TR_VRVis_2002_013_Full.pdf

Pickhardt P.J.; Taylor A.J. & Gopal D.V. (2006). Surface Visualization at 3D Endoluminac CT Colonography: Degree of Coverage and Implications for Polyp Detection. *Gastroenterology*. Vol. 130, No. 6 (May 2006) pp. 1582-1587, ISSN 0016-5085.

Phong B.-T. (1975). Illumination for computer generated pictures. *Communications of ACM* Vol. 18, No. 6, (June 1975), pp. 311–317, ISSN 0001-0782.

Preim B. & Bartz D. (2007). Visualization in Medicine: Theory, Algorithms, and Applications (The Morgan Kaufmann Series in Computer Graphics). (1 ed.) *Morgan Kaufmann Publishers Inc.*, ISBN 9-78012370-596-9, San Francisco, CA, USA.

Regge D., et al. (2009). Diagnostic accuracy of computed tomographic colonography for the detection of advance neoplasia in individuals at increased risk of colorectal cancer. *JAMA*, Vol. 301, No. 23, (June 2009), pp. 2453-2461, ISSN 1538-3598.

Sadleir R. & Whelan P. (2005). Fast colon centreline calculation using optimised 3D topological thinning. *Computerized Medical Imaging and Graphics*. Vol. 29, No. 4, (December 2004), pp. 251-258, ISSN 0895-6111.

Schroeder W., Zarge J., & Lorensen W. (1992). Decimation of triangle meshes, *ACM SIGGRAPH Computer Graphics*, Vol. 26, No. 2, (July 1992), pp.65-70, ISSN 0097-8930.

Schroeder W., Martin K. & Lorensen B. (2006). Visualization Toolkit: An Object-Oriented Approach to 3D Graphics. (4th ed.) *Kitware*, ISBN 1-930934-19-X .

Serlie I, et al. (2001). Maximizing Surface Visibility in Virtual Colonoscopy. *ASCI 2001 Proceedings of the Seventh Annual Conference of Advanced School for Computing and Imaging*. ISBN 90-803086-6-8, *Heijen, The Netherlands*, pp. 196-201, May/June 2001.

Serlie I, et al. (2010). Electronic cleansing for computed tomography (CT) colonography using a scale-invariant three-material model. *IEEE Transactions on Biomedical Engineering*, Vol. 57, No. 6, (June 2010), pp. 1306-1317, ISSN 0018-9294.

Sezille N.; Sadleir R. & Whelan P.F. (2003). Automated synthesis, insertion and detection of polyps for CT colonography. *Opto-Ireland 2002, Proceedings of the SPIE,* Vol. 4877, ISBN 9-78081944-658-9, Galway, Ireland, pp. 183-191, September 2002.

Skalski A., et al. (2007a). Colon cleansing for virtual colonoscopy using non-linear transfer function and morphological operations. *Proceedings of the 2007 IEEE international workshop on Imaging systems and techniques.* ISBN 1-4244-0965-9, Krakow, Poland, pp. 1-5, May 2007.

Skalski A., et al. (2007b). CT data processing and visualization aspects of virtual colonoscopy. *EUSIPCO 2007, 15th European signal processing conference,* ISBN 978-83-921340-2-2, Poznań, Poland, pp. 2509–2513, September 2007.

Summers R, et al. (2005). Computer-aided detection of polyps on oral contrast-enhanced CT colonography. *American Journal Roentgenology,* Vol. 184, No. 1, (January 2005) pp. 105-108, ISSN 0361-803X.

The Visible Human Project. U.S. National Library of Medicine *http://www.nlm.nih.gov/research/visible/visible_human.html,* accessed on April 2, 2011.

Wang Z., et al. (2006). An improved electronic colon cleansing method for detection of colonic polyps by virtual colonoscopy. *IEEE Transaction on Biomedical Engineering,* Vol. 53, No. 8, (August 2006), pp. 1635-1646, ISSN 0018-9294.

Wang J., et al. (2008). Virtual Colonoscopy Screening With Ultra Low-Dose CT and Less-Stressful Bowel Preparation: A Computer Simulation Study. *IEEE Transactions on Nuclear Science,* Vol. 55, No.5, (October 2008), pp. 2566-2575, ISSN 0018-9499.

Wax M., et al. (1998). Electronic colon cleansing for virtual colonoscopy. *Proc. 1st Symposium on Virtual Colonoscopy,* Boston, USA, pp. 94-94, 1998.

Van Uitert R.L. & Bitter I., (2007). Subvoxel precise skeletons of volumetric data based on fast marching methods, *Medical Physics,* Vol. 34, No. 2, (January 2007), pp. 627–638, ISSN 0094-2405.

Van Uitert R.L. et al. (2008). Temporal and multiinstitutional quality assessment of CT Colonography. *American Journal of Roentegenology* Vol. 191, No. 5, (November 2008) pp. 1503-1504, ISSN 1546-3141.

Vilanova A.; König A & Gröller E. (1999). VirEn: A Virtual Endoscopy System. *Machine Graphics & Vision.* Vol. 8 No. 3, (1999),pp. 469-487, ISSN 1230-0535.

Vincent L. & Soille P. (1991). Watersheds in digital spaces: An efficient algorithm based on immersion simulations. *IEEE Transactions on Pattern Analysis and Machine Intelligence.* Vol. 13, No. 6, (June 1991), pp. 583-598, ISSN 0162-8828.

VTK – Visualzation Toolkit, *http://www.vtk.org,* accessed on April 2, 2011.

Xie W.; Thompson R.P. & Perucchio R. (2003). A topology-preserving parallel 3D thinning algorithm for extracting the curve skeleton. *Pattern Recognition,* Vol. 36, No. 7, (July 2003), pp. 1529-1544, ISSN 0031-3203.

Yoshida H. et al. (2002) . Computer-aided Diagnosis Scheme for Detection of Polyps at CT Colonography. *Radiographics,* Vol. 22, No. 4, (July/August 2002), pp. 963- 979. ISSN 0271-5333.

Zalis M.E., Perumpillichira J. & Hahn P.F. (2004). Digital substraction bowel cleansing for CT colonography using morphological and linear filtration methods. *IEEE*

Transactions on Medical Imaging, Vol. 23, No. 11, (November 2004), pp. 1335-1343, ISSN 0278-0062.

Zhou Y. & Toga A.W., (1999). Efficient skeletonization of volumetric objects. *IEEE Transactions on Visualization and Computer Graphics,*, Vol. 5, No. 3, (July - September 1999) pp. 196–209, ISSN 1077-2626.

18

Robotic Colonoscopy

Felice Cosentino[1], Emanuele Tumino[2], Giovanni Rubis Passoni[3], Antonella Rigante[1], Roberta Barbera[1], Antonella Tauro[1] and Philipp Emanuel Cosentino[4]
[1]*San Giuseppe Hospital, Milan*
[2]*Pisana University Hospital, Pisa*
[3]*San Carlo Borromeo Hospital*
[4]*Veterinary Medicine, University of Milan*
Italy

1. Introduction

This chapter is focused on emerging robotic techniques for improving conventional colonoscopy.

Video-colonoscopy is considered the gold-standard for the diagnosis of colonic diseases, and it is included as first line choice in colon-rectum cancer screening program in high-risk populations. However, this diagnostic technique shows some technical limitations, such as invasiveness and patient discomfort, which limit the adherence to the procedure.

To facilitate the conventional colonoscopy procedure, robotic colonoscopy solutions have been proposed. State of the art of robotic colonoscopy has been thus summarized. In details, Endotics System and Invendoscope are presented.

The *Endotics System* is composed of a disposable probe and a workstation. The probe has a steerable tip, a flexible body and a thin tail. The head hosts both a vision system and channels for water jet and air in order to provide rinsing and suction/insufflation, respectively. The workstation allows the endoscopist to fully control the disposable probe by means of a hand-held console and to visualize on a screen real time images. The operator can steer the head of the robotic colonoscope in every direction, elongate the body of the probe in order to move it forward following the shape of the intestine, and control rinsing, insufflation and suction. This technology thanks its extremely flexible and disposable probe is highly safe and painless (Cosentino et Al, 2009).

The *Invendoscope*, a single-use, combines a flexible endoscope and the proprietary "inverted sleeve" technology that enables a potentially safe and sedactionless colonoscopy. The instrument is steered by a hand-held device and propelled by a motorized drive unit.

Limitations and advantages of the two devices are reported compared to conventional colonoscopy. In the last part of the chapter are presented data of pilot studies both in healthy volunteers and patients in terms of technical aspects (cecal intubation, pain score, sedation) and clinical results (lesions detection).

2. Why and how robotic systems in colonoscopy?

The first colonoscopy procedures go back to the 1960's, when in Japan a device for the examination of the left colon was developed (Niwa et Al, 1969). In the 1970's further progresses were made, and colonoscopy devices able to explore the whole colon were available (Classen et Al., 2010).

Since then, research efforts were focused towards improvements of the vision system, of the degrees of flexibility and of the localization systems. Nevertheless, the main characteristics of the devices, based on a CCD camera or a fiber optic camera on a flexible tube passed through the anus, remained unchanged till the 1990's. In those years, robotic technologies grew up enough to allow an increasing number of robots to be realized and used in various fields of medicine. The main reasons for including colonoscopy were to try to overcome the existing limitations of the standard devices, quite rigid, requiring high experience of the doctor to perform difficult maneuvers to proceed along the tortuous colon walls, and constructed of materials that could be damaged by heat, pressure, and moisture used during the decontamination processes. (Sturges & Laowattana, 1993) The stated above limitations made, and still make, standard colonoscopy a quite invasive technique, with risks related to perforation, sedation and cross-infections, far for being accepted by massive percentages of patients as needed in colorectal cancer screening programs. Screening as a matter of fact can find non-cancerous colorectal polyps and remove them before they become cancerous. If colorectal cancer does occur, early detection and treatment dramatically increase chances of survival. The relative 5-year survival rate for colorectal cancer when diagnosed at an early stage before it has spread is about 90%, but since screening rates are low, less than 40% of colorectal cancers are found early. Once the cancer has spread to nearby organs or lymph nodes, the 5-year relative survival rate goes down, and if cancer has spread to distant organs (like the liver or lung) the rate is about 11%, and as many as 60% of deaths from colorectal cancer could be prevented if everyone age 50 and older were screened regularly.

Moreover, painless colonoscopy, besides being a remarkable achievement for the patient, and avoiding any risk related to sedation, has major fallout in terms of prevention. As matter of fact, colonoscopy could be largely used for screening purposes of healthy and asymptomatic patients, less willing to feel pain because of an invasive procedure. Nowadays, colonoscopy is used as screening test just in first-level demonstrative studies and pilot projects. One of the main limitations to use this survey as primary screening, besides the feasibility related to allocation of facilities and complications rates, is the acceptance of the procedure. Participation in the first-level FOB (faecal occult blood) screening test is always above 50% (Faivre et Al., 2004), while the few available data in literature about compliance to colonoscopy as primary screening is in a range from 15% to 90% (Swaroop et Al., 2002). Compliance for second level screening programs, which in principle should be very high since this second examination takes place after positive results of the first one, is in a range from 30 to 60%, as reported in a study of from AIGO - Oncology Group Study.

For the above listed reasons, it appears clear how big can be the impact, in terms of survival rate, of new devices able to perform painless and safe diagnostic colonoscopic procedures. Thus robotics, as a science that tries to find and develop methodologies that enable machines to perform specific tasks, could make the difference in developing endoscopes that pulled themselves, with no risk for stretching the colonic wall outward and causing painful cramps. The main challenge to building such devices involved clutching onto the slippery walls of the colon in a way that did not damage them. The new endoscopes had to be disposable, highly flexible, with a particularly suited internal locomotion, and with a direct vision of the colon tissue, to solve acceptance problems and maintain quality of gold standard.

2.1 Robotic colonoscopy: state of the art

As for robotic colonoscopy, first studies go back to 1995, with the locomotion system "inch-worm". Subsequently, a lot of research work was carried out aiming at devising several robotic colonoscopes based on different types of locomotion such as "snake", "earthworm", "continuum" and "caterpillar", or other different concepts.

The Inchworm robots were inspired to the caterpillar Geometridae, whose mode of locomotion is to firmly attach the rear portion of its body to a surface via its foot pads, extending the remainder of its body forward, attaching it to the surface and bridging the rear part of its body to meet the forward part. On this principle is based the Endotics system. (Slatkin et Al., 1995)

The **Endotics System** is composed of a sterile, disposable probe and a workstation. The probe has a head, a steerable tip and a flexible body. The head hosts both a vision system and channels for water jet and air. The locomotion is achieved by two clampers that are located in the proximal and distal part of the probe. The proximal clamper adheres to the mucosa and the central part of the body is elongated; the distal clamper adheres to the mucosa and the proximal clamper is released; the central part of the body is contracted so that the proximal clamper may adhere to the mucosa; and finally, the distal clamp is released. The sequence is repeated several times allowing the probe to move in a worm-like fashion. (Perri et Al., 2010)

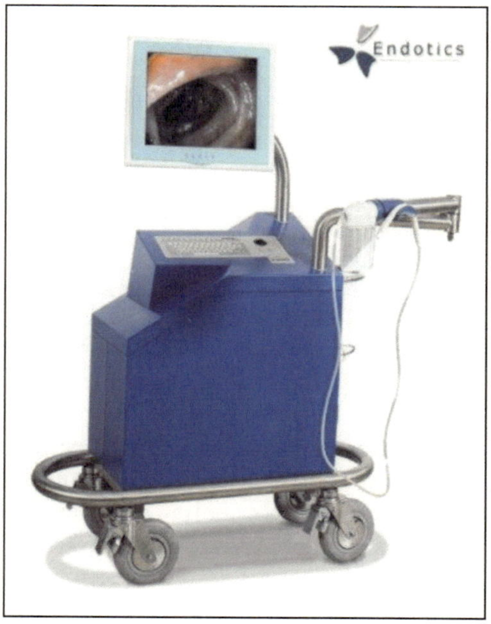

Fig. 1. Endotics Workstation and disposable probe

The Snake robots took inspiration from the sinuous movement of the snake, based on the temporal shifting of positions and angles of subsequent parts of its body. Movements starts from the head that, bending and moving forward, is able to avoid obstacles. In robotics, this is translated in devices with a finite number of independent segments where, during the progress, the position and the angle of the distal part is encoded by an algorithm and then associated with the next segment. All segments are associated with the same geometrical parameters of the previous segment. NES, the NeoGuide System is based on this principle of functioning.

The **NeoGuide Endoscopy System** (NES) has many features in common with standard colonoscopes. In addition to these, there is a "tip position sensor" that continually records the tip–steering commands of the endoscopist, and an external position sensor placed at the anus that records the insertion depth of the colonoscope. The scope also contains additional control elements in multiple segments following the tip of the scope. Each segment is the same basic length as the tip segment itself, and the orientation of each segment is separately controlled by the system's computer. The NES combines data on the depth of insertion of the scope and the orientation of the tip at each depth, to actively articulate each segment so that the scope follows the natural shape of the colon. The insertion tube is advanced manually into the colon and has a conventional CCD for visualization. The device includes a handle air insufflation7suction and rinsing systems similar to conventional scopes. (Eickhoff et Al. 2006)

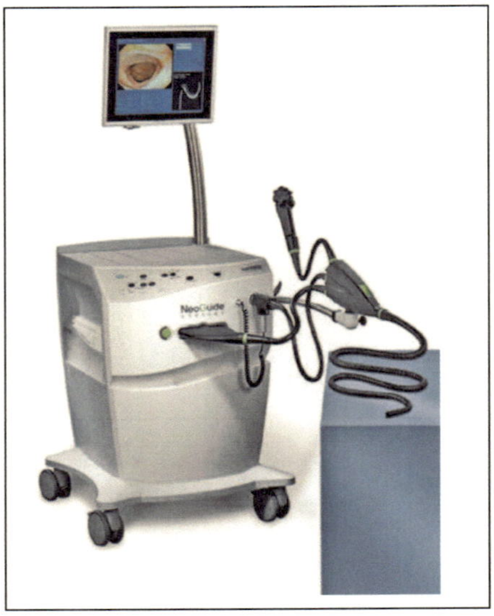

Fig. 2. NeoGuide Endoscopic device

Peristalsis motion like an earthworm has attracted attention because the movement is useful to progress in small spaces (Saito et Al., 2009). The Earthworm robots were based on the earthworm's locomotion, thus moving not only changing length, but also changing thickness (Zuo et Al., 2005). The Continuum robots worked according to the moving principle of the elephant trunk or the tongue, i.e. structures without rigid constraints able to perform complex movements (Hu et Al., 2009). Finally, the Caterpillar robots were characterized by wheels and caterpillar tracks and their locomotion was similar to a tank.

Other technique of locomotion not based on bio-mimicking, but having relations with robotics in terms of sensors or automated movements have been developed (Swain, 2009).
The **Aer-O-Scope system**, is a disposable, self-propelling, self-navigating, endoscope incorporating a CMOS camera with "omni-directional viewing system".
A rectal introducer, consisting of a hollow tube with a stationary balloon attached to its outer surface, is inserted through the anus and, when the stationary balloon is inflated, seals the orifice. An electro-optical capsule is embedded in the front of a lightweight balloon vehicle, while low pressure colon insufflation with $CO2$, between stationary and vehicle balloon, propels the vehicle balloon, causing it to glide along the 'slippery' colon walls. Computer controlled pressure management, coupled with sensors in the workstation, adjust balloon size and shape to changing bowel anatomy, thus allowing the pressure-propelled balloon to find its path. The Aer-O-Scope visual system provides simultaneous 360 degree viewing of the colon mucosal surface. (Pfeffer et Al., 2006)

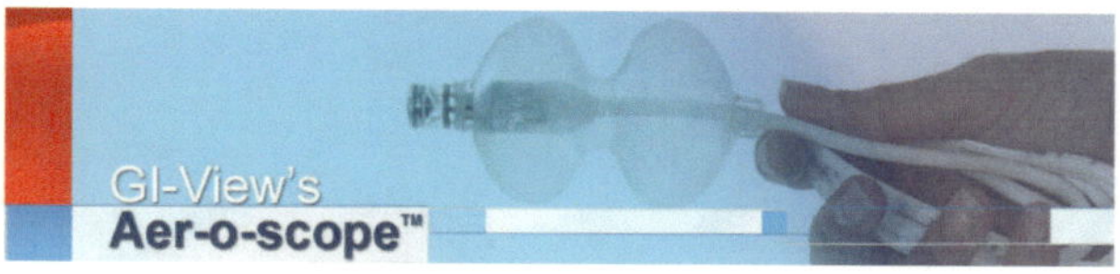

Fig. 3. Aer-O-scope disposable device

The **ColonoSight system** uses air pressure assisted pull technology to pull the scope into the colon. A disposable device consisting of a plastic sleeve, wrapped on a loader, is unfolded gradually through insufflation of air. The forward force of the device is generated by a pneumatic mechanism just below the tip of the scope. This force draws the scope in, and the operator then navigates with the handles, drastically reducing the need to push from the back. Aside from making the procedure safer, it also reduces the amount of local anesthetic required. (Shike et Al. 2005)

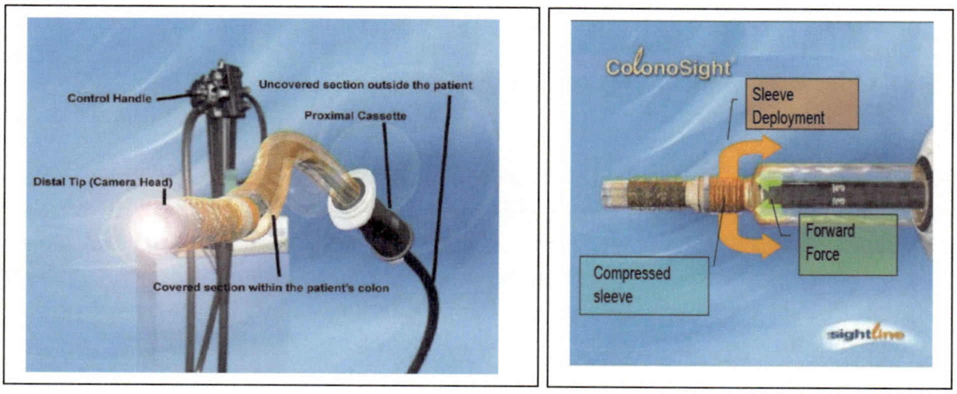

Fig. 4. The ColonoSight system and scheme of working principle

The **InvendoScope system** is a single-use, hand-held controlled computer-assisted colonoscope. A sleeve is pulled over this inner sheath, inverted at each of the respective ends, and attached to a propulsion connector. The outer wall of the sheath is motionless and the intubation is achieved by the eversion of an inner portion of the sleeve which carries the optical system and the instrument channel. The physician controls the device by activating the "Forward drive" and the "Backward drive" keys on the handheld control unit. By manipulating the joystick of the hand control unit the physician can electro-hydraulically deflect the endoscope tip, steering the colonoscope during the drive through the colon (Waye et Al., 2009).

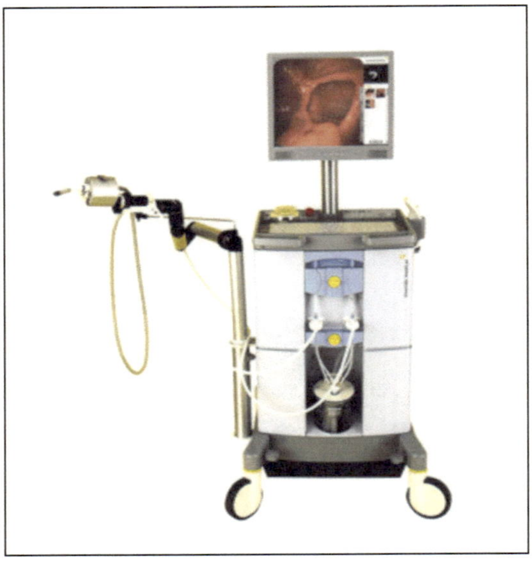

Fig. 4. Invendoscope workstation and disposable probe

The above stated overview of the state of the art of robotic devices developed for colonoscopy procedures shows that the main priority was to realize a system with an internal locomotion action, able to advance in a hostile environment. The movement of the device is always under computer control by means of mechanical, electrical, or computer-algorithm based sensors. Moreover, the robotic colonoscopes generally include the following sub-systems:

- A probe, with at least a disposable part (the one in contact with the colonic mucosa);
- A vision system located at the tip of the device;
- A PC-based workstation or a hand-held unit which controls the propulsion of the probe in the colon.

Some of the characteristics of the above listed sub-systems, as well as other aspects related to personnel and sedation during the procedures have of course an impact on the cost saving issue. Moreover, also the related timings have to be considered, including e.g. the preparation which non-disposable devices have to undergo to prevent from cross-infections, the duration of the procedures themselves, the gaining of time in the turn-over of patients and the recovery time for the patients to go back to work.

Even if several robotic colonoscopes have been tested in vitro and seemed to be ready to be used in pilot studies on human beings, very few completed the engineering phase and went through the certification steps, and only one became available off-the-shelf as a real product. In particular, in the following further details will be presented on the Endotics System, whose core component is a disposable probe with inchworm locomotion, currently used in clinical practice in a few hospitals, and on the Invendoscope, based on inverted sleeve technology, not yet commercially available, but with most recent news than others.

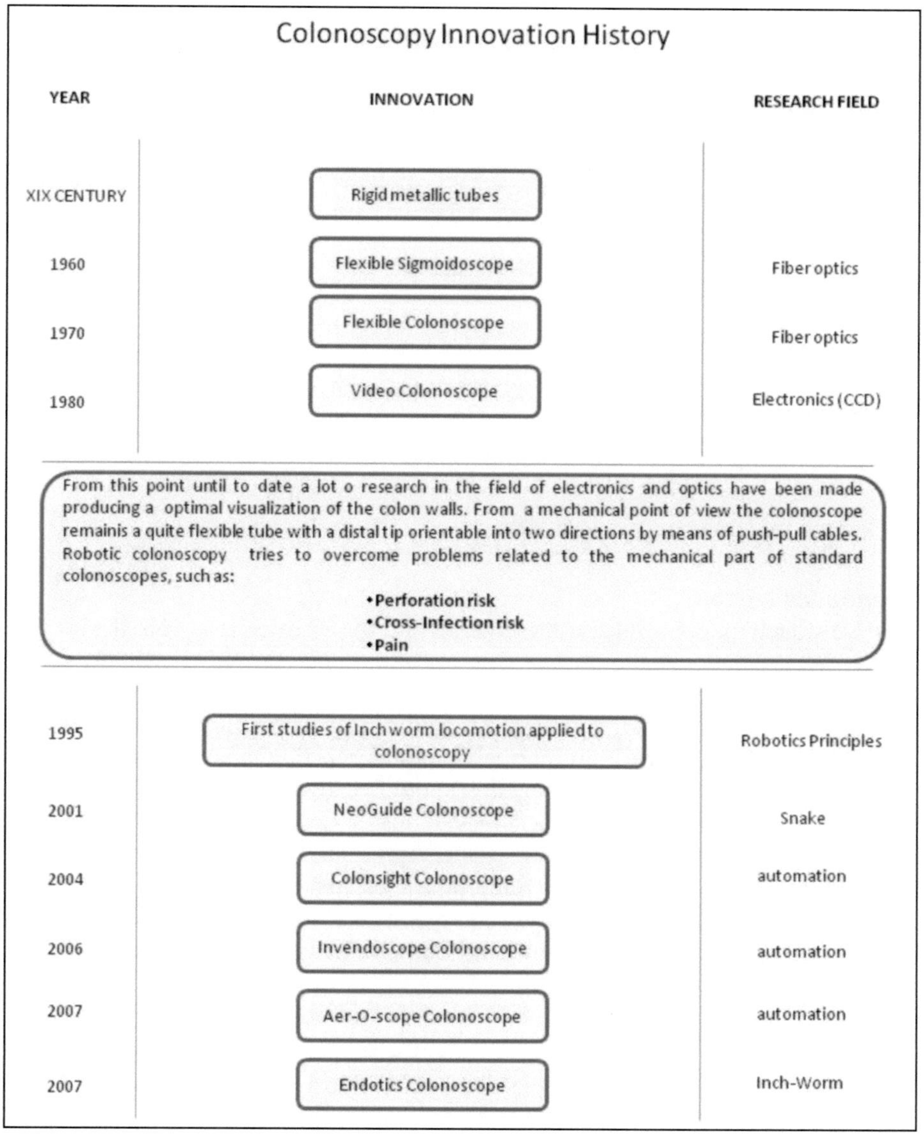

Fig. 5. Colonoscopy innovation history diagram

PRODUCT NAME	LATEST PUBLICATION	LATEST EVENT	COMMERCIALLY AVAILABLE
Neoguide	2006	Transformed in laparoscopic device	No
Aer-o-Scope	2007	DDW 2007	No
Colonosight	2007	Closed business 2008	No
Endotics	2011	Fismad 2011	Yes
Invendoscope	2011	-	No

Table 1. Publication & event blatancy

PRODUCT NAME	DEVELOPER/ COMPANY NAME	NATIONALITY	DEVELOPMENT STATUS	INITIAL COMMERCIAL FOCUS
Neoguide	NeoGuide Systems Inc	USA	Abandoned *	n.a
Aer-o-Scope	GI View Ltd	Israel	Almost abandoned *	n.a.
Colonosight	Sightline Technologies Ltd	Israel	Almost abandoned *	n.a.
Endotics	Era Endoscopy Srl	Italy	Off the shelf product	Europe
Invendoscope	invendo medical GmbH	Germany	Filed 510(K) notice submission with the FDA (08/03/2010)	USA

Table 2. Commercial information * (Ell, 2008)

2.2 The endotics system

The excessive stretching of bowel and mesenteries and the air insufflation are the main reasons of the pain felt by the patient during this uncomfortable procedure. In order to avoid perforation risks, addressed both to pushing action exerted by the endoscopist during the intubation phase and to the rigidity in the pushing direction of the traditional colonoscope, it is essential to realize a system with an internal locomotion action, able to advance in a hostile environment. The ideal screening investigation should be as non invasive as possible and safe while maintaining a high diagnostic accuracy. Thus, a device extremely flexible and soft, which gently deforms just locally the colon tissue, represents the optimal solution.

The innovative systems require a lower amount of insufflations and do not stress on mesenteries resulting in a real painless colonoscopy. Moreover, infective risks, due to sterilization procedure's limits, are definitively eliminated by disposable endoscopes.

From a technical point of view, the simplest inchworm device consists of two clampers at the ends, used to adhere securely onto the "terrain", and one extensor as its midsection that brings about a positive displacement. The device of the robot was focused towards a disposable device, totally pneumatically driven, and very soft and flexible, able to adapt its shape to the configuration of the bowel. The probe is composed of two main parts: an active one, including the head, the steering and the flexible extensible body, and the passive components of the devise including the tail and the tank containing eventual body fluids, and the connector used to fix the disposable probe to the workstation. The overall dimensions of the active part are: a diameter of 17 mm and a variable length from 24 to 40 cm, considering the inchworm movements. The head hosts both a vision system, including a CMOS camera and LED light sources, and channels for water jet and air in order to provide rinsing and suction/insufflations, respectively. As the Endotics system requires air insufflations only in the immediate proximity of the head lens, an accurate automatic insufflations-suction balance prevents painful bowel stretching.

The passive component, a very thin and extremely flexible plastic tail, has a diameter of 7,5 mm and a length of 180 cm. The workstation allows the endoscopist to easily and fully control the disposable probe by means of a hand-held console and to visualize on a screen real time images. Thanks to the electro-pneumatic steerable tip, the operator can steer the head of the robotic colonoscope of 180° in every direction, elongate the soft body of the probe in order to move it forward and backward following the shape of the intestine, and control rising, insufflations and suction.

The locomotion phase begins with the automatic adherence of the proximal clamper of the probe to the colon walls. The next phases can be described as follows:

1. the midsection is elongated under control of the operator;
2. the distal clamper adheres to the colon walls (automatic);
3. the proximal clamper is released (automatic);
4. the midsection is contracted (automatic);
5. the proximal clamper adheres to the colon walls (automatic);
6. the distal clamp is released (automatic).

The purposely developed patented clamping system allows to hold the colonic tissue by means of a combined vacuum-mechanical action. The clamping mechanism does not create neither lesions in the bowel wall, nor mucosal lacerations.

Diagnostic accuracy and patient acceptance of robotic colonoscopy have been evaluated in a first pilot multicentre study, in 40 consecutive volunteers (27 men and 13 women) who underwent standard colonoscopy also. This pilot study showed that the Endotics System has a diagnostic accuracy equivalent to the one achievable through the standard colonoscope. Moreover, the Endotics System was able to visualize two small polyps (sized below 2 mm), in two different cases, not seen using standard colonoscopy. This probably due to the fact that during standard colonoscopy a bigger amount of air was insufflated causing a flattening of the small polyps. Considering the patient acceptance issue, the Endotics colonoscopy was unanimously rated strongly better than conventional colonoscopy: in a scale from 0 to 10 for pain and discomfort the procedure performed by means of the Endotics System scored on average 0.9 and 1.1 (mode 0 for both), compared to 6.9 and 6.8 (mode 9 and 8) of the standard colonoscopy, respectively. (Cosentino et Al., 2009)

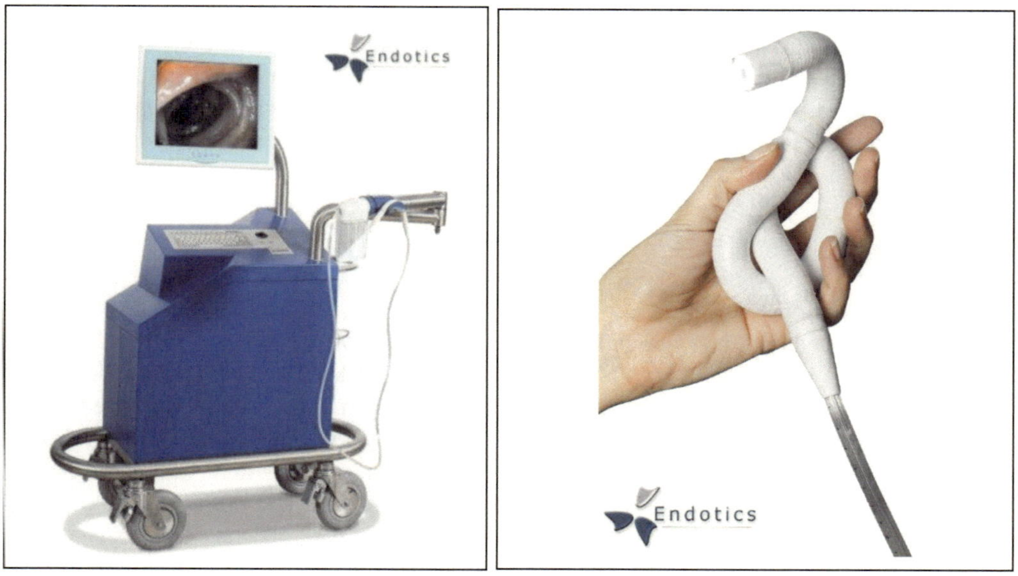

Fig. 6. Workstation and disposable probe Endotics

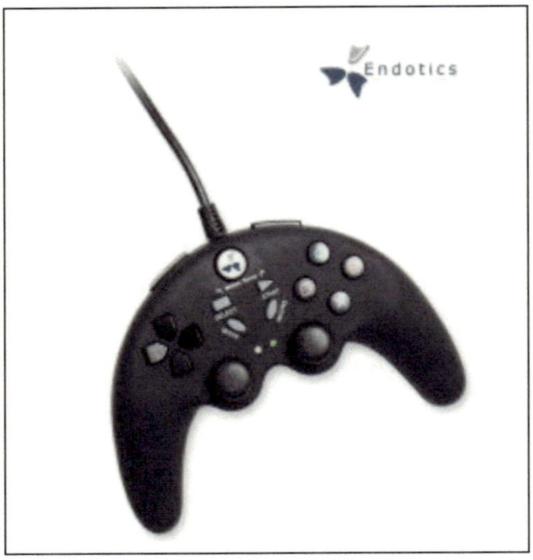

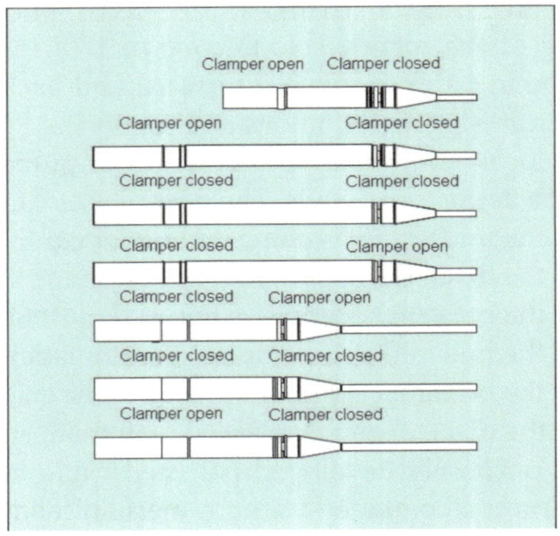

Fig. 7. Hand-Held device and locomotion sequence of Endotics probe

In a second pilot study which involved 71 patients (40 men and 31 women), diagnostic accuracy and enhanced patient acceptance of Endotics system compared with standard colonoscopy, was confirmed showing a sensitivity equal to 93,3% (95% C.I.:68.0-99.0), a specificity equal to 100% (95% C.I.:88.0-99.9), a predictive positive and negative values, PPV and NPV respectively, equal to 100% and 97.7%. No patients requested sedation during the Endotics procedure, while 14 subjects (19.7%) requested the administration of midazolam and meperidine during standard colonoscopy. In this study has been used a slightly different Endotics probe version from the one used in the previous pilot study (25 cm length in the contracted form and 43 cm in the elongated form, with respect to 23 and 37 cm, respectively, of the previous version) (Tumino et Al., 2010)

In a third study 12 patients with inflammatory bowel diseases were enrolled in order to compare the diagnostic performance and tolerability of the Endotics System with standard colonoscopy for the staging of ulcerative colitis. Mean pain/discomfort on a 0-10 scale was 2.08 (SD 1.67) for Endotics system and 4.17 (SD 1.74) for standard colonoscopy, with a statistically significant difference ($p = 0.066$) favoring Endotics system.

In conclusion, the Endotics System is a diagnostic instrument comparable to the gold standard and highly suitable for screening purposes due to the extremely high level of patients acceptance. (Pallotta et Al., 2011)

2.3 The invendoscope

This computer-assisted colonoscope is based on inverted sleeve technology, where the outer side of the inverted sleeve stays in position, and the inner side is pulled forward below the distal tip, moving the colonoscope into the colon by 10 cm each time. Wheels are rolled on the inner side of an inverted sleeve, so that the sleeve is rolled inside out, drawing the colonoscope deeper into the colon. With this mechanism there is no relative movement to the colon wall, and in combination with the small bending diameter minimizes the forces on the colon walls and prevents looping, minimizing pain and discomfort for the patient. The device is equipped with a centralized 3.2 mm working channel with the support of the deflectable electrohydraulic tip; therefore it can be also used for routine therapeutic procedures such as

polypectomy. Both the vision capabilities and the working channels are similar to those of conventional colonoscopes. All endoscopic activities are controlled by a hand-held unit.
First pilot study (Roesch et Al, 2007) was focused on capability of the device of reaching cecum measuring time needed and pain/discomfort rate. Were enrolled 24 patients reaching cecum in 79% of cases, with a mean time 26 minutes. Participants rated the examination on an overall score (1.77 points; range, 1-3), using a self assessed pain scale (pain scale range was from 1 = no discomfort to 6 = severe pain).

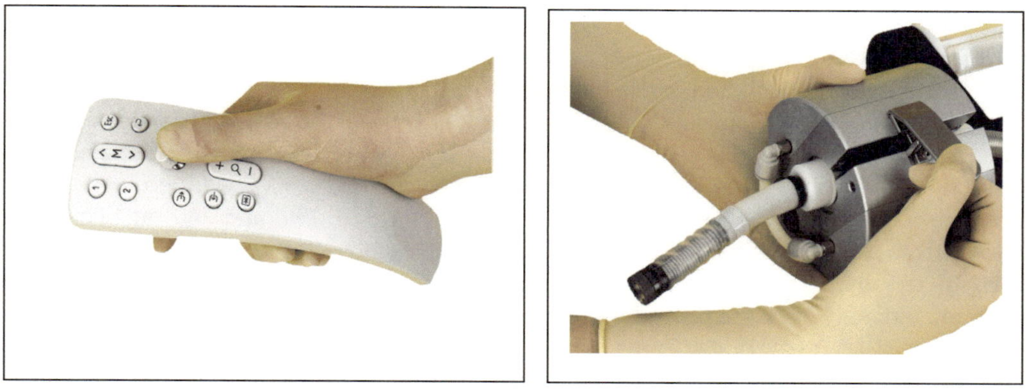

Fig. 8. Hand-Held device and the instrument tip in the driving unit.

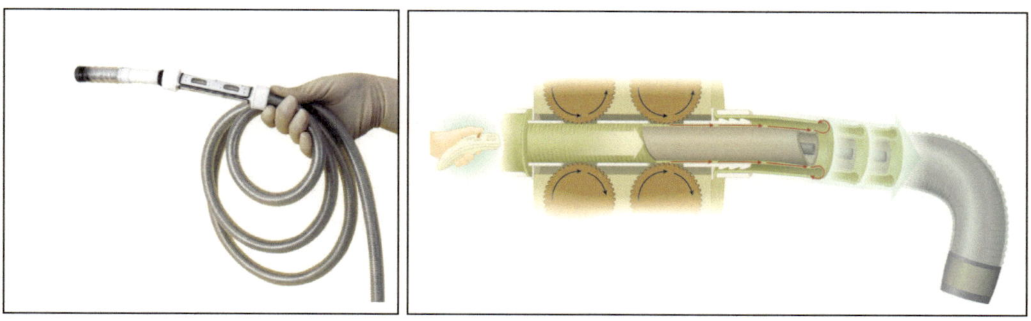

Fig. 9. Disposable probe and scheme of working principle of Invendoscope system.

A second single-arm, pilot study (Invendoscope 1st) on 39 paid healthy volunteers was carried out. Again, cecum reaching rate and time were the focus of study, with some attention towards the patient acceptance. The cecal intubation rate was of 82% (95% C.I., 66-92). Two incomplete colonoscopies had to be stopped at the sigmoid colon because of pain, and in other four volunteers the procedure was terminated at the hepatic flexure. Bloating was reported in four volunteers after that an endoscopy intravenous administration of 20 to 40 mg of hyoscine butylbromide was allowed to facilitate endoscope passage. It should be noted that only limited time was spent on inspection of the mucosa while withdrawing the instrument. The volunteer rating showed a mean score of 1.96 (range 1-6; 1 = no discomfort). Study was divided into two phases. On the basis of experience during phase 1, the instrument was made longer (from 170 to 180 or 200 cm) and a few other modifications (e.g., stiffening below the endoscope tip, improved coating) were also made to achieve better performance in the right colon, however, a comparison between the two instruments was

not the main aim of the pilot study. To date, no data concerning diagnostic accuracy and comparison with conventional colonoscopy are available.
Moreover, a third prospective single-arm study (Invendoscope 2nd) on 61 paid healthy volunteers was conducted. There were 34 men and 27 women with a mean age of 57.5 years (range 50 - 70) and a mean body mass index of 26.3 kg/ m 2 (19.5 - 36.8). Main outcome parameters were safety, as measured by the frequency and severity of device related adverse events, and device effectiveness, as shown by cecal intubation rate. Secondary outcome parameters were utility of the device in the documentation and biopsy of pathological findings, and pathological findings. Pain/discomfort rating and introduction/withdrawal timing were also recorded. Comparison with standard colonoscopy was not included in the parameters of the study. Cecal intubation was reached in 60 volunteers (98,4%): introduction mean time was 16.4 min as also withdrawal mean time. Abdominal compression and/or position change were used in approximately two-thirds (66%) of the patients, to help in further advancing the scope. Sedation was used in three participants (4.9%); the Propofol doses used were 120, 130, and 180 mg. The mean ratings from the screenees, immediately after colonoscopy, for overall assessment and pain/discomfort were 1.6 (range 1- 3) and 2.3 (range 1- 6). A rating of 6 was automatically given immediately after the procedure in cases where sedation was used. CO_2 was used for insufflation in all cases. Water immersion, administered via a foot pump, was used during insertion at the discretion of the endoscopist. Follow-up at 24 h and 7 days was complete for all the study participants. The mean overall ratings at 24 h and at 7 days were 1.4 and 1.3 (range 1-5). The mean pain/discomfort ratings at 24 h and at 7 days were 1.5 and 1.3 (range 1-6). Only three screenees had previous colonoscopy. (Groth et Al., 2011)

2.4 Endotics Vs Invendoscope: a data comparison coming from published results

Before to compare the two technologies it is mandatory to uniform data recovered from studies:

- In the calculation of cecum reaching rate Endotics included procedures where device had technical problems, while Invendoscope not. For the calculation, procedures with technical failures are excluded also for Endotics.
- Both systems presented two models, where the second one was intended as a ameliorative system. For the calculation of caecum reaching rate and time for both devices is considered the second device
- According to observational studies (Rex et Al., 2002 - a) and as reported in guidelines (National Guidelines Clearinghouse-NGC 4969, 2006) , cases in which procedures are aborted because of poor preparation or severe colitis need not be counted in determining cecal intubation rates. Thus, such procedure are not counted in the presented data. Moreover, because of the protocol of third study afferent Endotics system is focused on the assessment of ulcerative colitis endoscopic activity with Endotics system, related data are not included in the comparison.
- Pain score is calculated on the basis of different ranges, from 0 to 10 for Endotics and from 1 to 6 for Invendoscope. Pain score is indicated in the following table as percentage of maximum value of the respective range. Moreover, should be noted that Endotics system used air for insufflation, while Invendoscope, in the last paper, described the use of advanced reduction discomfort techniques, such as CO_2 insufflation instead of air and water immersion during insertion.

- For all devices, comprising standard colonoscope, "time to cecum" does not include the time spent to carefully analyze the colonic mucosa with diagnostic purposes, except for Endotics, that, due to its working principle, makes observations useful for diagnosis while proceeding towards cecum. Thus, to make a consistent comparison, data related to colonoscopy completion timing should be taken into account. As regards the Endotics system, time to cecum and time to complete diagnosis is slightly different, while for other colonoscopes that make diagnosis during withdrawal is substantially different. According to ASGE guideline, physicians performing a colonoscopy should have an average withdrawal time of six minutes or more for a thorough exam (ASGE-Media Backgrounder, 2010). Moreover, colonoscopist with a low miss rate of lesions have a mean withdrawal time of about nine minutes (Rex et Al., 2000) (Simmons et Al, 2006) (Barclay et Al., 2006) (Overholt et Al, 2010)

	Endotics	Invendoscope	
Disposable	Yes	Yes	
Tool channel	No	Yes	
# Studies	3	3	
# Patients enrolled	123	124	
For the following data comparison, Tumino, Roesch and Groth papers are considered			
	Endotics	Invendoscope 1st	Invendoscope 2nd
Comparison with Standard Colonoscopy	Yes	No	No
Asymptomatic volunteers	No	Yes	Yes
Paid volunteers	No	Yes	Yes
Mean Age	51.9	49.7	57.5
One to One procedure*	Yes	No	No
Sedation (Propofol)	0%	0%	4.9%
Antispasmodic given	0%	79%	Not mentioned
Insufflation of CO_2	No	No	Yes
Water immersion technique	No	No	Yes
Pain range	9% fs	32.6% fs	26.6% f.s.
Discomfort range	11% f.s.	Not mentioned	38.3% f.s.
Abdominal compression	0%	Occasionally	66%
Sensitivity	93.3%	n.a.**	n.a.**
Specificity	100%	n.a.**	n.a.**
NPV	97.7%	n.a.**	n.a.**
PPV	100%	n.a.**	n.a.**
Cecal intubation rate	93,6%	90%	98.4 %
Mean time to cecum (min)	n.a.	23	16.4
Mean completion time procedure (min)	45,3	n.a.	32.8

* One to one procedure is intended procedure conducted without any additional personnel
** Data are not applicable because they require a comparison with standard colonoscopy

Table 3. Data comparison: Endotics Vs Invendoscope

- Moreover it has to be considered that studies carried out with Endotics have eligibility criteria that include mainly people with prior diagnosis of colorectal diseases (about 70% of patients in the second study) thus procedures' timing should be compared with a similar study population where completion of the procedure is reached in a mean time of 33 min (range 10-80) (Rex. et Al. 2002 – b).

The problem with studies reporting a very high completion rate is that they are screening endoscopies in asymptomatic individuals. These populations are different from normal daily practice. Patients undergo colonoscopy for all kinds of clinical indications (Loffeld et Al., 2009). For this reason it is very important, in order to fully understand carry out an exhaustive comparative analysis a comparison between different clinical trials, to study also eligibility and exclusion criteria adopted. The Endotics and Invendoscope systems are described and compared with parameters advocated to predict a difficulty colonoscopic procedure. Parameters are listed in table 3 (Anderson et Al., 2001). Sometimes difficulty's parameters could be described in different ways, e.g. *"previously failed colonoscopies can usually be characterized as an angulated sigmoid colon or redundant colon "* (Rex, 2008). In people with high BMI, percentage of redundant colon is much higher than people with lower BMI, whereas people with low BMI has probably very angulated bends.

	Exclusion Criteria		
Difficulty's parameters	Endotics	Invendoscope 1st	Invendoscope 2nd
Age > 50	No	Not described	No
History of abdominal surgery	No	Not described	Yes
History of pelvic surgery	No	Not described	Yes
History of diverticular disease	No	Not described	Yes
Body mass index	No	Not described	Yes
Inflammatory bowel disease	Yes	Not described	Yes

Table 4. Difficulty's parameters and exclusion criteria

3. Conclusion

In this chapter main reasons for including robotic colonoscopy in common practice of colonoscopy screening have been considered. Standard devices are quite rigid, require high experience of the doctor to perform difficult maneuvers to proceed along the tortuous colon walls, and are constructed of materials that could be damaged by heat, pressure, and moisture used during the decontamination processes. The stated above limitations, that could be overcome with robotic colonoscopies, made, and still make, standard colonoscopy a quite invasive technique, with risks related to perforation, sedation and cross-infections, far for being accepted by massive percentages of patients as needed in colorectal cancer screening programs. Nowadays, colonoscopy is used as a matter of fact as screening test just in first-level demonstrative studies and pilot projects. Participation in the first-level FOB (fecal occult blood) screening test is above 50%, and compliance for second level screening

programs, is very low compared to expected values, since it is in a range from 30 to 60%. Other important issues that have to be taken into account are related to timing and personnel. As a matter of fact, timing affects all the procedure phases, starting from the preparation which not-disposable devices have to undergo to prevent from cross-infections, and including the duration of the procedures themselves, the gaining of time in the turn-over of patients and the recovery time for the patients to go back to work. As for the personnel, both the number of operators needed and their specific competences.
A state of the art related to working principles of robotic devices have been described as well as main robotic devices proposed for pilot studies. Among these devices two robotic colonoscopes are deeply described and compared: Endotics System and Invendoscope. The comparison included:

- If the device is disposable or not
- Age of the patients and if they are asymptomatic and/or paid
- Presence of tool channel
- Number of studies, with related number of patients enrolled
- Comparison with standard colonoscopy, in terms of pain range, sensitivity, specificity, NPV and PPV
- Sedation or antispasmodic administration
- Procedure details, such as cecal intubation rate and timing, abdominal compression maneuvers

An additional table related to the difficulty's parameters in colonoscopy and exclusion criteria adopted in clinical trials has been filled. In this table parameters related to the age of patients, their surgical and/or colonic disease history, and their BMI are considered.
Endotics system appears to be a promising diagnostic instrument comparable to the gold standard and highly suitable for screening purposes due to the extremely high level of patients' acceptance even without the adoption of advanced discomfort reducing techniques like CO_2 insufflation and water immersion during insertion.
The introduction of this diagnostic instrument in clinical practice could facilitate the adoption of colonoscopy as first-level screening, with a further reduction in the incidence of the colon cancer, estimated in the order of 76-90%. In conclusion a painless colonoscopy, besides being a remarkable achievement for the patient and avoiding any risk related to sedation, has major fallout in terms of prevention.

4. References

Anderson J. C., Messina C.R., Cohn W., Gottfried E., Ingber S., Bernstein G., Coman E. & Polito J. (2001) Factors predictive of difficult colonoscopy, Gastrointestinal Endoscopy Volume 54, N. 5, 2001

Berclay R.L., Vicari J.J., Doughty A.S., Johanson J.F. & Greenlaw R.L. (2006) Colonoscopic Withdrawal Times and Adenoma Detection during Screening Colonoscopy N Engl J Med 2006;355:2533-41.

Classen M., Tygat G.N.J. & Lightdale C.J. (2010) Two Centuries of digestive tract endoscopy: a concise report. Gastroenterological Endoscopy, Thieme, 2010

Cosentino F., Tumino E., Rubis Passoni G., Morandi E. & Capria A. (2009) Functional evaluation of the Endotics System, a new disposable self-propelled robotic colonoscope: in vitro tests and clinical trial. The International Journal of Artificial Organs / Vol. 32 / no. 8, 2009 / pp. 517-527

Eickhoff A., Jakobs R., Kamal A., Mermash S., Riemann J.F. & van Dam J. (2006) In vitro evaluation of forces exerted by a new computer−assisted colonoscope (the NeoGuide Endoscopy System), Endoscopy 2006; 38: 1224±1229

Ell C., Riemann J.F., Pochon T., Sakai P. & Yamamoto H. (2008) GI Endoscopy - Standards and Innovations. Proceedings of the Falk Symposium 166 held in Mainz, Germany, September 18-19, 2008. Published by Springer, Dordrecht, The Netherlands, 2009, 154 pages

Faivre J., Dancourt V., Lejeune C., Tazi MA, Lamour J., Gerard D., Dassonville F & Bonithon-Kopp C. (2004) Reduction in colorectal cancer mortality by fecal occult blood screening in a French controlled study. Gastroenterology. 2004 Jun;126(7):1674-80.

Groth S., Rex D.K., Rösch T. & Hoepffner N. (2011)High Cecal Intubation Rates With a New Computer-Assisted Colonoscope: A Feasibility Study. American Journal of Gastroenterology advance online publication, 8 March 2011; doi: 10.1038/ajg.2011.52

Hu H., Li M. Wang P.i, Feng Y. & Sun L. (2009) Development of a continuum robot for colonoscopy, High Technology Letters, 2009 , Issue 2 , Page 115-119

Levin B., Lieberman D.A., McFarland B., MD, Smith R.A., Brooks D., Andrews K.S., Dash C., Giardiello F.M., Glick S., Levin T.R., Pickhardt P., Rex D.K., Thorson A. & Winawer S.J. (2008)Screening and surveillance for the early detection of colorectal cancer and adenomatous polyps, 2008: a joint guideline from the American Cancer Society, the US Multi-Society Task Force on Colorectal Cancer, and the American College of Radiology. Gastroenterology 2008; 134:1570–1595.

Loffeld R.J.L.F. & van der Putten A.B.M.M. (2009) The Completion Rate of Colonoscopy in Normal Daily Practice: Factors Associated with Failure. Digestion 2009; 80:267–270

Niwa H., Utsumi Y., Nakamura T., Yoshida A., Yoshitoshi Y., Fujino M., Kaneko E., Kasumi A. & Matsumoto M. (1969). Clinical experience of colonic fiberscope. Gastroent. Endosc. 1969 Tokyo, 11, 163-173.

Overholt B.F., Brooks-Belli L., Grace M., Rankin K., Harrell R., Turyk M., Rosenberg F.B., Barish R. & Gilinsky N.H. (2010) Withdrawal times and associated factors in colonoscopy: a quality assurance multicenter assessment. Journal of clinical Gastroenterology-April 2010-Volume 44 - Issue 4 - pp e80-e86

Pallotta S., Tumino E., Manes G., Sacco R., Ardizzone S., Bresci G. & De Franchis R. (2011) Assessment of ulcerative colitis endoscopic activity with novel robotic colonoscope: the Endotics system. XVII Congresso Nazionale delle malattie digestive Torino, 5-9 Marzo 2011

Perri F., Iacobellis A., Gentile M., Tumino E. & Andriulli A. (2010) The intelligent, painless, "germ free" colonoscopy: A Columbus' egg for increasing population adherence to colorectal cancer screening? Dig Liver Dis (2010), doi:10.1016/j.dld.2010.06.007

Pfeffer J., Grinshpon R., Rex D.K., Levin B., Rösch T., Arber N. & Halpern Z. (2006) Proof of New Colonoscope Concept in a Pig Model ´ Endoscopy 2006; 38: 144±148RexD.K.

(2000) Colonoscopic withdrawal technique and adenoma miss rates. Gastrointestinal Endoscopy Volume 51, No. 1, 2000

Rex D.K., Bond J.H., Winawer S., Levin T.R., Burt R.W., Johnson D.A., Kirk L.M., Litlin S., Lieberman D.A., Waye J.D., Church J., Marshall J.B. & Riddell R.H. (2002) Quality in the Technical Performance of Colonoscopy and the Continuous Quality Improvement Process for Colonoscopy: Recommendations of the U.S. Multi-Society Task Force on Colorectal Cancer The American Journal of Gastroenterology Vol. 97, No. 6, 2002 - a

Rex D.K. & Goodwine B.W. (2002) Method of Colonoscopy in 42 Consecutive Patients Presenting After Prior Incomplete Colonoscopy. The American Journal of Gastroenterology Vol. 97, No. 5, 2002 – b

Rex D.K. (2008) Achieving cecal intubation in the very difficult colon. Gastrointestinal Endoscopy Volume 67, No. 6 : 2008

Roesch T, Adler A., Pohl H., Wettschureck E., Koch M., Wiedenmann B. & Hoepffner N. (2007)A prospective pilot study to assess technical performance of a new single use colonoscope with inverted sleeve technology. Gastrointest Endosc 2007, 65, AB340.

Saito T., Kagiwada T., Harada H. & Kawamura Y. (2009) Development of an Earthworm Robot with a Shape Memory Alloy and Braided Tube. Advanced Robotics, Volume 23, Numbers 12-13, 2009 , pp. 1743-1760(18) Publisher: VSP, an imprint of Brill

Shike M., Fireman Z., Eliakim R., Segol O., Sloyer A., Cohen L.B., Goldfarb-Albak S. & Repici A. (2005) New Technology ColonoSight OMED Colorectal Cancer Screening Meeting May 15, 2005

Simmon D.T., Harewood GC, Baron TH, Petersen BT, Wang KK, Boyd-Enders F & Ott BJ (2006)Impact of endoscopist withdrawal speed on polyp yield: implications for optimal colonoscopy withdrawal time. Alimentary pharmacology & therapeutics-2006-Sep; vol 24 (issue 6) : pp 965-971

Slatkin B.A. & Burdik J. (1997)The development of a robotic endoscope, Experimental Robotics IV, The 4th International Symposium, Stanford, California, June 30 – July 2, 1995, Volume 223/1997pp 161-169

Sturges R. H. & Laowattana S. (1993) A flexible, tendon-controlled device for endoscopy, 1993 - The International Journal of Robotics Research 12(2): 121–131.

Swain P. (2009) Colonoscopy: New Designs for the Future Gastrointestinal Endoscopy Clinics of North America, Volume 15, Issue 4, Pages 839-863

Swaroop V.S. & Larson M.V. (2002)Colonoscopy as a Screening Test for Colorectal Cancer in Average-Risk Individuals. Mayo Clin Proc. 2002;77:951-956

Tumino E, Sacco R., Bertini M., Bertoni M., Parisi G. & Capria A. (2010)Endotics system vs colonoscopy for the detection of polyps. World J Gastroenterol 2010; 16(43): 5452-5456

Waye J.D., Rex D.K. & Williams C.B. (2009)Colonoscopy: Principle and practice. Second edition. 2009 Published by Wiley-Blackwell

Zuo J., Yan G. & Gao Z. (2005) A micro creeping robot for colonoscopy based on the earthworm, J Med Eng Technol. 2005 Jan-Feb; 29(1):1-7

Guideline

Media Backgrounder. American Society for Gastrointestinal Endoscopy, 2010
Quality indicators for colonoscopy. Guideline summary NGC-4969, 2006

19

Experimental Small Animal Colonoscopy

Terrah J. Paul Olson and Richard B. Halberg
University of Wisconsin-Madison
United States of America

1. Introduction

Diseases of the colon and rectum produce a large burden of morbidity and mortality. Inflammatory bowel disease (IBD), such as Crohn's disease and ulcerative colitis, affects as many as 1.4 million people in the United States and 2.2 million people in Europe and leads to significant utilization of healthcare resources (Loftus, 2004). Crohn's disease (CD) is a chronic inflammatory disease that can affect the entire gastrointestinal tract from mouth to anus, and typically manifests itself with abdominal pain, diarrhea, and weight loss, as well as intestinal strictures, obstruction, perforation, or fistulae formation. CD most often manifests in the second to third decade of life. The usual disease course is periods of abdominal pain and diarrhea alternating with relatively asymptomatic periods. Over time, the symptomatic periods become longer, more frequent, and more severe. Ulcerative colitis (UC) is limited to the colon and occasionally the terminal ileum, and typically presents with diarrhea, passage of mucus, and rectal bleeding. UC is also most commonly diagnosed in patients younger than 30 years of age. IBD and colorectal cancer (CRC) are intimately linked, as long-standing IBD leads to an increasing risk for CRC over time. In patients with UC, the risk for CRC begins to increase after approximately 10 years of disease. The estimated risk of CRC is 25% after 25 years with the disease, 35% at 30 years, 45% at 35 years, and 65% at 40 years (reviewed in Townsend, 2008).

CRC is the third most commonly diagnosed cancer and the third-leading cause of cancer-related death in the United States in both men and women (American Cancer Society, 2011). In 2010, the American Cancer Society estimated that there were 142,579 new cases of CRC and 51,370 deaths attributed to this disease in the US (National Cancer Institute, 2011). The incidence of CRC is rising in many countries, in part because a western-style diet is being widely adopted (Center et al., 2009). CRC is currently the fourth leading cause of cancer deaths in the world (World Health Organization, 2011).

IBD and CRC are active areas of research, and a number of useful animal models of these diseases have been generated. Some of the most widely studied are rodent models, including various rat and mouse models. Mouse models are particularly attractive. Mouse genetics have been extensively studied, and there is a detailed knowledge base describing hundreds of inbred mouse strains as well as a variety of transgenic, knockout, and knockin models (reviewed in Rosenberg et al., 2009). Both genetic and chemically induced models of IBD and CRC have been validated (reviewed in Kanneganti et al., 2011; Rosenberg et al., 2009). These models are continually used to more fully understand the natural history of colonic diseases as well as test strategies for prevention and treatment. See Table 1 for an overview of genetic and chemically induced mouse models of IBD and CRC.

Models of Inflammatory Bowel Disease			
Genetic			
Model	**Human Disease**	**Mechanism**	**Phenotype**
SAMP-Yit	CD	High IFN-γ production	Spontaneous terminal ileitis, occasional perianal ulcers and fistulae
C3H/HejBir	UC	Increased IFN-γ and IL-2 production	Spontaneous ileocecal and right-sided colonic ulcers and crypt abscesses
$TNF^{\Delta ARE}$/TNF 3′ $UTR^{-/-}$	CD	Increased constitutive and inducible TNF	Polyarthritis and transmural intestinal inflammation
T-cell receptor-$\alpha^{-/-}$	UC	Increased aberrant T_H2-type T-cells producing IL-4	Pancolitis with soft stools
STAT4 transgenic	UC	Overproduction of STAT-4, leading to CD4+ T-cell production of TNF-α and IFN-γ	Severe transmural colitis
STAT3 deficient	CD	Disruption of STAT3 in macrophages and neutrophils, decreased IL-10	Enterocolitis with high incidence of colorectal adenocarcinomas
IL-$10^{-/-}$/CRF2-4 deficient	CD	Decreased IL-10 with increased IL-12 and TNF-α, loss of downregulation of T_H1-type T cells, NK cells, macrophages	Chronic enterocolitis with lesions in duodenum, proximal jejunum, and ascending colon primarily
IL-$2^{-/-}$/IL-2 receptor $\alpha^{-/-}$	UC	Decreased IL-2 (key regulatory immune cytokine)	Pancolitis with ulcers and wall thickening, crypt abscesses, mucin depletion, and epithelial dysplasia
IL-7 transgenic	UC	Initial IL-7 increase, then IL-7 deficiency	Initial acute colitis, followed by chronic colitis with proctoptosis and anal bleeding
$CD4^+CD45RB^{Hi}$ T-cell transfer	UC	Decreased IL-10, increased IFN-γ	Diarrhea, weight loss, transmural colonic inflammation, and death
Heat shock protein 60-specific $CD8^+$ T-cell transfer	CD	Presentation of bacterial protein on MHC class 1 with action of TNF-α	Severe small intestinal inflammation, death

Model	Human Disease	Mechanism	Phenotype
A20 deficient	CD	Lack of inhibition of TNF-induced NFκB activity	Intestinal inflammation, cachexia, death
IKK-γ (NEMO)/IKKαβ deficient	UC	Complete shutdown of NFκB signaling, leading to massive inflammatory cell infiltration	Severe chronic pancolitis
MDR1 deficient	UC	Spontaneous inflammatory response triggered by intestinal bacterial flora	Intestinal inflammation
Keratin $8^{-/-}$	UC	Primary intestinal epithelial cell defect leading to inflammation from intestinal bacterial flora	Colitis and colonic hyperplasia
Double negative N-cadherin transgenic/chimeric	IBD	Disrupted intestinal mucosal barrier leading to inflammation from contact with intestinal bacterial flora	Chronic inflammation in chimeric regions of intestinal epithelium
Chemical			
Model	**Human Disease**	**Mechanism**	**Phenotype**
Acetic acid	UC	Enema; epithelial inflammation and damage	Epithelial necrosis and edema extending from lamina propria to as deep as muscularis layer
Iodoacetamide	UC	Enema; sulfhydryl blocker that decreased amount/action of protective sulfhydryl groups	Diarrhea, dilation, adhesions, mucosal erosions to deep ulcerations, inhibited weight gain
Indomethacin	CD	In diet; inhibition of protective prostaglandin synthesis (PGE1, PGE2, prostacyclin)	Ulceration and transmural inflammation of mid-small intestine
Trinitrobenzene sulfonic acid (TNBS)	UC	Enema; haptenization of colonic autologous or microbial proteins making them immunogenic - delayed hypersensitivity response	Acute and chronic colitis

Model	Human Disease	Mechanism	Phenotype
Oxazolone	UC	Enema; haptenization of colonic autologous or microbial proteins making them immunogenic - delayed hypersensitivity response	Distal colitis
Dextran sodium sulfate (DSS)	UC	Drinking water; directly toxic to epithelial cells in basal crypts	Colitis with bloody diarrhea, ulcerations, granulocytic infiltration, weight loss, shortening of intestines
Models of Colorectal Cancer			
Genetic			
Model	**Human Disease**	**Mechanism**	**Phenotype**
Apc$^{Min/+}$ mutations	FAP	Truncating mutations of *Apc* (codons 850, 716, 1638, and others)	Multiple small intestinal adenomas
Mismatch repair gene mutations (*Msh2, Msh3, Msh6, Mlh1, Mlh3*)	HNPCC	Mutations in various mismatch repair genes	Adenomas and adenocarcinomas of entire GI tract, some mutations prone to lymphomas, squamous or basal cell carcinomas
β-catenin stabilizing mutations	FAP	Stabilization of β-catenin leading to activation of *c-Myc* and *cyclin D*	Hundreds of small intestinal adenomas
Smad3$^{-/-}$	CRC	Loss of cellular signaling protein in TGF-β pathway	CRC with occasional metastasizes to regional lymph nodes
K-ras^{V12G}	CRC	Activation of mutated *K-ras*	Colorectal tumors ranging from microadenomas to invasive adenocarcinomas without metastasis
Muc2$^{-/-}$	IBD-related CRC	Mutation of *Muc2*, which controls gastrointestinal mucin	Adenomas and adenocarcinomas in the intestines without distant metastasis, rectal cancers
IL-2$^{-/-}$/ β_2-microglobulin$^{-/-}$	UC-related CRC	Chronic inflammation from decreased IL-2 and β2-microglobulin	Adenocarcinoma of colon and rectum

Model	Human Disease	Mechanism	Phenotype
IL-10-/-	CD-related CRC	Chronic inflammation with decreased IL-10 in setting of colonic bacterial infection	Adenocarcinomas without metastasis or mutations in *K-ras*, *p53*, *Apc*, and *Msh* genes
RAG2-/-	Inflammation-related CRC	Induced with *Helicobacter hepaticus* infection	Intestinal dysplasia, tubular adenomas, and adenocarcinomas of cecum and colon
RAG2-/-/*Tgfβ1*-/-	Colitis-related CRC	Downregulation of TGF-β signaling pathway	Locally invasive adenocarcinomas in cecum and colon
TCRβ-/-/*p53*-/-	UC-related CRC	Dysregulation of T-cell function with lack of p53 tumor suppression	Dysplasia and adenocarcinoma of ileum and cecum
Gpx1-/-/Gpx2-/-	Ileo-colitis-related CRC	Loss of glutathione peroxidase 1 and 2 leading to peroxidative stress with bacteria-associated inflammation	Dysplasia, adenocarcinomas, signet ring cell carcinoma seen in ileum and colon
$G_{\alpha i2}$-/-	UC-related CRC	Loss of G protein function	Colonic ulcerations, atypical colonic glands
Conditional *Apc*-/-	Metastatic CRC	Floxed *Apc* mutation activated by adenovirus-delivered cre recombinase	Invasive colorectal cancers with metastases to liver
Xenografts	Metastatic CRC	Implantation of human CRC tumor cells in immunocompromised mice	Invasive CRC with metastases
Chemical			
Model	**Human Disease**	**Mechanism**	**Disease/Pathology**
1,2-dimethylhydrazine (DMH)/ Azoxymethane (AOM)/methyl-azoxymethanol (MAM)	CRC	Intraperitoneal injection; procarcinogens activated to DNA-reactive products which alkylate molecules in liver and colon	Distal colon tumors
Heterocyclic amines (PhIP, IQ, etc.)	CRC	In diet; mutagenic and tumorigenic agents in broiled food	Colon cancers, mammary tumors, prostate tumors

Model	Human Disease	Mechanism	Phenotype
Aromatic amines (DMAB)	CRC	Subcutaneous injection; tumorigenic agent	Adenomas, invasive adenocarcinomas of colon and mammary glands, salivary gland sarcomas, skin and ear squamous cell carcinomas, stomach squamous cell papillomas, sarcomas/lymphomas/ urothelial carcinomas of bladder
Alkylnitrosamides (MNNG, MNU)	CRC	Enema; direct alkylating agent	Sessile and polypoid adenomas and adenocarcinomas, rare metastases

Table 1. Mouse models of inflammatory bowel disease (IBD) and colorectal cancer (CRC). This table provides a summary of currently utilized mouse models of IBD and CRC. In addition to these singly listed models, various models are often combined, e.g. DSS and AOM or DSS in *Apc*$^{Min/+}$ mice. (Reviewed in Hung, 2010; Jurjus et al., 2004; Kanneganti et al., 2011; McCart et al., 2008; Rosenberg et al., 2009; Taketo, 2006; Taketo & Edelmann, 2009; Wirtz & Neurath, 2007)
Abbreviations: CD: Crohn's disease; IFN: interferon; UC: ulcerative colitis; IL: interleukin; TNF: tumor necrosis factor; UTR: untranslated region; STAT: signal transducer and activating transcription; MHC: major histocompatibility complex; IBD: inflammatory bowel disease; *Apc*: *Adenomatous polyposis coli*; *Min: Multiple intestinal neoplasia*; FAP: familial adenomatous polyposis; HNPCC: hereditary nonpolyposis colon cancer; CRC: colorectal cancer; TGF: transforming growth factor; PhIP: 2-amino-1-methyl-6-phenylimidazo[4,5-*b*]pyridine; IQ: 2-amino-33-methylimidazo[4,5-*f*]quinoline; DMAB: 3,2′-dimethyl-4-aminobiphenyl; MNNG: *N*-methyl-*N*′-nitro-*N*-nitrosoguanidine; MNU: methylnitrosourea

Although murine models of colonic diseases are powerful, one limitation has been the large number of animals needed to complete an adequately powered study. Traditionally, experiments had a cross-sectional design in which mice from different groups were sacrificed at a set point in time, and the intestinal tract was examined at necropsy. This limitation has been overcome with recent advances in technology. A variety of imaging tools have been developed, allowing longitudinal assessment of the large intestine in animal models. Currently utilized methods include computed tomography (CT), magnetic resonance imaging (MRI), and direct visualization with colonoscopy. The ability to serially assess changes in the large intestine allows more detailed information about diseases to be gathered with a smaller cohort of experimental animals (Durkee et al., 2009).

This chapter will discuss the use of colonoscopy in rodent models of IBD and CRC. The method of performing colonoscopy in experimental animals will be described as well as the various adjuncts that can be combined with colonoscopy to enhance the amount of data that can be gathered. The strengths and limitations of colonoscopy will be discussed. Finally, colonoscopy will be compared and contrasted with alternative methods of imaging the large intestine, such as CT and MRI.

2. Colonoscopic technique

Colonoscopy is the gold standard for screening, evaluating, and potentially treating diseases of the colon, including IBD and CRC. In humans, this procedure in its current manifestation involves inserting a flexible endoscope through the anus, using compressed gas to insufflate the colon, and carefully advancing to the cecum and terminal ileum. The camera at the tip of the colonoscope displays images on a monitor. As the colonoscope is withdrawn, the colonic mucosa is carefully inspected. The colonoscope has channels allowing insertion of various tools (biopsy forceps, snare cautery, needles for injection, etc.), allowing collection of biopsies, removal or destruction of potentially neoplastic lesions, or other interventions.

The power of this tool was recognized by researchers, and various groups have attempted to adapt it for use in animal models of IBD and CRC. Colonoscopy has been successfully adapted for use in rat models. Using modified bronchoscopes (Hull et al., 1990) or other small-caliber flexible endoscopes (Haughn et al., 2006), total colonoscopy of the rat has been performed successfully, as well as other variations of this procedure (Zhang et al., 1994). Colonoscopy in mice was first attempted with a pediatric cystoscope with good results, although because of anatomic and instrumental limitations, the entire colon to the cecum could not be visualized (Huang et al., 2002). High resolution endoscopy can now be performed with colonoscopes designed specifically for work with rat and mouse models of colonic disease.

Becker, Fantini, and Neurath published a description of high-resolution colonoscopy in live mice (Becker et al., 2006). This procedure is followed by our lab with modifications. We use the Coloview miniendoscope system (Karl Storz, Tuttlingen, Germany), which includes an colonoscope (0 degree, 1.5 mm, rigid) with operating sheath and light source, video monitor, and camera with the capability to record video as well as obtain still images during colonoscopy, and a small air pump. See Figure 1 for an illustration of the set-up that we use. The mouse is anesthetized with inhaled isoflurane, and is placed ventral-side down on an operating platform. An oral gavage needle on a syringe is used to introduce Dulbecco's phosphate buffered saline (PBS) via the anus as a pre-procedure enema for bowel preparation to ensure adequate visualization. This step can be repeated as needed to ensure adequate clearing of colonic contents prior to colonoscopy. We do not fast the mice prior or provide any additional bowel preparation other than the PBS enema, and we are nearly always able to obtain adequate visualization of the colonic mucosa. Note that we initially did fast the mice and provide oral NuLytely (an osmotic bowel preparatory agent), but we found that this step was unnecessary to obtain excellent visualization of the colon. The PBS enema also serves as lubrication prior to insertion of the colonoscope. The air pump is attached to the colonoscope to provide insufflation of the colon for adequate visualization throughout the procedure. Figure 2 shows an experimental mouse undergoing colonoscopy while under general anesthesia.

The mouse colon has relatively simple geometry, unlike the tortuosity that is associated with the human colon. The mouse colon extends in a fairly straight line for approximately 4 cm cranially from the anus toward the left kidney, where it turns approximately 90 degrees and

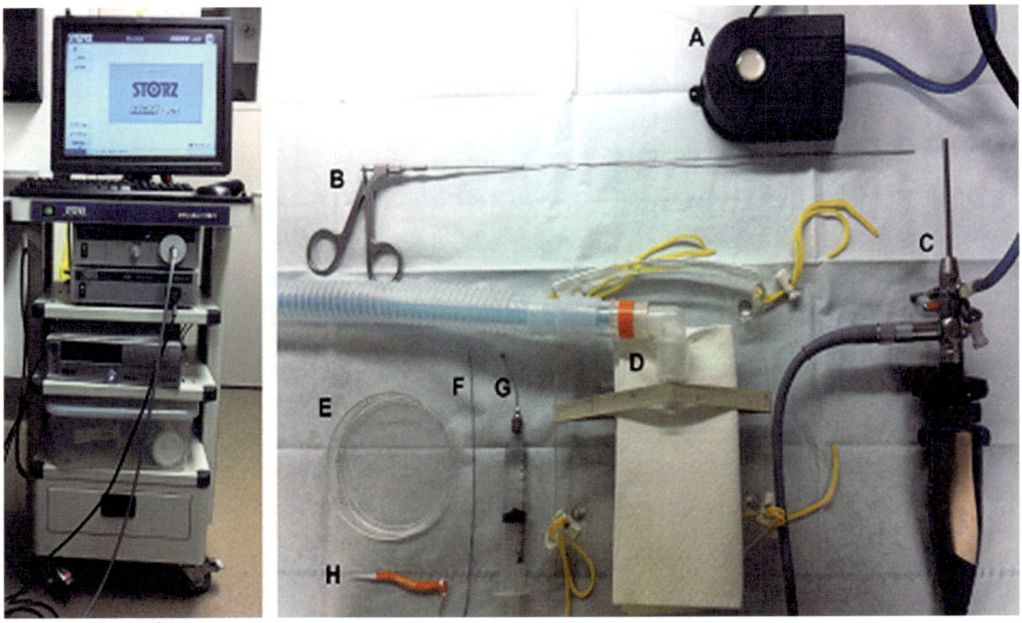

Fig. 1. Colonoscopy set-up.
On the left is the portable tower containing the monitor, light source, camera, and computer used for recording and saving videos and still images. On the right is the benchtop set-up for colonoscopy in mice. A: air pump for insufflation of the colon. B: biopsy forceps. C: colonoscope with working sheath in place, connected to air pump (blue tube) and light source (gray cable). D: nose cone for administration of inhaled anesthetic attached to operating platform. E: PBS for pre-operative enemas. F: flexible catheter to be inserted through working channel of colonoscope with scale markings for standardization of images and in situ measurments. G: gavage needle attached to syringe with PBS for administration of pre-procedure enemas. H: soft brush for cleaning lens of colonoscope.

extends across the upper abdominal cavity, connecting with the generous mouse cecum near the right kidney. The colonoscope is carefully introduced into the anus and advanced about 4 cm, or until the first area of curvature of the colon (corresponding to the splenic flexure) while observing progress on the monitor. We typically record video and obtain still images as the colonoscope is slowly withdrawn. The entire procedure takes approximately 5 minutes or less. The mouse is then allowed to awake from anesthesia. Figure 3 demonstrates the appearance of normal mucosa on colonoscopic examination.

This procedure is very well tolerated by experimental animals. However, some complications should be mentioned. Mice that are ill or moribund may not tolerate general anesthesia, so careful assessment of the animal's overall state of health should be made prior to the procedure. The wall of the colon is quite thin, so care must be taken not to cause perforation. Perforation can occur at the time of enema with the gavage needle or with the colonoscope. This injury is most likely to happen at the time of insertion, as inadvertent trauma to the colon becomes less likely under direct visualization. Care needs to be taken during insufflation as two potential complications could occur. Over-insufflation can cause air to travel throughout the length of the gastrointestinal tract to the point that gastric

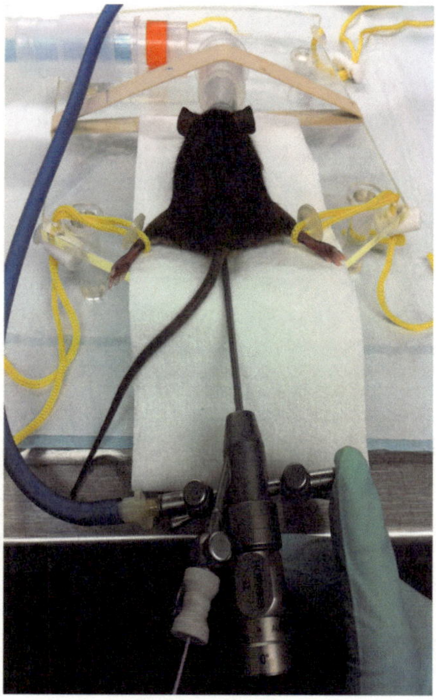

Fig. 2. Mouse colonoscopy. Image of colonoscopy being performed in a living mouse under general anesthetic. Insufflation is provided by air via the blue tube shown above. The amount of insufflation is controlled by placing a finger over the opposite opening of the working sheath. The graduated flexible measuring catheter is seen protruding from the working channel of the colonoscope.

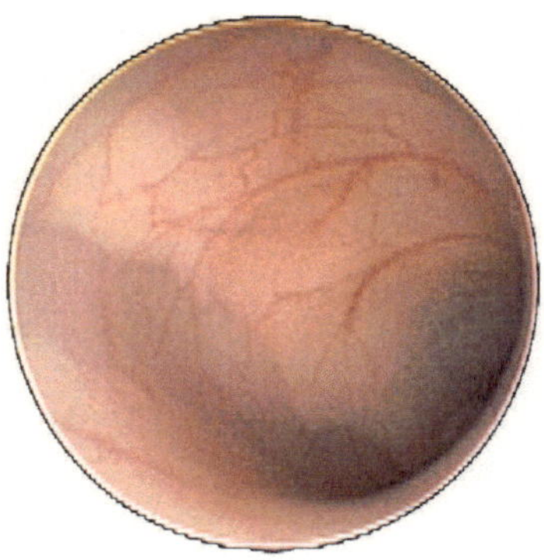

Fig. 3. Normal intestinal muscosa. Colonoscopy image showing normal intestinal mucosa.

contents are forced up the esophagus and lead to aspiration. In addition, over-distention of the intestines can lead to respiratory compromise if the abdomen becomes sufficiently distended to affect diaphragmatic function. Such complications are rare for experienced operators. Incorporation of additional procedures, such as biopsies, during the colonoscopy has the potential to increase complications. Reported mortality rates range from <1% to 2.9% (Becker, 2005; Hensley, 2009).

2.1 Experimental uses and adjuncts

Colonoscopy allows visual grading of colitis and repeat assessment over time. Both video and still images can be obtained and stored for analysis. Scoring systems of colitis have been developed and published. The criteria that can be easily visualized include the thickness of the colon, changes in vascular pattern, presence of fibrin, mucosal surface granularity, and stool consistency (Becker et al., 2005, 2006). In order to better visualize crypt patterns and detect aberrant crypt foci, which some consider early neoplastic lesions, the colonic epithelium can be stained with a 1% solution of methylene blue and then examined with the colonoscope. By performing this procedure, termed chromoendoscopy, according to previously published protocols, aberrant crypt foci can be identified that would be undetectable without staining, potentially enabling early recognition of pre-neoplastic lesions prior to tumor formation (Becker et al., 2005, 2006).

Colonic tumors that are at or distal to the splenic flexure (approximately the distal 3-4 cm of colon) can be followed serially by colonoscopy. This allows study of the natural history of tumors. Figure 4 demonstrates the progression of a single tumor in one mouse over the course of four months. Several groups have published methods of visually grading the size of tumors assessed on colonoscopy. Becker and colleagues have published a method of scoring tumor size relative to the lumen of the insufflated colon (Becker et al., 2005). However, the still images must be taken at a consistent distance from the tumor and the colon must be consistently insufflated in order for meaningful comparisons to be made between time-points. Hung and colleagues describe using the relative lumen size of a fully insufflated colon as a normalization factor when obtaining images (Hung et al., 2010). Various tools can be inserted through the working channel of the colonoscope to provide a visual frame of reference and guide for standardization of view. A tool that has a known diameter and has markings

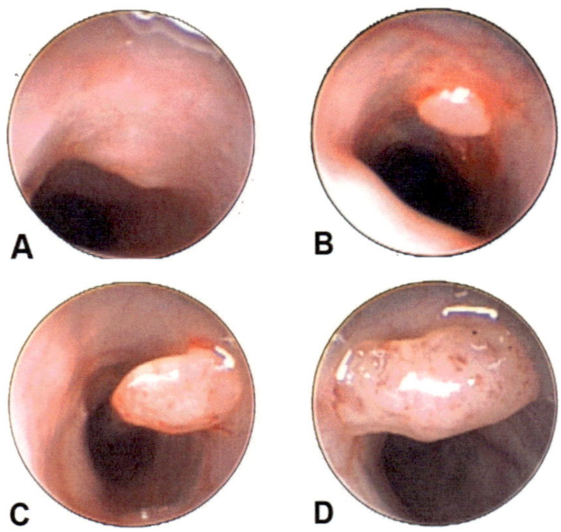

Fig. 4. Intestinal tumor development. Colonoscopy images showing the development of an intestinal tumor in a single mouse over time. Panel A: Early neoplastic lesion. Panel B: Small flat tumor approximately 1 month after image in A. Panel C: The tumor has continued to increase in size and is now pedunculated after 10 weeks. Panel D: The same tumor after an additional 4 weeks, with noticeable increase in size.

at set intervals can be used to quantify the size of tumors seen on endoscopy. Hensley and collegues have described a method using biopsy forceps. The 1-mm-diameter flexible metal biopsy forceps was inserted through the working channel of the colonoscope and advanced until it was visible in the field of view adjacent to the tumor. Still images were taken in this configuration, and the images were analyzed using a specifically written software program that allowed estimation of the tumor size by performing geometric reconstruction based on the position of the cylindrical forceps relative to the adenoma (Hensley et al., 2009). We use a flexible embolectomy catheter that has been marked at 1 mm intervals to standardize our images (see item F in Figure 1).

Biopsy forceps are available from Karl Storz which can be passed through the instrument channel of the operating sheath. Using these small, flexible forceps, tissue can be taken from tumors or areas of colon wall thickened by colitis. Figure 5 demonstrates the endoscopic biopsy of a single tumor in an experimental mouse. Care must be taken, however, not to biopsy normal colonic mucosa as the colon wall in the mouse is quite thin, and biopsies of this tissue would have an unacceptably high rate of perforation. Biopsies can be snap frozen with liquid nitrogen, placed in stabilizing media, or fixed in formalin for immunohistochemistry, molecular analysis, hematoxylin-eosin staining, or other biomolecular studies (Becker et al., 2005, 2006). In addition, Becker and colleagues have described directly injecting individual tumors with reagents via a small-gauge needle under endoscopic guidance. They inserted a 26-gauge needle mounted on a small tube through the working channel of their endoscope and injected fluorescein isothiocyanate into a tumor under direct visualization. On necropsy, the tumor was dissected free from the mouse colon and cryosections were analyzed by immunofluorescence, which showed fluorescein isothiocyanate throughout the tumor (Becker et al., 2005).

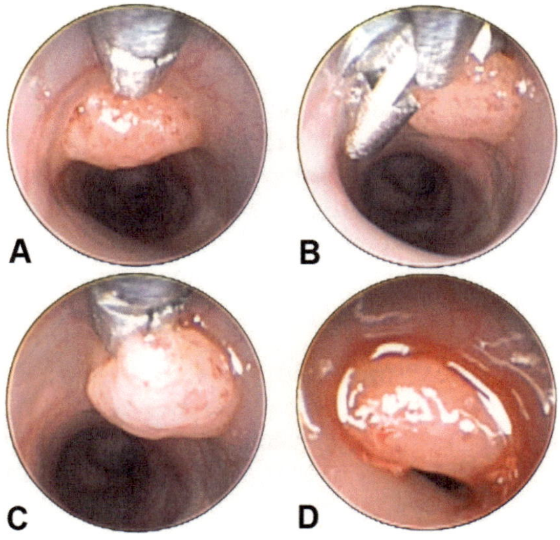

Fig. 5. Colonoscopic tumor biopsy. This series of images shows the steps in obtaining a biopsy of a tumor during colonoscopy. Panel A: insertion of biopsy forceps. Panel B: opening biopsy forceps. Panel C: grasping tumor with forceps. Panel D: bleeding from the tumor after biopsy ensures that adequate tissue was obtained.

An exciting recent development in small animal research is the use of bioluminescent and fluorescent molecules to image diverse cellular, molecular, and tissue processes. Fluorescent probes have been developed for specific antibodies, protein ligands, and other substrates (see Citrin & Camphausen, 2004, and Luker & Luker, 2008, for reviews of these techniques). These technologies can be combined with endoscopy to provide real-time imaging of fluorescent probes to detect perfusion and protease activity, as was demonstrated by Funovics and colleagues with their miniaturized multichannel near-infrared endoscope. They designed an endoscope that also allowed simultaneous fluorescent imaging of murine colonic tumors, allowing them to superimpose fluorescent perfusion and protease activity over white-light images (Funovics et al., 2003). This method has been shown to be useful for imaging adenomas as well as adenocarcinomas (Funovics et al., 2006). Hung and colleagues have reported using protease-activated synthetic probes to identify colonic lesions with near-infrared colonoscopy (Hung et al., 2010). Fluorescent probes such as this may prove useful in identifying early neoplastic lesions that are not easily visible on white-light endoscopy or in monitoring action of novel preventive or therapeutic agents.

3. Strengths and limitations

3.1 Strengths

Utilizing colonoscopy in mice has a number of distinct advantages. One of the most striking is the ability to monitor changes in colonic pathology over time. Within the same mouse, the initiation and evolution of colitis as well as response to treatment can be followed. Similarly, tumors can also be followed longitudinally, potentially from their earliest manifestation and as they progress from a benign to invasive state over time. This allows the study of a single tumor in a single mouse over time. Researchers are able to gain valuable information about the morphology of the tumor, i.e. flat vs. pedunculated, smooth vs. lobulated, as well as visualize vascular patterns in and around the tumor mucosa. Small sessile lesions that are missed on other *in vivo* imaging modalities can be easily identified on colonoscopy. Additionally, tissue can be obtained by biopsy at multiple time points for histology as well as for molecular analysis. Prior to use of colonoscopy, in order to study the natural history of colonic disease, multiple mice would have to be sacrificed at various time points, and the results of the examinations aggregated. With colonoscopy, diseases such as colitis or colon neoplasm can be studied at multiple time points in the same mouse, allowing the mouse to serve as its own control, thereby eliminating variation owing to genetic and environmental effects. In addition, being able to serially study the same mouse greatly reduces the number of mice needed in order to design an adequately powered study (Becker et al., 2005, 2006; Durkee et al., 2009; Hensley et al., 2009).

Colonoscopy in mice is a relatively simple and cost-effective procedure that is well-tolerated by experimental animals. Colonoscopy is portable and relatively inexpensive, although there is an initial cost to purchase the equipment. Other methods of imaging murine colonic disease, such as microCT colonography or MRI, require more expensive scanners as well as a dedicated space for the necessary equipment.

3.2 Limitations

There are significant limitations of colonoscopy that deserve discussion. Although colonoscopy is a relatively safe procedure, there is still an associated morbidity and mortality, as discussed earlier in the section on colonoscopic technique. There are also limitations inherent in the procedure itself. The quality of the data gathered by colonoscopy is operator-dependent, and there is a learning curve before the scope can be safely and effectively used. The images that are obtained are two-dimensional, so estimating the volume of a tumor is difficult. Most significantly, current technology only allows visualization of the distal half (3-4 cm) of the mouse colon. A flexible colonoscope that can be used safely in mice is unavailable, which means that any lesions proximal to the splenic flexure are inaccessible *in vivo*.

4. Comparison to other imaging modalities

4.1 Micro-computed tomography colonography

A number of methods for imaging the colons of experimental mice are becoming available. Micro-computed tomography (mCT) colonography is a useful tool for examining colonic disease, in particular neoplasia. Also known as virtual colonoscopy, this modality uses x-rays to image the colon and surrounding tissues, and can be used to generate either two-dimensional or three-dimensional reconstructions of individual tumors. Virtual colonoscopy has been shown to be an accurate screening tool for detecting colon polyps in humans (Kim et al., 2007), making its utilization in murine experiments very clinically relevant. Several groups have modified this technology for use in the mouse, allowing longitudinal study of mouse models of colonic disease (Durkee et al., 2010). Choquet and colleagues have used mCT with luminal and intraperitoneal contrast to detect azoxymethane-induced cecal heterotypia and colon tumors. They identified 9 of 9 areas of heterotypic thickened cecal wall and 11 of 11 colon tumors with no false positives (Choquet et al., 2007). Pickhardt and colleagues showed that by modifying feed and providing bowel preparation with an osmotic agent, mCT could detect colonic tumors ≥2mm in maximum diameter with 93.3% sensitivity and 92% specificity (Pickhardt et al., 2005). These investigators went on to demonstrate tumor volume measurements by mCT were accurate predictors of actual tumor size (Durkee et al., 2008). Good quality mCT scans had a mean standard deviation in tumor volume measurements of 8%, meaning that changes in tumor volume of >16% are detectable with a 95% confidence interval. Thus, colon tumors can be reliably identified and followed over time by mCT in order to determine if they grow, regress, or remain static either spontaneously or in response to therapy (Durkee et al., 2009). This imaging platform is very powerful when testing therapeutic interventions.

mCT colonography offers several advantages over colonoscopy. This is a non-invasive procedure, so there is minimal risk of morbidity or mortality to the experimental animals, although general anesthesia and colonic insufflation are not without risk. Current technology allows three-dimensional rendering of tumors, allowing accurate measurement of volume, as opposed to the size estimates that can be made using flat two-dimensional images from colonoscopy (Durkee et al., 2008). Importantly, the entire colon from cecum to anus can be assessed by mCT colonography, rather only the distal 4 cm as is currently visible on colonoscopy. In addition, extracolonic manifestation of disease, specifically metastatic lesions, can be seen on mCT *in vivo*.

There are advantages offered by colonoscopy, however. Compared to mCT colonography, colonoscopy is faster (an average of 5 minutes versus 20 minutes), requiring less time under anesthesia for experimental animals (Durkee et al., 2009). The equipment and set-up for colonoscopy are also less expensive than mCT, both in terms of actual hardware required as well as the dedicated space needed for a CT scanner. Colonoscopy is also able to detect small or sessile tumors that are not visible on mCT colonography, which relies on the contrast between the appearance of colonic contents and tissue structures, and is thus unable to detect lesions <2mm or flat lesions. Colonoscopy can also be used to monitor colonic inflammation, which is not easily appreciated on mCT colonography. mCT colonography does employ ionizing radiation, and the length of the scan currently exposes experimental animals to approximately 0.25 Gray, which is to up to 10 times the amount used on humans. The effects of this level of radiation on mice are unknown. Finally, colonoscopy offers the opportunity to perform additional procedures concurrently under direct visualization. mCT colonography does not offer the opportunity to obtain biopsies, perform *in vivo* staining as with chromoendoscopy, or add any of the other adjunctive procedures discussed above.

4.2 Magnetic resonance imaging

Another imaging modality used to study colonic disease is magnetic resonance imaging (MRI). Hensley and colleagues described a protocol whereby the entire colon is visualized by MRI. Using this imaging platform, polypoid tumors 1.5 mm in largest dimension could be reliably identified, with 17 correctly identified tumors, 2 false negatives, and 2 false positives. Volumes of the tumors were estimated from MRI and correlated well with tumor weight (Hensley et al., 2004). Young and colleagues were able to accurately measure the volume of polypoid colonic tumors at multiple time points (Young et al., 2009). Estimates of cross-sectional area made on colonoscopy, MRI, and necropsy were compared by Hensley and colleagues, and were found to have a strong correlation (Hensley et al., 2009). In addition to colon tumors, numerous investigators have demonstrated that colitis can be visualized on MRI. A number of groups have been able to appreciate acute experimentally induced colonic inflammation when imaging mice after treatment with dextran sodium sulfate, a commonly used agent to model acute colon inflammation in the mouse. Acute inflammation seen on MRI was confirmed on histological examination of the colon after sacrifice (Larsson et al., 2006; Melger et al., 2007; Mustafi et al., 2010; Young et al., 2009). The colon wall thickness, T2-weighted imaging, and quantitative analysis of contrast uptake and wash-out were all significantly different in inflamed colons. These studies show that MRI colonography is a viable option for longitudinal study of experimentally induced colitis, allowing the longitudinal study of inflammatory colon diseases (Larsson et al., 2006; Melger et al., 2007; Mustafi et al., 2010; Young et al., 2009).

MRI colonography offers the same advantages over colonoscopy that mCT colonography does with the additional advantage that no ionizing radiation is used. However, there are reasons to choose colonoscopy over MRI. MRI colonography requires the use of contrast agents, either intravenously, intramuscularly, or rectally; in addition to being difficult to administer, the exact effects of these agents on experimental mice are unknown. As with mCT, set-up and maintenance of an imaging facility are expensive. MRI is also less than ideal for identifying flat tumors when compared to colonoscopy as these are not as readily apparent as polypoid tumors. Table 2 compares and contrasts these modalities for imaging colon tumors *in vivo* in mice.

Imaging Platform	Advantages	Disadvantages
Colonoscopy	Quick Relatively safe for experimental animals Relatively inexpensive Serial examinations Direct visualization of colonic mucosa Visualization of flat or polypoid lesions Ability to perform *in vivo* staining Ability to obtain tissue biopsies Ability to combine with fluorescent probes for protease or vascular imaging	Occasional mortality in experimental animals Initial cost of equipment Unable to visualize proximal to splenic flexure Unable to visualize extra-luminal disease 2-dimensional images only, so difficult to accurately assess tumor size and volume Quality of images operator-dependent
mCT colonography	Non-invasive with minimal risk of mortality in experimental animals Ability to measure tumors in 3 dimensions, resulting in accurate and precise measurements of tumor volume Ability to image entire length of colon Visualization of extracolonic lesions, i.e. metastases	More time required for procedure Ionizing radiation with unknown effects Expensive Inability to identify sessile lesions or lesions <2 mm Unable to perform additional procedures (biopsy, staining, etc.)
MRI colonography	Noninvasive with minimal risk of mortality No ionizing radiation Ability to visualize inflammation Ability to measure tumors in 3 dimensions Ability to visualize extracolonic lesions	Contrast required More time required Expensive Inability to identify small or sessile lesions Unable to perform additional procedures

Table 2. Comparison of imaging modalities.
This table compares and contrasts colonoscopy, mCT colonography, and MRI colonography for colorectal cancer in mouse models.

5. Conclusion

Colonoscopy is a powerful tool for studying pathology in mouse models of colonic disease. This is a safe, relatively quick procedure that enables researchers to study the natural history of colonic diseases, to visually assess response to therapeutics or interventions, and to obtain tissue from living animals. By allowing serial examinations of the colon, it decreases the number of mice needed to adequately power a study. Colonoscopy can be combined with staining techniques or fluorescent probes to gather data about a variety of cellular, molecular, or tissue processes simultaneously. Colonoscopy is comparable to other imaging modalities available to study the murine colon, such as mCT or MRI colonography.

6. Acknowledgements

The authors would like to thank Linda Clipson for critical review of the manuscript and Brian Olson for technical help and critical review.

7. References

American Cancer Society. *Colorectal Cancer Facts & Figures 2011-2013.* Atlanta: American Cancer Society, 2011.

Becker, C.; Fantini, M.C.; Wirtz, S.; Nikolaev, A.; Kiesslich, R.; Lehr, H.A.; Galle, P.R.; Neurath, M.F. (2005). In vivo imaging of colitis and colon cancer development in mice using high resolution chromoendoscopy. *Gut*, Vol. 54, No. 7, (July 2005), pp. 950-954, ISSN 0017-5749

Becker, C.; Fantini, M.C. & Neurath, M.F. (2006). High resolution colonoscopy in live mice. *Nature Protocols*, Vol. 1, No. 6, (December 2006), pp. 2900-2904, ISSN 1754-2189

Center, M.M.; Jemal, A. & Ward, E. (2009). International trends in colorectal cancer incidence rates. *Cancer Epidemiology, Biomarkers, and Prevention*, Vol. 18, No. 6, (June 2009), pp. 1688-1694, ISSN 1055-9965

Choquet, P.; Calon, A.; Breton, E.; Beck, F.; Domon-Dell, C.; Freund, J-N.; Constantinesco, A. (2007). Multiple-contrast X-ray micro-CT visualization of colon malformations and tumours in situ in living mice. *Comptes Rendus Biologies*, Vol. 330, No. 11, (November 2007), pp. 821-827, ISSN 1631-0691

Citrin, D. & Camphausen, K. (2004). Optical imaging of mice in oncologic research. *Expert Review of Anticancer Therapy*, Vol. 4, No. 5, (October 2004), pp. 857-864, ISSN 1473-7140

Durkee, B.Y.; Mudd, S.R.; Roen, C.N.; Clipson, L.; Newton, M.A.; Weichert, J.P.; Pickhardt, P.J.; Halberg, R.B. (2008). Reproducibility of tumor volume measurement at microCT colonography in living mice. *Academic Ragiology*, Vol. 15, No. 3, (March 2008), pp. 334-341, ISSN 1076-6332

Durkee, B.Y.; Shinki, K.; Newton, M.A.; Iverson, C.E.; Weichert, J.P.; Dove, W.F.; Halberg, R.B. (2009). Longitudinal assessment of colonic tumor fate in mice by computed tomography and optical colonoscopy. *Academic Radiology*, Vol. 16, No. 12, (December, 2009), pp. 1475-1482, ISSN 1076-6332

Durkee, B.Y.; Weichert, J.P. & Halberg, R.B. (2010). Small animal micro-CT colonography. *Methods*, Vol. 50, No. 1, (January 2010), pp. 36-41, ISSN 1046-2023

Funovics, M.A.; Alencar, H.; Su, H.S.; Khazaie, K.; Weissleder, R; Mahmood, U. (2003). Minaturized multichannel near infrared endoscope for mouse imaging. *Molecular Imaging*, Vol. 2, No. 4, (October 2003), pp. 350-357, ISSN 1535-3508

Funovics, M.A.; Alencar, H.; Montet, X.; Weissleder, R.; Mahmood, U. (2006). Simultaneous fluorescence imaging of protease expression and vascularity during murine colonoscopy for colonic lesion characterization. *Gastrointestinal Endoscopy*, Vol. 64, No. 4, (October 2006), pp. 589-597, ISSN 0016-5107

Haughn, C.; Uchal, M.; Raftopoulos, Y.; Rossi, S.; Santucci, T.; Torpey, M.; Pollice, A.; Yavus, Y.; Marvik, R.; Bergamaschi, R. (2006). Development of a total colonoscopy rat model with endoscopic submucosal injection of the cecal wall. *Surgical Endoscopy*, Vol. 20, No. 2, (February 2006), pp. 270-273, ISSN 0930-2794

Hensley, H.H.; Chang, W. & Clapper, M.L. (2004). Detection and volume determination of colonic tumors in *Min* mice by magnetic resonance micro-imaging. *Magnetic Resonance in Medicine*, Vol. 52, No. 3, (September 2004), pp. 524-529, ISSN 0740-3194

Hensley, H.H.; Merkel, C.E.; Chang, W.L.; Devaragan, K.; Cooper, H.S.; Clapper, M.L. (2009). Endoscopic imaging and size estimation of colorectal adenomas in the multiple intestinal neoplasia mouse. *Gastrointestinal Endoscopy*, Vol. 69, No. 3 pt 2, (March 2009), pp. 742-749, ISSN 0016-5107

Huang, E.H.; Carter, J.J.; Whelan, R.L.; Liu, Y.H.; Rosenberg, J.O.; Rotterdam, H.; Schmidt, A.M.; Stern, D.M.; Forde, K.A. (2002). Colonoscopy in mice. *Surgical Endoscopy*, Vol. 16, No. 1, (January 2002), pp. 22-24, ISSN 0930-2794

Hull, C.C.; Stellato, T.A.; Ament, A.A.; Gordon, N.; Galloway, P. (1990). Endoscopic and radiographic evaluation of the murine colon. *Cancer*, Vol. 66, No. 12, (December 1990), pp. 2528-2532, ISSN 0008-543x

Hung, K.E.; Maricevich, M.A.; Georgeon Richard, L.; Chen W.Y.; Richardson, M.P.; Kunin, A.; Bronson, R.T.; Mahmood, U.; Kucherlapati, R. (2010). Development of a mouse model for sporadic and metastatic colon tumors and its use in assessing drug treatment. *Proceedings of the National Academy of Sciences of the United States of America*, Vol. 107, No. 4, (January 2010), pp. 1565-1570, ISSN 0027-8424

Jurjus, A.R.; Khoury, N.N. & Reimund, J-M. (2004). Animal models of inflammatory bowel disease. *Journal of Pharmacological and Toxicological Methods*, Vol. 50, No. 2, (September-October 2004), pp. 81-92, ISSN 1056-8719

Kanneganti, M.; Mino-Kenudson, M. & Mizoguchi, E. (2011). Animal models of colitis-associated carcinogenesis. *Journal of Biomedicine and Biotechnology*, Vol. 2011, pp. 1-23, ISSN 1110-7243

Kim, D.H.; Pickhardt, P.J.; Taylor, A.J.; Leung, W.K.; Winter, T.C.; Hinshaw, J.L.; Gopal, D.V.; Reichelderfer, M.; Hsu, R.H.; Pfau, P.R. (2007). CT colonography versus colonoscopy for the detection of advanced neoplasia. *New England Journal of Medicine*, Vol. 357, No. 14, (October 2007), pp. 1403-1412, ISSN 0028-4793

Larsson, A.E.; Melgar, S; Rehnström, E.; Michaëlsson, E.; Svensson, L.; Hockings, R.; Olsson, L.E. (2006). Magnetic resonance imaging of experimental mouse colitis and association with inflammatory activity. *Inflammatory Bowel Disease*, Vol. 12, No. 6, (June 2006), pp. 478-485, ISSN 1078-0998

Loftus, E.V., Jr. (2004). Clinical epidemiology of inflammatory bowel disease: incidence, prevalence, and environmental influences. *Gastroenterology*, Vol. 126, No. 6, (May 2004), pp. 1504-1517, ISSN 0016-5085

Luker, G.D. & Luker, K.E. (2008). Optical imaging: current applications and future directions. *Journal of Nuclear Medicine*, Vol. 49, No. 1, (January 2008), pp. 1-4, ISSN 0161-5505

McCart, A.E.; Vickaryous, N.K. & Silver, A. (2008). *Apc* mice: models, modifiers, and mutants. *Pathology – Research and Practice*, Vol. 204, No. 7, (July 2008), pp. 479-490, ISSN 0344-0338

Melgar, S.; Gillberg, P-G.; Hockings, P.D.; Olsson, L.E. (2007). High-throughput magnetic resonance imaging in murine colonic inflammation. *Biochemical and Biophysical Research Communications*, Vol. 355, No. 4, (April 2007), pp. 1102-1107, ISSN 0006-291x

Mustafi, D.; Fan, X.; Dougherty, U.; Bissonnette, M.; Karczmar, G.S.; Oto, A.; Hart, J.; Markiewicz, E.; Zamora, M. (2010). High-resolution magnetic resonance colonography and dynamic contrast-enhanced magnetic resonance imaging in a murine model of colitis. *Magnetic Resonance in Medicine*, Vol. 63, No. 4, (April 2010), pp. 922-929, ISSN 0740-3194

National Cancer Institute. (n.d.). Colon and Rectal Cancer Home Page, 16.03.2011, Available from: www.cancer.gov/cancertopics/types/colon-and-rectal

Pickhardt, P.J.; Halberg, R.B.; Taylor, A.J.; Durkee, B.Y.; Fine, J.; Lee, F.T., Jr.; Weichert, J.P. (2005). Microcomputed tomography colonography for polyp detection in an *in vivo* mouse tumor model. *Proceedings of the National Academy of Sciences of the United States of America*, Vol. 102, No. 9, (March 2005), pp. 3419-3422, ISSN 0027-8424

Rosenberg, D.W.; Giardina, C. & Tanaka, T. (2009). Mouse models for the study of colon carcinogenesis. *Carcinogenesis*, Vol. 30, No. 2, (February 2009), pp. 183-196, ISSN 0143-3334

Taketo, M.M. (2006). Mouse models of gastrointestinal tumors. *Cancer Science*, Vol. 97, No. 5, (May 2006), pp. 355-361, ISSN 1347-9032

Taketo, M.M. & Edelman, W. (2009). Mouse models of colon cancer. *Gastroenterology*, Vol. 136, No. 3, (March 2009), pp. 780-798, ISSN 0016-5085

Townsend, C.M.; Beauchamp, R.D.; Evers, B.M.; Mattox, K.L. (Eds.) (2008). *Sabiston Textbook of Surgery: the Biological Basis of Modern Surgical Practice*, 18th Ed. Saunders Elsevier, ISBN 978-1-4160-5233-3, Philadelphia, PA, USA

Wirtz, S. & Neurath, M.F. (2007). Mouse models of inflammatory bowel disease. *Advanced Drug Delivery Reviews*, Vol. 59, No. 11, (September 2007), pp. 1073-1083, ISSN 0169-409X

World Health Organization. (n.d.) World Health Organization Cancer Fact Sheet No. 297, In: *World Health Organization Media Center*, 16.03.2011, Available from http://www.who.int/mediacentre/factsheet/fs297/en/

Young, M.R.; Ileva, L.V.; Bernardo, M.; Riffle, L.A.; Jones, Y.L.; Kim, Y.S.; Colburn, N.H.; Choyke, P.L. (2009). Monitoring of tumor promotion and progression in a mouse model of inflammation-induced colon cancer with magnetic resonance colonography. *Neoplasia*, Vol. 11, No. 3, (March 2009), pp. 237-246, ISSN 1522-8002

Zhang, J. & Lam, L.K.T. (1994). Colonoscopic colostomy model in rats for colon tumorigenesis studies. *Carcinogenesis*, Vol. 15, No. 8, (August 1994), pp. 1571-1567, ISSN 0143-3334